Pharmacology for
Veterinary Technicians

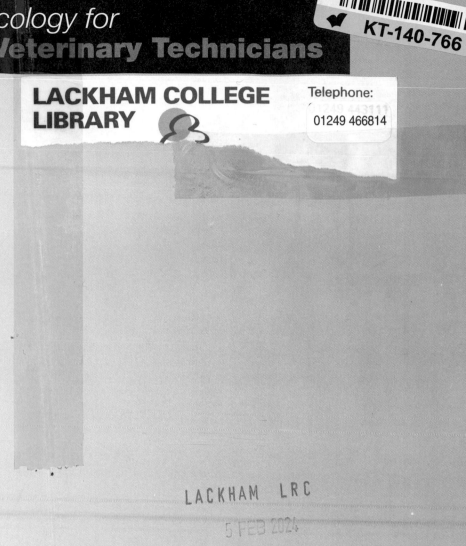

Pharmacology for Veterinary Technicians

Second Edition

Robert L. Bill, DVM, PhD

Veterinary Physiology and Pharmacology
School of Veterinary Medicine
Purdue University
West Lafayette, IN 47907

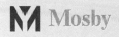 Mosby

St. Louis   Baltimore   Boston   Carlsbad   Chicago   Naples   New York   Philadelphia   Portland
London   Madrid   Mexico City   Singapore   Sydney   Tokyo   Toronto   Wiesbaden

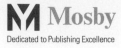

Mosby
Dedicated to Publishing Excellence

A Times Mirror
Company

Publisher: Don Ladig
Editor: Paul W. Pratt
Senior Developmental Editor: Teri Merchant
Project Manager: Linda McKinley
Production Editor: Julie Zipfel
Designer: Elizabeth Fett
Manufacturing Supervisor: Don Carlisle

A NOTE TO THE READER:
The author and publisher have made every attempt to check dosages and nursing content for accuracy. Because the science of pharmacology is continually advancing, our knowledge base continues to expand. Therefore we recommend that the reader always check product information for changes in dosage or administration before administering any medication. This is particularly important with new or rarely used drugs.

Second Edition

Printed in the United States of America
Composition by The Clarinda Co.
Printing/binding by RR Donnelly & Sons Co.

Mosby-Year Book, Inc.
11830 Westline Industrial Drive
St. Louis, Missouri 63146

Library of Congress Cataloging-in-Publication Data

Bill, Robert.
   Pharmacology for veterinary technicians / Robert (Pete) Bill. — 2nd ed.
      p. cm.
   Includes bibliographical references and index.
   ISBN 0-8151-0902-4
   1. Veterinary pharmacology.   I. Title
   [DNLM: 1. Veterinary Drugs—pharmacology.   SF 915 B596p 1997]
   SF915.B55   1997
   636.089'57—dc21
   DNLM/DLC
   for Library of Congress   97-11
                                                                      CIP

97 98 99 00 01 9 8 7 6 5 4 3 2 1

This second edition is dedicated to
Lorita, Chelsea, and *Christopher.*

Acknowledgment

Many thanks to Dr. Joann Colville for the work she put into the illustrations. A sincere thank you to Dr. Paul Pratt for his patience and persistent, yet gentle, nagging to get this edition completed. Thanks also to my friends for their encouragement and reminders to not be such a perfectionist.

Contents

Chapter **1**

Introduction to Veterinary Pharmacology and Therapeutic Applications, 1

Prudent Use of Therapeutic Agents, 2
Terminology Used in Describing Therapeutic Agents, 2
  Drug Names, 2
  Dosage Forms, 4
Sources of Drug Information, 6
Information Listed in Drug References, 6

Chapter **2**

Pharmacy Procedures, Drug Handling, and Dosage Calculations, 11

Preparing Prescriptions and Dispensing Medication, 12
  Guidelines for Writing Prescriptions, 12
  Components of a Prescription, 12
  Abbreviations Used in Prescriptions, 13
  Medication Dispensing, 13
Calculating Drug Doses, 14
  The Ratio Method, 14
  Factor Label Method (Stoichiometry), 15
  Other Calculation Used with Drugs, 17
Storing and Handling Drugs in the Pharmacy, 19
  Environmental Considerations, 20
  Storage and Handling of Controlled Substances, 20
  Handling of Antineoplastic Agents, 22
Drug Compounding, 24

Chapter **3**

Pharmacokinetics and Principles of Pharmacology, 29

The Therapeutic Range, 30
  Maintaining Drug Concentrations Within the Therapeutic Range, 31
Dosage Regimen and Routes of Administration, 32
  Drug Dose, 32
  Dosage Interval, 33
  Routes of Administration, 34

Movement of Drug Molecules in the Body, 35
  Passive Diffusion, 35
  Facilitated Diffusion, 36
  Active Transport, 36
  Physical Transport, 36
  Effect of Transport Mechanisms on Drug Molecule Movement, 37
  Effect of a Drug's Lipophilic or Hydrophilic Nature on Drug Molecule
    Movement, 38
Pharmacokinetics, 38
  Drug Absorption, 39
  Effect of Route of Administration on Absorption, 39
  Effect of Lipophilic/Hydrophilic Properties on Absorption, 41
  Effect of pH of the Environment on Absorption, 41
  Ion Trapping and Absorption of Drugs, 44
  Factors Affecting Absorption and Bioavailability of Orally Administered
    Drugs, 45
  Factors Affecting Absorption of Parenteral Drugs, 49
Drug Distribution, 50
  Barriers to Drug Distribution, 50
  Effect of Tissue Perfusion on Drug Distribution, 51
  Effect of Plasma Protein Binding on Drug Distribution, 53
  Volume of Distribution, 54
The Way Drugs Exert Their Effects, 56
  Antagonists and Agonists, 57
  Nonreceptor Mediated Reactions, 60
Biotransformation: The Way the Body Alters Drugs, 61
  Drug Interactions Affecting Biotransformation, 61
  Species and Age Differences in Drug Biotransformation, 62
Drug Elimination, 64
  Routes of Drug Elimination, 64
  Renal Elimination of Drugs, 64
  Hepatic Elimination of Drugs, 65
  Halflife and Clearance: Measures of Drug Elimination Rates, 66
  Relationship of Halflife to Steady-state Concentrations, 67
  Drug Withdrawal Times, 68
Using Concepts of Pharmacokinetics, 69

Chapter **4**

Drugs Affecting the Gastrointestinal Tract, 74

Function and Control of the Gastrointestinal Tract, 75
Emetics, 77
  The Vomiting Reflex, 77
  Induction of Vomiting, 79
  Types of Emetics, 80
Antiemetics, 81
Antidiarrheals, 83
  Antidiarrheals that Modify Intestinal Motility, 84
  Antidiarrheals that Block Hypersecretion, 85
  Adsorbents and Protectants, 86
Laxatives, Lubricants, and Stool Softeners, 87

Antacids and Antiulcer Drugs, 88
Ruminatorics and Antibloat Medications, 91
Other Drugs Used for Gastrointestinal Problems, 91
    Antimicrobials, 91
    Oral Electrolyte Replacements, 92
    Pancreatic Enzyme Supplements, 92
    Corticosteroids, 93

Chapter **5**

Drugs Affecting the Cardiovascular System, 99

Normal Cardiac Function, 100
    Cardiac Anatomy and Dynamics of Blood Flow, 100
    Electrical Conduction Through the Heart, 101
    Depolarization, Repolarization, and Refractory Periods, 103
    Role of the Autonomic Nervous System in Cardiovascular Function, 106
Antiarrhythmic Drugs, 108
    Antiarrhythmic Drugs That Inhibit Sodium Influx, 109
    β-Blocker Antiarrhythmic Drugs, 111
    Calcium Channel Blocker Antiarrhythmic Drugs, 112
Positive Inotropic Agents, 113
Vasodilators, 115
    Vasoconstriction in Heart Disease, 115
    Vasodilator Drugs, 117
    Hydralazine, 117
    Nitroglycerin, 118
    Angiotensin-Converting Enzyme Inhibitors, 118
    Prazosin, 119
Diuretics, 119
    Loop Diuretics, 120
    Thiazide Diuretics, 121
    Potassium-Sparing Diuretics, 121
    Osmotic Diuretics, 122
    Carbonic Anhydrase Inhibitors, 122
Other Drugs Used in Treating Cardiovascular Disease, 122
    Aspirin, 122
    Bronchodilators, 122
    Sedatives and Tranquilizers, 123

Chapter **6**

Drugs Affecting the Respiratory System, 128

Antitussives, 129
    Butorphanol, 130
    Hydrocodone, 131
    Codeine, 131
    Dextromethorphan, 131
Mucolytics, Expectorants, and Decongestants, 131
    Mucolytics, 132
    Expectorants, 133

Decongestants, 133
Precautions in Using OTC Products, 133
Bronchodilators, 134
β-Adrenergic Agonists, 136
Methylxanthines, 136
Other Drugs Used to Treat Respiratory Problems, 139
Corticosteroids, 139
Antihistamines, 139
Antimicrobials, 140
Diuretics, 141
Oxygen, 141

Chapter **7**

Drugs Affecting the Endocrine System, 144

The Negative Feedback System, 145
Drugs Used to Treat Thyroid Disease, 146
Drugs Used to Treat Hypothyroidism, 146
Drugs Used to Treat Hyperthyroidism, 149
Endocrine Pancreatic Drugs, 151
Drugs Affecting Reproduction, 153
Hormonal Control of the Estrous Cycle, 153
Types of Reproductive Drugs, 156
Drugs Used to Control Estrous Cycling, 158
Drugs Used to Prevent, Maintain, and Terminate Pregnancy, 160
Other Uses of Reproductive Drugs, 163

Chapter **8**

Drugs Affecting the Nervous System, 168

Anesthetics, 169
Barbiturates, 169
Propofol, 172
Dissociative Anesthetics, 173
Inhalant Anesthetics, 174
Tranquilizers and Sedatives, 177
Acepromazine, 177
Droperidol, 178
Diazepam, Zolazepam, Midazolam, and Clonazepam, 178
Xylazine, Detomidine, and Medetomidine, 178
Analgesics, 181
Narcotic or Opioid Analgesics, 181
Neuroleptanalgesics, 184
Anticonvulsants, 184
Phenobarbital, 185
Primidone, 186
Phcnytoin, 187
Diazepam, 187
Clonazepam, 188
Potassium Bromide, 188
Valproic Acid, 189

Central Nervous System Stimulants, 189
  Methylxanthines, 189
  Doxapram, 190
  Yohimbine and Tolazoline, 190

Chapter 9

Antimicrobials, 196

Types of Antimicrobials, 197
Goals of Antimicrobial Therapy, 198
Resistance of Microorganisms to Antimicrobial Therapy, 199
Concern Over Antimicrobial Residues, 200
Mechanisms of Antimicrobial Action, 201
  Effects Against the Cell Wall, 201
  Effects Against the Cell Membrane, 202
  Effects Against Ribosomes, 202
  Effects Against Cell Metabolism, 203
  Effects Against Nucleic Acids, 203
CLASSES OF ANTIMICROBIALS, 203
Penicillins, 203
  Mechanism of Action, 204
  Pharmacokinetics of Penicillins, 204
  Bacterial Resistance to Penicillins, 205
  Precautions for Use of Penicillins, 206
  Considerations for Use of Specific Penicillins, 206
Cephalosporins, 208
  Mechanism of Action, 209
  Pharmacokinetics of Cephalosporins, 209
  Precautions for Use of Cephalosporins, 210
Bacitracins, 210
Aminoglycosides, 211
  Mechanism of Action, 211
  Pharmacokinetics of Aminoglycosides, 211
  Precautions for Use of Aminoglycosides, 212
Quinolones, 215
  Mechanism of Action, 215
  Pharmacokinetics of Quinolones, 216
  Precautions for Use of Quinolones, 216
Tetracyclines, 217
  Mechanism of Action, 218
  Pharmacokinetics of Tetracyclines, 218
  Precautions for Use of Tetracyclines, 219
Sulfonamides and Potentiated Sulfonamides, 220
  Mechanism of Action, 221
  Pharmacokinetics of Sulfonamides, 221
  Precautions for Use of Sulfonamides, 222
Other Antimicrobials Used in Veterinary Medicine, 223
  Lincosamides, 223
  Macrolides, 223
  Metronidazole, 224
  Nitrofurans, 225

Chapter 1

Introduction to Veterinary Pharmacology and Therapeutic Applications

Prudent Use of Therapeutic Agents
Terminology Used in Describing
   Therapeutic Agents
   Drug names
   Dosage forms

Sources of Drug Information
Information Listed in Drug References

Key Terms

adverse reaction
ampule
chemical name
contraindication
controlled substance
dosage form
elixir
emulsion
enteric-coated tablet
extract
extra-label use
generic equivalent
indication
injectable drug
liniment
lotion
multidose vial
nonproprietary name
off-label use
ointment
overdose
paste
precaution
proprietary name
repository form
side effect
single-dose vial
solution
suspension
sustained-release
   formulation
syrup
topical application
trade name
warning

Learning Objectives

*After studying this chapter,
the veterinary technician should know the following:*

The types of drug names

The dosage forms of drugs

The sources of drug information

The terminology used in drug references

The information listed on drug package inserts and in drug references

The increasing number of therapeutic agents available to the veterinarian necessitates an expanding responsibility to use these drugs safely and reasonably. The effects of this responsibility on food-animal producers, companion animal practitioners, and regulatory veterinarians can be affirmed in professional publications and the daily press. The general public is more demanding that meat products be free of harmful drug residues and is increasingly knowledgeable about medications used in companion animal practice.

The veterinary technician plays an important role in ensuring that therapeutic agents are dispensed properly, clients are correctly informed about medication side effects or withdrawal times, and in-hospital drug administration is performed so that patients and staff are protected.

An informed veterinary technician can help the veterinarian in detecting adverse reactions to drugs, alert the veterinarian to possible drug incompatibilities, and be aware of potential problems that might result from using certain common medications. The technician has the responsibility to help reduce the number of unfortunate therapeutic accidents that can occur with inappropriate administration of veterinary drugs.

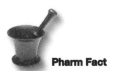

Pharm Fact

Every drug is a potential poison.

PRUDENT USE OF THERAPEUTIC AGENTS

Every drug is potentially a poison. Often the only difference between drugs being lifesavers or potentially lethal poisons depends on administration: the correct amount and method of administration are critical. Complacency about the potential lethality of drugs often results because people commonly use medications such as aspirin or vitamins themselves without considering the possible adverse effects. This complacency occurs when veterinary medications are routinely dispensed or administered without adverse reactions in the patient. However, such complacency may result in a therapeutic accident if the veterinary professional does not know or remember the conditions that make the administration of the drug inappropriate or dangerous to the health of an animal.

Drugs are not "silver bullets" to be dispensed in a "cookbook" manner such that disease X is always treated with drug A. The veterinarian cannot assume that when treating disease X or clinical sign Y, drug Z should be dispensed. Each animal is different, and as is discussed in Chapter 3, each animal may require an adjustment of dosage or kind of medication based on breed, gender, disease state, and various preexisting conditions. When dispensing of medication becomes routine, a veterinary professional may often have to explain to an owner why a beneficial therapeutic agent resulted in loss of life.

TERMINOLOGY USED IN DESCRIBING THERAPEUTIC AGENTS

Drug Names

Drugs are generally referred to by three different names (Fig. 1-1). The **chemical name,** such as *D*-α-amino-p-hydroxybenzyl-penicillin trihy-

Chemical Name	Nonproprietary name	Proprietary/trade name
D-(-)α-amino-p-hydroxybenzyl penicillin trihydrate	Amoxicillin	Amoxi-Drop® Biomox® Robamox-V®
[(3-phenoxyphenyl) methyl *cistrans*-3-(2, 2-dichloroethenyl)-2, 2-dimethylcyclopropanecarboxylate)]	Permethrin insecticide	Basus® Defend® Flysect®
dl 2-(σ-chlorophenyl)-2-(methylamino)cyclohexanone hydrochloride	Ketamine hydrochloride	Ketaset® Vetalar®

Fig. 1-1 Examples of the chemical name, nonproprietary name, and trade name for three drugs.

drate, describes the chemical composition of a drug and is of use to chemists and pharmacologists but of little practical use for the veterinary professional. The **nonproprietary name,** also called the *generic name,* is a more concise name given to the specific chemical compound. Examples of nonproprietary names are aspirin, acetaminophen, and amoxicillin. The **proprietary,** or **trade, name** is a unique name a manufacturer gives to its particular brand of a drug. Examples of proprietary or trade names include Excedrin®, Tylenol®, and Amoxitabs®. These trade names identify the drug as being manufactured by a particular company. Because the trade name is a proper noun, it is capitalized, and the superscript ® or ™ is added to signify that the trade name is a registered trademark and cannot be legally used by other manufacturers. Because many drug manufacturers produce similar products, a single generic drug can be sold under multiple trade names. For example, the antibiotic amoxicillin is manufactured by several different companies, each of which uses its own trade name (for example, Amoxi-Tabs®, Robamox-V®, Utimox®, Amoxil®).

When a drug company develops, patents, and obtains FDA approval to sell a new drug (that is, a new chemical, not just a new name for trade name for an old drug), the company has the exclusive rights to manufacture this drug for a number of years. During that time, no other drug manufacturer can produce this same drug. This allows the drug company to recover from the consumer the costs of the research, development, and testing performed to bring this drug to market.

After a certain number of years, the exclusive rights to manufacture the drug expire, and other companies are then permitted to produce the drug. These drugs are called **generic equivalents** because they have properties equivalent to those of the original compound. Generic equivalents are usually sold at a much lower price than the original manufacturer's product because the generic manufacturer did not have to underwrite development of the original drug.

As a general rule, generic drugs are equivalent drugs and are as effective as the original patented compound. On occasion, however, differences in the manufacturing process produce minor fluctuations in the physical char-

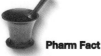

Pharm Fact

A specific drug can be marketed under various trade names by several manufacturers.

Pharm Fact

Most generic drugs are equivalent in efficacy to the original patented compound.

acteristics of the generic drug's dosage form (for example, a tablet, a capsule, and so on). Although the exception, some generic drugs have not performed as consistently as the original compound in veterinary patients, in contrast to equivalent performances of the same generic and original drug in humans. These differences may be associated with the rapid transit of orally administered drug through the gastrointestinal tract of animals or other physiologic anomalies unique to the veterinary patient.

Dosage Forms

Drugs are also described by their **dosage forms.** Solid dosage forms for delivering the drug include tablets, which are powdered drug compressed into disks, or gel caps, which are powdered drug enclosed within gelatin capsules. Compressed tablets shaped like capsules are commonly referred to as caplets.

Tablets may be simply the compressed powdered drug, or they may be coated with a glossy sugar compound to make administration or identification of the tablet easier. **Enteric-coated tablets** contain a special covering over the powdered drug that protects the drug from the harsh acidic environment of the stomach and prevents dissolution of the tablet until it enters the intestine. Molded tablets are soft, chewable tablets in which the powdered drug is mixed with lactose, sucrose, or dextrose and a "flavoring" to encourage the patient to chew the tablet. Examples of molded tablets include chewable vitamins and chewable heartworm preventive.

Troches, or lozenges, are powdered drug that is incorporated into a hard, candylike tablet. These dosage forms are intended to be held in the mouth and slowly dissolved, releasing small amounts of drug in the mouth as they dissolve (such as cough tablets and sore throat lozenges). Because a veterinary patient is unlikely to hold a lozenge in its mouth, this dosage form is not used in veterinary medicine. Suppositories are designed to be placed into the rectum, where they dissolve and release the drug to be absorbed across the membranes of the intestinal wall.

Sustained-release formulations of oral drugs are tablets, capsules, or caplets that are specially formulated to release small amounts of drug into the intestinal lumen over an extended time. In humans, this allows the drug to be absorbed over a longer period, thereby reducing the number of times the drug must be administered each day. Unfortunately, many oral sustained-release medications fail to work as planned because the intestinal tract transit time, which is the time it takes for a drug to pass along the length of the digestive tract, varies among species and among individual species. Thus an animal with a rapid intestinal transit time might pass a sustained-release tablet all the way through the intestines before all drug can be released for absorption. Some tablets have an enteric coating, which prevents destruction of the drug by gastric acid during its passage through the stomach. The enteric coating then dissolves in the intestines, where the drug is absorbed. If sustained-release or enteric-coated forms of oral medication are used in animals, these tablets or caplets should not be broken into halves or sections because this negates the enteric coating or sustained-release nature of the formulation, which depends on uniform dissolution of the tablet from the outside surface inward.

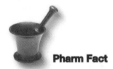

Pharm Fact

Enteric-coated or sustained-release tablets should not be broken into pieces before administration.

Liquid forms of drugs are usually divided into solutions and suspensions. A **solution** means that the drug is dissolved in a liquid vehicle and does not settle out, or precipitate, if left standing. In contrast, a **suspension** contains drug particles that are suspended but not dissolved in the liquid vehicle. These drug particles usually settle to the bottom when the container is undisturbed; before drug administration, the veterinary technician shakes the container to ensure the drug is evenly resuspended in the liquid and provides accurate drug dosing. Suspensions can also be subdivided into **emulsions,** a mixture of a drug and a liquid fat or an oil; and gels, a semi-solid or jellylike suspension of drug such as toothpaste.

Solutions can also be described as **syrups,** such as cough syrups, which are solutions of drug with water and sugar (for example, 85% sucrose). Syrups often disguise the unpleasant taste of a drug and are a popular drug form for children's medications. **Elixirs** are solutions of drug dissolved in sweetened alcohol. Because elixirs are used for drugs that do not readily dissolve in water, they should not be diluted with water because the alcohol and water will separate into distinct layers.

Whereas elixirs and syrups are intended for oral administration, tinctures are alcohol solutions meant for **topical application.** Topical products are available as **liniments,** which contain a drug in an oil base that is rubbed into the skin, or **lotions** such as poison ivy medications, which are drug suspensions or solutions that are dabbed, brushed, or dripped onto the skin without rubbing.

Semisolid dosage forms include **ointments** and creams, which are applied onto the skin, and **pastes,** which are given orally. Ointments and creams are designed to liquefy at body temperatures, whereas pastes tend to keep their semisolid form at body temperature. Pastes are commonly packaged in large plastic syringes for administering oral deworming medications to horses, cattle, sheep, and occasionally dogs.

Injectable drugs, as the name implies, are administered via a needle and syringe. Injectables are often referred to by the type of container in which they are supplied. **Ampules** are small, airtight glass containers; the neck of the ampule is broken to access the drug. Drugs contained within ampules are used completely at one time; the ampule cannot be resealed. Vials are glass bottles with rubber stoppers. The drug is withdrawn from the vial by inserting a needle through the rubber stopper. Vials may be **multidose vials,** in which multiple doses can be withdrawn over time, such as most injectable antibiotics, or **single-dose vials,** in which all the drug is used at one time, such as vaccines. The rubber stopper on multidose vials should be kept clean because reinsertion of needles through a contaminated stopper can introduce bacteria or other contaminants.

Repository forms of injectable drugs are formulated to prolong absorption of the drug from the site of administration and thus provide a more sustained, effective drug concentration in the body. Implants are solid dosage forms that are injected or inserted under the skin. Implants are designed to dissolve or release medication over an extended period.

An **extract** is a therapeutic agent composed of specially prepared plant or animal parts rather than manufactured from chemicals. Examples of extracts include thyroid supplements made from ground-up pig or cattle thy-

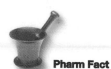

Pharm Fact

The rubber stopper of multidose vials must be disinfected before needle insertion to prevent contamination of the vial's contents.

roid glands and pancreatic enzyme powder derived from prepared livestock pancreas. Although many extracts provide reasonably consistent effects among different bottles, the potency of different batches may vary as a result of variation in amounts of extracted natural drug contained in the plant or animal part. Although extracts might be less expensive to purchase, they may not provide as consistent a clinical effect as a compound developed by conventional manufacturing processes.

SOURCES OF DRUG INFORMATION

Because information on appropriate and safe drug use in veterinary medicine is constantly changing, the veterinary professional must have access to a current drug reference guide. This information may come from package inserts, which are included with each container of drug sent to a veterinarian; formularies, which are small booklets containing drug dosages; or larger resource books, such as *Veterinary Pharmaceuticals and Biologicals, Mosby's Veterinary Drug Reference, Compendium of Veterinary Products,* and *Veterinary Drug Handbook by Donald C. Plumb.*

Because information on pharmaceuticals changes so rapidly, the veterinary technician should have the most current edition of any drug references used. Information on human drugs not contained in the veterinary resources may be found in *Physician's GenRx* and *Physicians' Desk Reference (PDR),* the latter of which also has several smaller spin-off publications such as *Nonprescription Drugs* and *Ophthalmic Drugs.* Both references are also available on CD-ROM. Although these publications contain detailed information on thousands of drugs and their effects in humans, they do not provide any information about effects in veterinary patients. Therefore the technician should consult current veterinary drug references.

Manufacturers are also required to provide certain information on the package label and in the package insert. The information in drug references is often derived directly from these package inserts.

The veterinary technician should have and correctly use a current drug information resource. The technician must understand terms used to describe drug effects, know adverse reactions that may occur, and be aware of any risks associated with administration of a drug to use it safely and effectively.

Pharm Fact

Before administering any drug, the veterinary technician should be familiar with its effects, possible adverse reactions, and risks associated with its use.

INFORMATION LISTED IN DRUG REFERENCES

The information in most drug references and package inserts conveys a large amount of information in a readily accessible format. In drug references, each drug heading usually contains important information. (A typical heading for a fictitious drug listing is shown in Fig. 1-2.) The bold-face, capital letters with the circled R (®) indicate the copyrighted proprietary or trade (brand) name of the product (Goze-2-Sleep). In some cases the ® is replaced by a superscript ™, which indicates that the name is a registered trademark owned by the company and, like the copyrighted brand name, cannot be used by other manufacturers.

GOZE-2-SLEEP® ℞ ℂⅡ
(pentobarbital sodium injection, USP)
Single-dose vials

Fig. 1-2 Typical listing of a hypothetic brand of pentobarbital in a drug reference.

The nonproprietary name is printed in smaller type below the boldface name and usually includes the dosage form for this particular product (for example, tablets, syrup, or for injection). *Rx* indicates that this product is available by prescription or on the order of a licensed veterinarian. *C* and *II* indicate that this drug is a **controlled substance** and therefore has special requirements for dispensing, prescribing, or using within a veterinary facility. The II indicates the general level of abuse potential for the drug. Categories, or schedules, of controlled substances range from C-I to C-V. The higher the Roman numeral, the less potential for abuse of the drug. Drugs classified as C-I have the highest potential for abuse; drugs classified as C-V have the least.

The description, or composition statement, follows the drug heading and describes the physical characteristics and ingredients of the drug or drug combination. This section specifies which additives such as preservatives and solvents are included, some of which may be harmful to some veterinary patients. This information is especially important when using a drug approved for humans in an animal.

Indications are the approved uses for the drug. Many veterinary and human drugs are used in species or for purposes other than those intended by the drug's manufacturer. These uses are called **extra-label** or **off-label uses** of the drug; that is, these uses have not been approved by the Food and Drug Administration and are not listed on the drug's label (Sidebar 1-1).

Because of public concern over drug residues in the human food supply, food-animal producers and the veterinarians who serve these producers are facing increasing pressure to restrict or regulate the extra-label uses of drugs in cattle, sheep, swine, and other food animals. Veterinary professionals are obligated to be familiar with these issues as part of their responsibility to serve and protect the public.

Precautions, warnings, and contraindications are reasons the drug should be used with great care or not at all. **Precautions** usually relate side effects or adverse reactions in which the animal or person may experience some difficulties. A **side effect,** or an **adverse reaction,** is any effect of the drug other than its intended beneficial effect. Side effects may be listed within the *Warning, Contraindication,* or *Precaution* sections, or they may be listed under a separate *Adverse Reactions* section depending on the severity or life-threatening nature of the side effect. Generally, *Precaution* listings describe fairly rare adverse reactions or mild side effects. For example, a stomach upset caused by aspirin is considered a mild side effect and is included under *Precautions.* The veterinarian must then use clinical judgement to decide whether to administer the drug. By listing the precautions (including even mild side effects), the drug manufacturer has legally informed the veterinarian of the potential side effects or adverse reactions.

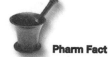

Pharm Fact

Extra-label drug use is *any* use of a drug not specifically approved by the Food and Drug Administration.

The Controversy of Extra-Label Drug Use*

The Food and Drug Administration (FDA) has the responsibility of ensuring the safety and effectiveness of all drugs and is charged with monitoring the safety of the food supply. This tremendous responsibility, as defined by the Federal Food, Drug, and Cosmetics Act, places the FDA in the role of watchdog over the ways veterinary drugs are used. Section 512 of the act states that an animal drug is considered unsafe unless it has been approved and the intended use of the drug conforms to that approval. This means that *any* use of a veterinary or human drug in species other than those approved, at dosages other than those approved, for uses other than the approved indications, or in ways that do not adhere to stated withdrawal times is considered extra-label use and is in violation of the law.

The intent of the law is primarily to keep drug residues out of the food supply. Therefore enforcement efforts are more directed toward the food-animal producing segment of the veterinary profession. A U.S. Department of Health and Human Services brochure, *FDA and the Veterinarian-HHS Publication No. (FDA) 94-6046 (1994)*, states the following in reference to non–food-producing animal practice: "under usual circumstances veterinary practitioners may consider the extra-label use of drug products in non–food-producing animal practice without ordinarily being subject to FDA enforcement actions."

Although the information from the FDA makes it clear that the "agency will consider regulatory action" if drugs are altered or extra-label use occurs in animals intended for food, they also acknowledge that extra-label drug use "may be considered by a veterinarian when the health of animals is immediately threatened and suffering or death would result from failure to treat affected animals." The FDA considers extra-label use in animals produced for food legitimate under the following conditions:

- Careful medical diagnosis is made by attending veterinarian within the context of a valid veterinarian-client-patient relationship.
- No drug is specifically labeled to treat the condition diagnosed, or drug therapy at the dosage recommended on the label has been found by the veterinarian to be clinically ineffective in the animals to be treated.
- Procedures are instituted to ensure that the identity of the treated animals is carefully maintained.
- A significantly extended period is assigned for drug withdrawal before marketing meat, milk, or eggs from treated animals; and steps are taken to ensure that the assigned time frames are met, and no illegal residues occur.
- The prescribed or dispensed extra-label drugs bear labeling information that is adequate to ensure the safe and proper use of the product (see Chapter 2).

*Additional information on this topic may be obtained by writing to the U.S. Department of Health and Human Services, FDA, Center for Veterinary Medicine, 7500 Standish Place, Rockville, MD 20855. Request *Bulletin 7125.06* and *HHS Publication No (FDA) 94-6046.*

Warnings are more serious or frequent side effects or adverse reactions than those found in the *Precaution* section. An example might include hallucinations as a possible side effect resulting from a person who is aspirin sensitive taking aspirin compounds. Because many of the adverse reactions in the *Warnings* section are potentially life threatening, veterinary professionals have a moral and ethical obligation to know the key points of *Warnings* and *Contraindications* for every drug they use.

Contraindications consist of situations in which the drug should not be used. Perhaps the most common example of a contraindication is hypersensitivity to a drug, which could result in a life-threatening allergic reaction if the drug is taken. Failure to heed a known contraindication for a drug, with subsequent death of the veterinary patient because of it, could constitute malpractice.

When possible or applicable, information on a drug **overdose** is also supplied in the drug inserts and drug information bulletins. This information is invaluable if miscalculation of a drug dose results in an animal receiving too much of a drug. This information is also valuable in an animal that because of illness or a change from its normal physiologic state, accumulates the drug in its body and subsequently shows signs of overdose even though it received a "correct" dose.

Dosage and *Administration* information must be followed closely. Drugs are designed to be given by a specific route and in a certain way (see Chapter 3). Failure to follow this procedure could result in insufficient or excessive medication being administered or harm to the patient. Failure to follow dosage and administration procedures is considered extra-label use and is subject to legal scrutiny.

Pharm Fact

Failure to heed a contraindication for use of a drug could result in death of the patient.

Review Questions

1. A drug is listed as Acepromazine®, acetylpromazine maleate. Which is the proprietary name and which is the nonproprietary name?
2. The doctor asks you to order a generic equivalent for Lasix®. Using a drug information resource, list two or three generic equivalents.
3. Why are generic forms of drugs so much less expensive than trade-name drugs? Are there any disadvantages to using generic drugs instead of the original manufacturer's brand?
4. What is the difference between a tablet and a caplet?
5. What is the function of an enteric coating on a tablet?
6. By what route of administration is a suppository drug given?
7. How does a sustained-release tablet differ from a standard tablet?
8. Which liquid formulation of a drug can be safely given intravenously, a solution or a suspension?
9. What is the difference between a syrup and an elixir?
10. How are topical drugs used?
11. What is the difference in the way a lotion is applied versus a liniment?
12. Ointments and pastes are semisolid dosage forms. Which form is more appropriate to medicate a dog's ear canal?
13. If the standard injectable form of a drug is given every 12 hours, is the repository form more likely to be given every 6 hours or every 96 hours?
14. Why are extracts fairly inexpensive? What is one potential problem with extracts?
15. The doctor tells you that a drug has a C-II rating. What does that signify about this drug? How does a C-II drug differ from a C-V drug?

16. What is the difference between a contraindication and an indication for use of a drug?

17. If a drug package insert lists "Safety of use in pregnancy has been un-determined" as a precaution, is the drug contraindicated for use in a pregnant animal?

18. Drug X will cause death if given to an animal with condition Z. Should this be considered a warning, a precaution, or a contraindication?

Chapter 2

Pharmacy Procedures, Drug Handling, and Dosage Calculations

Preparing Prescriptions and Dispensing
Medication
Guidelines for writing prescriptions
Components of a prescription
Abbreviations used in prescriptions
Medication dispensing
Calculating Drug Doses
The ratio method
Factor label method (Stoichiometry)

Other calculation used with drugs
Storing and Handling Drugs in the
Pharmacy
Environmental considerations
Storage and handling of controlled
substances
Handling of antineoplastic agents
Drug Compounding

Key Terms

antineoplastic agent
controlled substance
conversion factor
cytotoxic agent
DEA certification number
dosage
dose
drug compounding
drug manufacturing
expired drug
factor label method
(stoichiometry)
material safety data
sheet (MSDS)
percentage solution
prescription
ratio
ratio method
reconstituting
Sig

Learning Objectives

After studying this chapter,
the veterinary technician should know the following:

The circumstances for writing prescriptions

The components of a prescription

Methods of calculating drug doses

Procedures for handling and storing drugs

Guidelines for drug compounding

Because most veterinary practices have their own self-contained pharmacies and use of veterinary drugs has come under greater scrutiny by regulatory bodies such as the Drug Enforcement Administration (DEA), Food and Drug Administration (FDA), U.S. Department of Agriculture (USDA), and Environmental Protection Agency (EPA), veterinary professionals must be aware of their responsibilities to safely store medications, calculate doses, and prepare, dispense, and record medications they use.

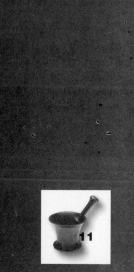

11

PREPARING PRESCRIPTIONS AND DISPENSING MEDICATION

Guidelines for Writing Prescriptions

A **prescription** is an order from a licensed veterinarian that directs a pharmacist to prepare a drug for use in an animal. When writing prescriptions, veterinarians must adhere to the following guidelines:

- Veterinary prescription drugs must be used only by or on the order of a licensed veterinarian.
- A valid relationship must exist between the veterinarian and the client and patient.
- Veterinary prescription drugs must meet proper requirements for labeling.
- Appropriate records must be maintained for all prescriptions issued.
- Veterinary prescription drugs must be appropriately handled and stored for safety and security.

Because veterinary technicians often help fill prescriptions, dispense medications, and keep records, they must understand the responsibilities and limitations of their actions. Veterinary technicians cannot legally write prescriptions but can fill them and dispense medications as instructed by veterinarians within their practice. (In several states, veterinarians and technicians from one practice cannot legally fill a prescription from another practice.) Technicians must understand the proper format of a typical prescription and the meaning of the abbreviations used in prescription writing to properly fill a prescription and dispense medicine.

Components of a Prescription

A hypothetical prescription is shown in Fig. 2-1. For a prescription to be valid, it must contain the following items:

- Name, address, and telephone number of the veterinarian who wrote the prescription
- Date on which the prescription was written

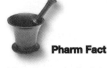

Pharm Fact

Veterinary technicians must understand the abbreviations commonly used in prescriptions.

Hometown Veterinary Associates
2000 West Chelsea Ave, Momack, PA
(324) 555-4313

Date: *November 22, 1995*
Patient: *Cricket*
Owner: *Lee Ann Wozniak*
Address: *929 Christopher Robin Ln, Brookside, PA 13235*

Species: *Canine*
Phone: *555-0127*

℞ *Amoxicillin tablets 100 mg #30 tabs*
Sig: *1 tab q8h PO PRN until gone*

Robert L. Bill DVM

Fig. 2-1 A typical prescription for a veterinary drug.

- Client's (owner's) name and address and species of animal (animal's name optional)
- *Rx* symbol (abbreviation of *recipe,* Latin for "take thou of")
- Drug name, concentration, and number of units to be dispensed
- **Sig** (abbreviation of *signa,* Latin for write or label), which indicates directions for treatment of the animal
- Signature of the veterinarian
- DEA registration number if the drug is a controlled substance

Other items frequently found on the prescription include refill status, which shows whether the client may obtain a refill of the prescription; and internal inventory or record-keeping numbers.

Abbreviations Used in Prescriptions

Although few veterinary technicians work in a commercial pharmacy setting, the same general information required by a registered pharmacist is required by a technician in a veterinary practice to correctly fill an in-house drug order. Frequently, the same abbreviations are used for prescriptions sent to a pharmacy and for filling in-house drug orders. (Fig. 2-2 shows common abbreviations used in prescriptions and their meanings.)

Abbreviations may be capitalized or lower case. The technician should check with the veterinarian when the writing on the prescription is difficult to interpret. Asking what you may think is a silly question is preferable to correcting a mistake that could have been avoided.

Pharm Fact

When in doubt, the technician should ask the veterinarian to clarify any abbreviations.

Medication Dispensing

When dispensing medication, the technician should keep in mind that children may have access to the container and could ingest the medication. To-

BID:	twice a day	PO:	by mouth
cc:	cubic centimeter	prn:	as needed
disp:	dispense	q:	every
g (or gm):	gram	q4h:	every 4 hours
gr:	grain	q8h:	every 8 hours
h (or hr):	hour	qd:	every day (daily)
IM:	intramuscular	QID:	four times daily
IV:	intravenous	QOD:	every other day
L:	liter	SID:	once a day
lb:	pound	SQ (or SC):	subcutaneous
mg:	milligram	STAT:	immediately
mL (or ml):	milliliter	TID:	three times daily
od:	right eye	tsp:	teaspoon
os:	left eye	TBL or Tbsp:	tablespoon
ou:	both eyes		

Fig. 2-2 Abbreviations commonly used in prescriptions. NOTE: SID is rarely used or recognized by pharmacists outside the veterinary profession.

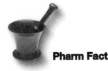

day, childproof containers are commonly used, but because they are more expensive, some veterinary practices continue to dispense medication in paper "pill envelopes."

The Poison Prevention Packaging Act of 1970 enabled the FDA to require special packaging for drugs that may be dangerous to children. Current regulations apply to drug manufacturers and pharmacists but not veterinarians; thus dispensing veterinary medication in pill envelopes is not illegal. However, if medication dispensed in a pill envelope is accessible to a child who ingests it, the veterinarian may be accused of negligence for placing the child at risk.

Sometimes dispensing of medication in nonchildproof containers is necessary, such as for elderly clients with arthritic hands. Veterinarians may give these clients medication packaged in dispensing vials with reversible lids that are childproof and nonchildproof depending on the position of the lid. Nevertheless, veterinary professionals are morally and ethically obligated to inform clients when containers are not childproof and advise them to keep medication out of the reach of children.

CALCULATING DRUG DOSES

Selection of a drug is the first step to properly medicating an animal. However, the wrong amount can make even the best drug ineffective or toxic. Therefore it is essential that the veterinary technician be able to calculate doses correctly.

Calculating a drug dosage includes the following steps:

1. Weigh the animal and convert the weight in lb to kg (if necessary).
2. If the veterinarian has not specified the dose to administer, consult the drug package insert or a drug reference to determine the correct **dosage,** based on mg/kg body weight or units/kg body weight administered according to a specified schedule. Then use the animal's weight to calculate the correct **dose,** which is measured in milligrams, milliliters, units, or grams.
3. Based on the drug concentration (for example, mg of drug/ml of solution or mg of drug/tablet), determine the volume or number of tablets to administer. This requires some basic algebra and a knowledge of metric conversions. (Common metric conversion factors are listed in Fig. 2-3. Abbreviations used in dosage calculations are shown in Fig. 2-4.)

Drug dosage can be calculated in several ways. This chapter discusses two: the **ratio method** and the **factor label method (stoichiometry).**

The Ratio Method

Equivalent fractions all represent the same number. Another way of describing this is: $\frac{1}{2} = \frac{8}{16}$. This equation, which describes a mathematical relationship among the numbers 1, 2, 8, and 16, allows you to determine one of the numbers if you know the other three. For example, because you

Weight or mass

1 kilogram	=	1000 grams
1 kilogram	=	1,000,000 milligrams
1 kilogram	=	2.2 pounds
1 gram	=	1000 milligrams
1 gram	=	0.001 kilogram
1 gram	=	15.43 grains
1 milligram	=	0.001 gram
1 milligram	=	1000 micrograms
1 pound	=	0.454 kilogram
1 pound	=	16 ounces
1 grain	=	64.8 milligrams
(rounded to 60 mgs)		

Volume

1 liter	=	1000 milliliters
1 liter	=	10 deciliters
1 milliliter	=	1 cubic centimeter
1 milliliter	=	1000 microliters
1 tablespoon	=	3 teaspoons
1 tablespoon	=	15 milliliters
1 teaspoon	=	5 milliliters
1 gallon	=	3.786 liters
1 gallon	=	4 quarts
1 gallon	=	8 pints
1 pint	=	2 cups
1 pint	=	16 fluid ounces
1 pint	=	473 milliliters

Fig. 2-3 Metric conversions.

know three of the four numbers, you can use the equation shown in Fig. 2-5 to determine which number represents *X*.

You can set up a similar equation to calculate a dog's weight in kilograms, given the dog's weight in pounds and a conversion factor, which is expressed as a fraction, or **ratio.** The ratios are set up so that the units (for example, kilograms or pounds) are the same on the top and bottom of both equations. As shown in Fig. 2-6, the kilogram units in the **conversion factor** (1 kg equals 2.2 lb) to the left of the equation are placed on top and the kilogram units on the right, which represent the dog's weight, also are placed on top. The pounds for both the conversion factor and the animal's known weight go on bottom. You can use the same algebraic steps as shown previously to solve for *X* kg of body weight.

When you have determined the animal's weight in the appropriate units (in this case, kilograms), use that number in another ratio to determine the quantity of drug for this particular animal. The conversion factor on the left of the equation in this second step is the drug dose, which is often expressed as milligrams of drug/kg body weight. *X* also is milligrams of drug (Fig. 2-7). Therefore the milligram values belong on top of both fractions.

When you have determined the drug dose, you calculate the volume such as milliliters or number of solid units such as tablets or capsules by using the concentration of drug in the solution (for example, mg of drug/ml of solution) or drug in each solid unit (for example, mg of drug/tablet) as the conversion factor, thereby solving for milliliters of liquid or number of tablets. Thus milliliters or tablets go on top (bottom half of Fig. 2-7).

Factor Label Method (Stoichiometry)

In the factor label, or stoichiometry, method, you set up a series of multiplication problems in which the units such as milligrams or kilograms in the numerators cancel the units in the denominators, leaving only the unit desired for the final answer. This method is similar to the ratio method with the exception of the initial configuration.

Weight or mass

kilogram: kg
gram: g
milligram: mg
pound: lb
grain: gr
ounce: oz

Volume

liter: L
milliliter: ml (or mL)
deciliter: dl
cubic centimeter: cc
tablespoon: TBL or Tbsp
teaspoon: tsp
gallon: gal
quart: qt
pint: pt
cup: c
fluid ounce: fl oz

Fig. 2-4 Common units of weight and volume and their abbreviations.

Set up the fraction: $\dfrac{2}{4} = \dfrac{X}{10}$

Rearrange the equation to solve for X by multiplying both sides of the equation by 10:

$$10 \times \dfrac{2}{4} = \dfrac{X}{10} \times 10$$

$$10 \times \dfrac{2}{4} = X \times 1$$

10/10 = 1, so X × 1 = X:

$$10 \times \dfrac{2}{4} = X$$

Multiply and divide the left side of the equation to find X:

$$\dfrac{20}{4} = X$$

$$5 = X$$

Plug 5 back into equation for X; thus 2/4 = 5/10:

$$\dfrac{2}{4} = \dfrac{5}{10}$$

Fig. 2-5 Simple algebraic calculation.

Set up the fraction with the conversion factor for kg/lb on the left, and the X to be solved on the upper right. Make sure the units are the same on the top and bottom:

$$\dfrac{1\ kg}{2.2\ lb} = \dfrac{X\ kg}{44\ lb}$$

Rearrange equation to solve for the X by multiplying both sides of the equation by 44 lb:

$$44\ lb \times \dfrac{1\ kg}{2.2\ lb} = \dfrac{X\ kg}{44\ lb} \times 44\ lb$$

The units on top will cancel with the same units below:

$$44\ \cancel{lb} \times \dfrac{1\ kg}{2.2\ \cancel{lb}} = \dfrac{X\ kg}{44\ \cancel{lb}} \times 44\ \cancel{lb}$$

$$44 \times \dfrac{1\ kg}{2.2} = \dfrac{X\ kg}{44} \times 44$$

44/44 = 1, so X × 1 = X:

$$44 \times \dfrac{1\ kg}{2.2} = X\ kg$$

Multiply and divide the left side of the equation to find X:

$$\dfrac{44\ kg}{2.2} = X\ kg$$

A 44-lb dog equals a 20-kg dog:

$$20\ kg = X\ kg$$

Fig. 2-6 Using the ratio method to convert 44 pounds to kilograms.

As shown in Fig. 2-8, typically the first element of the equation is the animal's weight in pounds. If the dose is given in mg drug/kg body weight, you must convert the animal's weight to kilograms. This results in a multiplication problem in which the pounds cancel each other, leaving just the kilograms on top. To determine the amount of drug in milligrams, you multiply by the dose, setting up the problem so that the kilograms of body weight

Set up the fraction with the dose (5 mg/kg) as the conversion factor:

$$\frac{5 \text{ mg drug}}{1 \text{ kg body wt}} = \frac{X \text{ mg drug}}{20 \text{ kg body wt}}$$

Determine the amount of drug a 20-kg dog needs:

$$20 \times \frac{5 \text{ mg drug}}{1} = X \text{ mg drug}$$

$$100 \text{ mg drug} = X \text{ mg drug}$$

Set up the fraction with the concentration of the drug in liquid (50 mg drug/ml liquid) to determine the volume to be administered (milliliters are on top):

$$\frac{1 \text{ ml liquid}}{50 \text{ mg drug}} = \frac{X \text{ ml liquid}}{100 \text{ mg drug}}$$

$$100 \times \frac{1 \text{ ml liquid}}{50} = X \text{ ml liquid}$$

Determine the volume of drug solution to inject:

$$2 \text{ ml liquid} = X \text{ ml liquid}$$

Fig. 2-7 Using the ratio method to calculate a drug dose for a dog that weighs 20 kg.

How many milliliters of a 50-mg/ml concentration of drug solution will a 44-lb dog receive if the dose is 5 mg/kg?

This is the same question as in Figs. 2-6 and 2-7

The equation will give the number of kilograms this 44-lb dog weighs:

$$44 \text{ lb} \times \frac{1 \text{ kg}}{2.2 \text{ lb}} = X \text{ kg}$$

This equation will give the number of milligrams of drug this 44-lb dog needs if the dose is 5 mg/kg:

$$44 \text{ lb} \times \frac{1 \text{ kg}}{2.2 \text{ lb}} \times \frac{5 \text{ mg}}{\text{kg}} = X \text{ mg}$$

The completed equation gives the number of milliliters of drug solution this animal is to be given (the answer is 2 ml):

$$44 \text{ lb} \times \frac{1 \text{ kg}}{2.2 \text{ lb}} \times \frac{5 \text{ mg}}{\text{kg}} \times \frac{1 \text{ ml}}{50 \text{ mg}} = X \text{ ml}$$

Fig. 2-8 Using the factor label method to calculate a drug dose.

units cancel each other, leaving the milligrams of drug on top. Finally, to determine the volume of drug, you set up the problem so that milligrams of drug cancel out, leaving milliliters (or number of tablets) on top. This method uses one long multiplication problem instead of a series of smaller steps as in the ratio method.

Other Calculations Used with Drugs

When determining the total number of tablets, capsules, or caplets to be dispensed, it is essential that the veterinary technician first calculate the number of tablets *per dose* to the nearest tablet or half tablet. The steps required for calculating a total number of tablets using the factor label method are shown in Fig. 2-9. You should be able to calculate total number of tablets to dispense and accurately assign the cost of the medication.

How many 25-mg tablets would you dispense for a 10-lb cat, using a dosage of 5 mg/lb twice daily for 7 days?

First calculate the mg dose:

$$10 \; \cancel{lb} \times \frac{5 \; mg}{\cancel{lb}} = 50 \; mg \; drug$$

Now figure how many tablets this would be (rounding to nearest tablet or half tablet):

$$50 \; \cancel{mg \; drug} \times \frac{1 \; tablet}{25 \; \cancel{mg}} = 2 \; tabs$$

Knowing how many tablets are needed per dose, figure the number of tablets needed based on how frequently and how long the doses are going to be given:

$$\frac{2 \; tablets}{\cancel{dose}} \times \frac{2 \; \cancel{doses}}{\cancel{day}} \times 7 \; \cancel{days} = 28 \; tablets$$

Fig. 2-9 Using the factor label method to calculate the number of tablets to dispense.

How many milliliters of drug should a 1000-lb horse receive if the dose is 2 mg/lb and the drug comes in a 15% solution?

Figure the dose for this horse as you do with all other dosage regimens:

$$1000 \; lb \times \frac{2 \; mg}{\cancel{lb}} = 2000 \; mg$$

Convert 15% solution into more familiar mg/ml concentration form:

$$15\% \; is \; \frac{15 \; g}{100 \; ml}$$

$$\frac{15 \; \cancel{g}}{100 \; ml} \times \frac{1000 \; mg}{1 \; \cancel{g}} = \frac{150 \; mg}{ml}$$

Set up dose/concentration equation so that milliliter unit (the answer) is on top:

$$2000 \; \cancel{mg} \times \frac{1 \; ml}{150 \; \cancel{mg}} = 13.3 \; ml$$

Fig. 2-10 Using the factor label method to calculate the required volume of solution.

Occasionally drug solutions are not described as a weight over volume such as mg/ml or g/L but instead are expressed as a **percentage solution** (for example, Tribrissen® 24% solution). When calculating a dose for this drug, you must first convert it to a mass over volume number. A 1% solution is equivalent to 1 g of drug in 100 ml of liquid. Therefore you can calculate a dose based on this conversion (Fig. 2-10).

For drugs that are administered via slow intravenous (IV) infusion (continuous flow of medication), you must determine the amount of drug needed, the appropriate volume for that quantity of drug, and the rate at which the solution is flowing through the IV set into the animal. To determine volume and rate, calculate the dose and the volume of drug as you did with the previous problems, and then determine how many drops per sec-

How fast would 360 ml of drug have to be administered to a horse by IV infusion to have it delivered in 30 minutes with an IV set that has a 10 drop : 1 ml calibration ratio?

The dose and volume to be administered for this horse have been calculated before this step. First set up the amount of drug to be delivered by this IV set:

$$360 \text{ ml} \times \frac{10 \text{ drips}}{1 \text{ ml}} = 3600 \text{ drips}$$

Because this amount of drug needs to be delivered within 30 minutes, set that up as a fraction:

$$\frac{3600 \text{ drips}}{30 \text{ minutes}}$$

Convert the drips/min into drips/sec using a min/sec conversion:

$$\frac{3600 \text{ drips}}{30 \text{ min}} \times \frac{1 \text{ min}}{60 \text{ sec}} = \frac{2 \text{ drips}}{\text{sec}}$$

Fig. 2-11 Calculating the drip rate for an IV infusion.

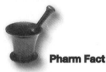

Pharm Fact

IV drip sets in veterinary medicine are usually calibrated so that 10, 15, or 60 drips equals 1 ml of solution.

ond or milliliters per minute must be given to deliver the calculated dose within a certain period.

An additional, necessary conversion factor relates to the transparent drip chamber on the IV set, where the drip rate is visible. In most standard IV sets, 10 drops equal 1 ml of solution. In pediatric or microdrip IV sets, 60 drops equal 1 ml of solution. In some other IV sets, 15 drops equal 1 ml. The appropriate conversion factor is normally listed on the box or container in which the IV set, is packaged. (Fig. 2-11 shows a typical calculation to determine the flow rate of a drug administered by IV infusion.)

Because calculating the correct dose is so critical, you should double-check your calculations and even spot check the dose in the syringe to further ensure that it is appropriate for the size of the animal. To spot check, compare one dose given to an animal of known weight with the dose you are about to administer to a second animal to see whether the doses are proportional. For example, if a 20-lb dog requires a 4-ml dose, a 10-lb dog should need half that amount, or 2 ml. This spot checking becomes easier as you become familiar with the drugs that are used often in your clinical setting.

STORING AND HANDLING DRUGS IN THE PHARMACY

Inventory control for drugs and other supplies used in veterinary practice is usually taught in conjunction with business management concepts. However, there are also medical and legal reasons for proper storage and handling of drugs. For example, drugs that are not stored in the proper temperature and light can degenerate or become inactivated, providing little or no benefit. Drugs that remain on the pharmacy shelf after the listed expiration date may be less effective. In some cases, such as with tetracycline, these **expired drugs** may actually be dangerous if they are used. Thus responsible storage and handling of therapeutic agents is essential to facilitate safe, effective veterinary care.

Pharm Fact

The veterinary technician must know the way to safely store and handle drugs to provide effective veterinary care.

Environmental Considerations

Drugs should be stored at their optimum temperature to prevent damage. According to label specifications, temperatures for drug storage are as follows:

Cold: not exceeding 8°C (46°F)
Cool: 8° to 15°C (46° to 59°F)
Room temperature: 15° to 30°C (59° to 86°F)
Warm: 30° to 40°C (86° to 104°F)
Excessive heat: greater than 40°C (104°F)

Large animal practitioners must be especially aware of environmental conditions because of the tendency to forget about drugs that are stored in the practice vehicle. These drugs can be subjected to wide variations of temperature. When frozen, some antibiotic preparations undergo a change in crystalline formation that inhibits suspension and causes injection of the drug to be much more painful than normal.

Drugs that are sensitive to light are usually kept in a dark amber container. Tablets and powders are sensitive to moisture, so their containers usually have silica packets to absorb moisture. Ionizing radiation can destroy some complex drug molecules. Other drugs are destroyed by physical stress such as vibrations. Some forms of insulin can be inactivated by violent shaking of the vial.

Drugs that must be **reconstituted** before use (for example, a powder to which a liquid is added) often do not contain preservative agents to prevent bacterial growth if the container becomes contaminated after reconstitution. Reconstituted drugs may be easily contaminated by repeated insertion of needles or because the reconstituted product is often chemically unstable; therefore it is inappropriate to keep reconstituted drugs for several days so that the contents may be completely used in several animals. The manufacturers of these products specify the time during which the product is considered safe and effective to use.

Storage and Handling of Controlled Substances

A **controlled substance** is defined by law as a substance that has the potential for physical addiction, psychologic addiction, and/or abuse. Within a veterinary practice or research facility, controlled substances should be kept in a locked storage cabinet of substantial construction such as a sturdy metal cabinet or a safe to prevent access by unauthorized personnel.

By law, a log must be kept stating the date, purpose, and amount of any controlled drug that was used. These records must include receipts for purchase or sale of controlled substances and must be maintained for 2 years. Because of the potential abuse for sale or resale of controlled drugs through medical, dental, or veterinary practices, the regulatory agencies of many states use computer systems to detect a higher-than-normal movement of controlled drugs through health facilities. If the DEA or other regulatory group detects an unusual flow of controlled substances and conducts an investigation, they will require the veterinary practice

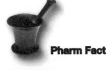

Pharm Fact

Some drugs can be inactivated by various physical agents, including heat, light, and excessive shaking.

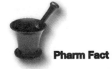

Pharm Fact

Veterinary professionals must keep records to document each use of controlled substances.

to provide accurate, reliable documentation of the way each dose of controlled medication was used in the clinic. Although ketamine, a drug that is commonly used in veterinary practices, is not listed as a controlled drug, its hallucinogenic characteristics increase the potential for abuse; therefore ketamine should be handled as a controlled substance.

Regulations for the prescribing, handling, and storing of controlled drugs are specified in the Controlled Substances Act of 1970 and enforced by the DEA. Drug manufacturers and distributors are required to identify a controlled substance on the drug's label with a *C* followed by a Roman numeral. The Roman numeral denotes the drug's theoretic potential for abuse (see Chapter 1):

C-I Has an extreme potential for abuse, has no approved medicinal purpose in the United States, includes such drugs as heroin, LSD, and marijuana

C-II Has a high potential for abuse, may lead to severe physical or psychologic dependence, includes such drugs as opium, pentobarbital, and morphine

C-III Has some potential for abuse but less than that of C-II drugs, may lead to low to moderate physical dependence or high psychologic dependence

C-IV Has a low potential for abuse, may lead to limited physical or psychologic dependence, includes such drugs as phenobarbital and diazepam (Valium®)

C-V Is subject to state and local regulation, has a low potential for abuse

Veterinarians must have a certification number from the DEA to legally use, prescribe, and buy controlled substances from an approved manufacturer or distributor. This **DEA certification number** must be included on all prescriptions or any order forms for Schedule (controlled) drugs. This means that veterinarians cannot order or prescribe phenobarbital for a convulsing dog unless they have a valid, current DEA number.

Even with a valid DEA number, veterinarians cannot prescribe Schedule I (C-I) drugs, which are illegal substances. Prescriptions for Schedule II (C-II) drugs, which have a high potential for abuse, must be in written form. Many states have special forms for C-II drug prescriptions. These prescriptions cannot be telephoned to a pharmacist except in an emergency, in which case the verbal prescription must be followed by a written order within 72 hours. Schedule II drug prescriptions may not be refilled; a new prescription must be written for each treatment period.

A controlled substance of Schedule II, III, or IV rating that is dispensed from the veterinary hospital pharmacy must be packaged in a childproof container, which must include on its label the following warning: *Caution: Federal law prohibits the transfer of this drug to any person other than the (client and) patient for whom it was prescribed.*

Additional information on storing and handling controlled substances may be obtained through the American Veterinary Medical Association (AVMA) or the DEA branch in your state.

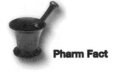

Pharm Fact

Cytotoxic agents must be stored and administered in a very different way from most other drugs.

Handling of Antineoplastic Agents

The safe handing of all drugs requires concentration on the task. However, this focus is especially important in the preparation, administration, and disposal of **antineoplastic agents,** which are used to treat cancer, and antifungal agents, which are used to treat fungal infections. At therapeutic doses, improper handling of antineoplastic drugs can cause birth defects (teratogenic or mutagenic effects) in the fetus of a pregnant veterinary professional or induce cancer or preneoplastic changes (carcinogenic effects) in animals and humans. Because little is known about the long-term effects of these drugs, the veterinary professional must handle mutagenic and carcinogenic drugs with great care.

Guidelines for safe handling of **cytotoxic agents,** which are toxic to cells and include antineoplastic drugs, have been published. The Occupational Safety and Health Administration (OSHA) has guidelines for safe storage, use, and disposal of chemicals and drugs. The American Animal Hospital Association* offers a series of videotapes on general hospital procedures, some of which relate to handling cytotoxic agents. The *ASHP Technical Assistance Bulletin on Handling Cytotoxic and Hazardous Drugs* contains guidelines for minimizing exposure to cytotoxic agents. Veterinary texts about oncology also contain guidelines and procedures for safe administration of antineoplastic agents.

Veterinary professionals may be exposed to toxic drugs during routine procedures:

- Absorption through skin via spillage from a syringe, vial, or other contact
- Inhalation of aerosolized drug as the needle is withdrawn from a vial that has been pressurized by the technician injecting air into the vile to facilitate removal of the drug
- Ingestion of food contaminated with drug via aerosolization or direct contact
- Inhalation resulting from crushing or breaking of tablets and subsequent aerosolization of drug powder
- Absorption or inhalation during opening of glass ampules containing antineoplastic agents

Because veterinary professionals routinely administer drugs to their patients, they often become complacent about safe hygiene practices. A veterinarian's or technician's lunch may often be found near a specimen jar containing formalin, a container with a fecal sample, or a container with antineoplastic medication. In a busy practice, veterinary professionals often quickly eat lunch between procedures and may briefly place food on a countertop while administering medication. These practices violate the basic rules of hygiene and can result in serious consequences.

The best way to avoid exposure to cytotoxic agents is to educate all involved personnel on safe handling and storage of these drugs. Training may be in-house or through workshops that are available in many communities. Safety training should be periodically repeated to emphasize the importance of handling precautions and serve as a refresher for staff members.

*PO Box 150899, Denver, CO 80215.

Within a veterinary practice, information on all cytotoxic agents should be compiled in a readily accessible format and should include the following items:

- A **material safety data sheet (MSDS)** for every cytotoxic agent used in the practice that contains guidelines for protective precautions, clean-up procedures, and first aid for accidental exposure
- A package insert for every drug used in the practice
- Hospital policies and descriptions of procedures for handling a spill or an exposure and routine disposal of drugs, contaminated syringes or equipment, and empty vials (based on manufacturer's recommendations in the MSDS and package insert)

The cytotoxic drugs should be stored separately from other drugs, with particular attention to environmental requirements such as temperature and exposure to light.

If preparation of the drug is required before administration, it should be done just before administration to the patient. In human hospitals, medications are often prepared ahead of time. The veterinary professional should adhere to some general guidelines for safe preparation, administration, and disposal of toxic drugs:

- Prepare and administer toxic drugs in a low-traffic, well-ventilated area.
- Wear proper protective attire when preparing and/or administering the drug. Such attire should include a high-efficiency filter mask (because surgical masks do not protect against inhalation of aerosols); some form of gloves, either two pairs of surgical-quality latex gloves (because all latex gloves are porous to some degree), or heavy-weight gloves that are commercially available for use with cytotoxic agents, or latex gloves with large animal obstetric sleeves to protect the arms; a long-sleeve, non-porous gown with close-fitting cuffs over which the gloves are worn; and goggles to prevent the eyes from being exposed to aerosols.
- Use syringes and IV lines with screw-on attachments to prevent spillage.
- Recheck the calculated dose.
- Confirm that the catheter is correctly placed within the vein and is still patent.
- Place all syringes, IV lines, catheters, and discarded vials in sealable plastic sandwich or freezer bags immediately after use.
- Place all items in a leakproof, puncture-proof container designed for and labeled as hazardous waste.

Veterinary professionals themselves should ensure that the treatment area is properly cleaned and decontaminated rather than depending on the lay staff to do so. A "chemotherapy spill kit" should be readily available. This kit should include a complete set of protective clothing as outlined above, absorbent pads with nonporous backing, a "sharps" container for needles and other sharp objects used, and a "hazardous materials" disposal bag. Because

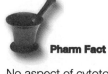

Pharm Fact

No aspect of cytotoxic drug administration or clean-up should be left to the lay staff.

of the potential for human and animal injury with use of these drugs, the time and effort spent on learning the way to safely store, prepare, administer, and dispose of these agents are well invested.

DRUG COMPOUNDING

A potentially controversial issue that veterinary professionals must be aware of is **compounding,** which is the practice of combining drugs to form a "new" drug, either approved or extra-label. Because a compounded drug is technically a new drug and has not been approved by the FDA for use in animals, it is subject to the regulations and restrictions of extra-label use (see Sidebar 1-1).

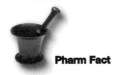

Pharm Fact

Mixing two drugs together creates a new drug that could cause unexpected effects.

Veterinary professionals often compound drugs without being aware that they are creating an unapproved drug according to the law. For example, the practice of creating "anesthetic cocktails" by combining various tranquilizers, analgesics, and anesthetic agents is an example of compounding. Other examples of compounding include diluting commercially prepared drugs with saline, another drug, or glycerol; crushing a tablet or emptying a capsule into a liquid to create a suspension or solution; and mixing two or more drugs in the same syringe.

Guidelines issued by the FDA and the AVMA acknowledge that drug compounding is an essential practice for the benefit, comfort, and safety of animals under veterinary care. However, any adverse reaction or undesirable effect from administration of the compounded drug could result in legal action against the veterinary professional and the practice. Veterinary professionals have an obligation to learn about the drugs they combine and must consider the physical properties of the drugs before compounding them to avoid producing a formulation that could cause severe side effects or even death.

Compounding is considered *acceptable* if done by a practitioner (or a pharmacist on the prescription by a veterinarian), if the resulting product will be used within the practice, and if the benefit to the animal is much greater than the health risk to the animal or public.

Compounding is considered *unacceptable* when the health risk to the general public is significant, such as from drug residues in food, regardless of potential benefit to the animal. Compounding a drug for use outside the practice is considered to be illegal **manufacturing** of a new drug. It is technically acceptable for veterinary professionals to compound different types of deworming medications for use in their own practices; however, they cannot legally sell those medications to another veterinary practice because that would constitute illegal manufacturing of a new drug.

According to the FDA, all the following criteria must be met for compounding to be considered legal:

- Compounding is done by a veterinarian or pharmacist. Veterinarians must decide whether compounding requires the skills of a pharmacist.
- A valid relationship exists between the veterinarian and the client and patient.

- The veterinarian or pharmacist must dispense the compound.
- No drug residue violations will occur with use of the compounded substance.
- The safety and efficacy of the compounded new drug are consistent with current standards of pharmaceutic and pharmacologic practices.
- Appropriate patient records are maintained.
- All compounds are labeled with the following information: name and address of the attending veterinarian, date on which the drug was dispensed and date of expiration (expiration date not to exceed the length of prescribed treatment), medically active ingredients, identity of treated animals, directions for use, cautionary statements if applicable, withdrawal times if needed, and the condition or disease for which the compound is being used.

Veterinary professionals *must* be aware of the regulations governing safe compounding of drugs in the veterinary practice. Failure to comply with regulations may result in public safety issues, litigation against the veterinary professionals involved (possibly including the technician who makes up the compounded material on the order of the veterinarian), and ultimately tighter government regulation of veterinary drug use in response to public demand for safe food and water.

Recommended Reading

American Veterinary Medical Association: *AVMA guidelines for veterinary prescription drugs,* Schaumburg, IL, 1993, The Association.

ASHP technical assistance bulletin on handling cytotoxic and hazardous drugs, *Am J Hosp Pharm* 47(5):1033, 1990.

Ballitch EJ: Labeling and record keeping for compounded drugs, *JAVMA* 205(2):249, 1994.

Boothe DM: Principles of drug therapy for the practicing veterinarian. In Bonagura JD, editor: *Kirk's current veterinary therapy XII,* Philadelphia, 1995, WB Saunders.

DEA: Following its "10 Commandments," *JAVMA* 205(10):1371, 1994.

Dickinson KL, Ogilview GK: Safe handling and administration of chemotherapeutic agents in veterinary medicine. In Bonagura JD, editor: *Kirk's current veterinary therapy XII,* Philadelphia, 1995, WB Saunders.

Extra-label use of new animal drugs in food-producing animals, FDA Compliance Policy Guides publication, Guide 7125.06, Form FDA 2678a, July 20, 1992.

Geyer RE: Legal restrictions on compounding, *JAVMA* 205(2):241, 1994.

Gloyd J: Compounding in veterinary anesthesiology, *JAVMA* 205(2):202, 1994.

Hannah HW: Direction and control of the veterinarian's assistants, *JAVMA* 205(1):43, 1994.

Lust EB: Compounding for veterinarians by pharmacists, *JAVMA* 205(2):261, 1994.

Mitchell GA, Spenser EL: Compounding of drugs for veterinary use in animals, *FDA Vet* Sept/Oct, 5, 1994.

Newton DW: Application of standards for compounding, *JAVMA* 205(2):232, 1994.

Papich MG, Davidson G: Unapproved use of drugs in small animals. In Bonagura JD, editor: *Kirk's current veterinary therapy XII,* Philadelphia, 1995, WB Saunders.

Raef TA: Flexible labeling, streamlined drug approval advocated at workshop, *JAVMA* 207(1):7, 1995.

Upson D: AVMA guidelines on compounding, *JAVMA* 205(2):199, 1994.

Webb AI, Aeschbacher G: Animal drug container labels—a guide to the reader, *JAVMA* 202(10):1591, 1994.

Why veterinary drugs are withdrawn from the market, *FDA Veterinarian* 8(5):1, 1993.

Review Questions

1. A pet owner is passing through town and stops by your veterinary clinic to see whether she can pick up some "car sickness" tablets for her dog. The owner is on a cross-country car trip and has no more of the motion sickness medication that was dispensed by her veterinarian. The doctor is not in the clinic at the moment. Is it legal to dispense the medication if you first telephone the doctor to obtain permission?

2. What deficiencies make the prescription illustrated in Fig. 2-12 legally invalid?

3. Make the following conversions:

2 g	=	_____ mg
5 mg	=	_____ g
14 lb	=	_____ kg
23 kg	=	_____ lb
83 kg	=	_____ mg
65 kg	=	_____ lb
0.4 kg	=	_____ g
0.003 lb	=	_____ mg
15 lb	=	_____ g
0.00043 kg	=	_____ mg
25,488 mg	=	_____ lb
0.0092 lb	=	_____ mg
25 ml	=	_____ L
43 cc	=	_____ ml
1.5 L	=	_____ ml
800 cc	=	_____ L
0.055 L	=	_____ ml
0.25 ml	=	_____ L

Veterinary Associates, Inc.
Oubache Plaza
Downtown Hancockville
(across from the Courthouse)

for Mrs. Knoertzer, "Fluffy"
1106 59th St.

Give 24 tablets of generic amoxicillin to be used until gone

Dr. L.S. Hemplock

Fig. 2-12 Hypothetical prescription pertaining to Review Question 2.

4. The doctor asks you to prepare a dose of ketamine sufficient to restrain a 15-lb cat. The drug formulary recommends using 15 mg/kg IV or IM. The concentration of ketamine in the vial is 100 mg/ml. What volume of ketamine is required for this cat?

5. The doctor asks you to fill a prescription for butorphanol for a coughing dog, dispensing sufficient tablets for 5 days of treatment. The dog weighs 55 lb. The recommended dose is 0.08 mg/kg. The tablets are available in 1-, 5-, and 10-mg sizes. The charge is $.35 per tablet. How many tablets are required for a single dose? If the dosage specifies use q6h, how many tablets are required for each day of treatment? How many tablets should you dispense for the total 5 days of treatment? What is the charge for the dispensed medication?

6. The veterinarian wants to medicate a 16-lb Chihuahua, a 27-lb terrier, and a 66-lb collie. The recommended dosage is 3 to 5 mg/kg given once daily. You are to dispense enough medication to last each dog 180 days (6 months). The 50-mg tablets cost $.03 each, the 100-mg tablets cost $.05 each, and the 200-mg tablets cost $.07 each. What are the minimum and the maximum daily doses (in mg) for each dog based on the recommended dosage range? How many tablets and what size are required for each dog each day? How much does the medication for the 180 days of treatment cost for each dog?

7. A diabetic dog is being treated in the clinic. The dog requires 3.2 units of insulin both in the morning and evening. U-100 insulin has a concentration of 100 units of insulin/ml and is supplied as 10-ml vials. At the insulin dosage listed above, how many full doses (3.2 units) of insulin for this dog are contained in this vial?

8. What is the concentration of drug (in mg/ml) in a 10% solution? In a 43% solution?

9. How many milligrams of drug are in 0.13 L of a 7.5% solution?

10. The doctor asks you to dispense digoxin for a client's dog. The recommended dose is 0.22 mg/m^2, where m^2 is the number of square meters of body surface area. The dog's body area is 0.8 m^2. The digoxin elixir is available in a concentration of 0.15 mg/ml. To prevent overdosing, the doctor instructs you to use 60% of the calculated normal dose for this dog. How many milliliters of digoxin elixir should this dog receive for each dose?

11. A 950-lb mare needs an IV drug infusion over the next 2 hours. The total dose to be given is 25 mg/kg. The drug concentration in the solution is 1.5%. The IV set is calibrated at 10 drops for each 1 ml. At what drip rate (in drops/second, rounded to the nearest drop) should you administer the solution to deliver the proper amount of drug in 2 hours?

12. A client wants to buy $10 worth of vitamins for his dog. The doctor asks you to dispense the medication but not to exceed the $10 value. The dog weighs 8 lb. The recommended dosage is 8 mg/kg given once daily. The medication is supplied as 15-mg tablets. A bottle of 1000 tablets costs $130. How many days' worth of tablets can you dispense for $10?

13. An IV fluid infusion is dripping medication into a 220-lb foal at 45 drops every 30 seconds. The IV set delivers 10 drops/1 ml. The recom-

mended dose is 18 ml/kg. You began the infusion at 1:00 PM. At what time should you stop the infusion?

14. A drug container's label states "Store in a dark, cool place." Is it appropriate to store the container in a closed cabinet at room temperature?

15. You are the technician who orders most of the drugs for your veterinary practice. Can you legally order drugs that are listed as C-II? Can any licensed veterinarian order such drugs?

16. Which drug has more potential for abuse, a C-III drug or a C-V drug?

17. What words must appear on the label of any container for C-II, C-III, or C-IV drugs dispensed from a veterinary clinic?

18. Generally, how long must records be retained that document use of controlled substances?

19. A fellow staff member routinely uses a surgical mask and a single pair of latex surgical gloves during preparation and administration of antineoplastic drugs. Is this adequate protection?

20. A veterinarian in another practice sees that there is a market for the "Blue Goo" concoction that he compounded as a teat dip to prevent mastitis. Can the doctor legally sell this product to your practice if he applies a label to each bottle stating "For use by or on the order of a licensed veterinarian"?

Chapter 3

Pharmacokinetics and Principles of Pharmacology

The Therapeutic Range
  Maintaining drug concentrations
    within the therapeutic range
Dosage Regimen and Routes of
  Administration
  Drug dose
  Dosage interval
  Routes of administration
Movement of Drug Molecules in the
  Body
  Passive diffusion
  Facilitated diffusion
  Active transport
  Physical transport
  Effect of transport mechanisms on
    drug molecule movement
  Effect of a drug's lipophilic or
    hydrophilic nature on drug
    molecule movement
Pharmacokinetics
  Drug absorption
  Effect of route of administration on
    absorption
  Effect of lipophilic and hydrophilic
    properties on absorption
  Effect of pH of the environment on
    absorption
  Ion trapping and absorption of drugs
  Factors affecting absorption and
    bioavailability of orally
    administered drugs

Factors affecting absorption of
    parenteral drugs
Drug Distribution
  Barriers to drug distribution
  Effect of tissue perfusion on drug
    distribution
  Effect of plasma protein binding on
    drug distribution
  Volume of distribution
The Way Drugs Exert their Effects
  Antagonists and agonists
  Nonreceptor-mediated reactions
Biotransformation: The Way the Body
  Alters Drugs
  Drug interactions affecting
    biotransformation
  Species and age differences in drug
    biotransformation
Drug Elimination
  Routes of drug elimination
  Renal elimination of drugs
  Hepatic elimination of drugs
  Half-life and clearance: measures of
    drug elimination rates
  Relationship of half-life to steady-
    state concentrations
  Drug withdrawal times
Using Concepts of Pharmacokinetics

Key Terms

absorption
active transport
agonist
antagonist
biliary excretion
bioavailability
biotransformation
clearance
distribution
elimination
enterohepatic circulation
facilitated diffusion
first-pass effect
half-life
hepatic excretion
induced
  biotransformation
ion trapping
loading dose
maintenance dose
metabolism
parenteral administration
passive diffusion
pharmacokinetics
pKa
protein-bound fraction
receptor
redistribution
renal excretion
route of administration
steady state
therapeutic range
tissue perfusion
volume of distribution
  (Vd)
withdrawal time

Factors to be considered in drug administration

Routes of drug administration

The way drugs move through the body

The way drugs are absorbed, distributed, metabolized, and excreted

The way drugs exert effects

Applications for the concepts of pharmacokinetics

Compounds such as strychnine, mercury, arsenic, and snake venoms were once considered useful drugs capable of curing a variety of ailments. Today, medical personnel know that these compounds if given in sufficient quantities can kill an animal or person. Although today's drugs are much safer, they can be just as deadly as strychnine or snake venom if given in excessive amounts or if administered inappropriately. A basic tenet of therapeutics is that all drugs are potential poisons. Only proper administration determines whether a compound is beneficial or deadly. To recognize clinical situations in which administration of certain drugs is inappropriate, the veterinary professional must have an understanding of the principles of **pharmacokinetics,** which is the study of the way drugs move into, through, and out of the body.

THE THERAPEUTIC RANGE

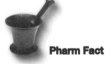

Pharm Fact

Drug doses and dosage

regimens are designed to

attain concentrations in

the therapeutic range.

Poisons like lead and arsenic are not toxic if given a single time in small quantities. In contrast, even very beneficial drugs can be toxic if given in quantities that exceed the normal recommended dose. Therefore the amount of drug administered and the concentration achieved in the body are very important in determining whether a drug is beneficial or detrimental to an animal. This ideal range of drug concentration within the body is referred to as the **therapeutic range,** or therapeutic window.

The "correct" dose of any drug should achieve concentrations within the therapeutic range. If an excessive dose results in accumulation of too much drug in the body, drug concentrations rise above the therapeutic range and signs of toxicity develop. Thus the top end of the therapeutic range usually marks the concentrations at which toxicity begins to develop (Fig. 3-1). Drug concentrations exceeding this point are at toxic concentrations, or at toxic levels.

An insufficient drug dose that does not produce drug concentrations within the therapeutic range will not achieve the drug's beneficial effect. Every drug has a specific minimum concentration at which beneficial effects

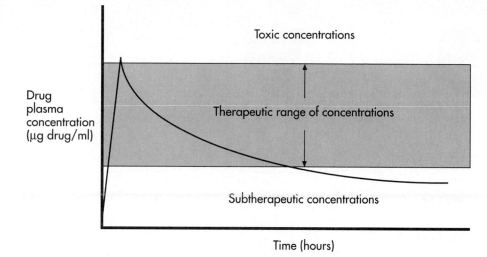

Fig. 3-1 The therapeutic range of concentrations of a drug in the plasma.

become evident. Below this lower end of the therapeutic range, drug concentrations are at subtherapeutic levels.

Maintaining Drug Concentrations Within the Therapeutic Range

The goal of pharmacologic therapy is to maintain drug concentrations in the body within the idealized therapeutic range; therefore the drug must enter the body at a rate that is balanced by the speed with which the drug leaves the body. Using a simple analogy, think of the body as a bucket with a small hole and an administered drug as water being poured into the leaky bucket. If you want the water in the bucket to remain at a particular level, you must continuously pour in water at a rate equal to that at which it leaks out of the hole.

To maintain therapeutic concentrations of a drug in an animal, the amount of the drug administered and the rate at which it is absorbed must match the rate at which it is eliminated from the body (Fig. 3-2).

If the hole in the bucket suddenly becomes smaller, you must decrease the rate at which you pour in water (administer the drug) to prevent overflow (toxicity). In animals the liver and kidneys are the primary organs involved in removing drugs from the body. If these organs are damaged and elimination of the drug is slowed, the drug dosage (rate of administration) must be slowed or the dose (drug amount) must be reduced to prevent accumulation to toxic levels.

In contrast, if the hole in the bucket is made larger and the rate of water addition remains constant, the water level falls. Similarly, if the rate of drug elimination is increased by diuresis, which is the administration of fluids or certain drugs to stimulate increased urine production, a drug normally eliminated through the kidneys is "flushed" from the body more rapidly, reducing drug concentrations in the body.

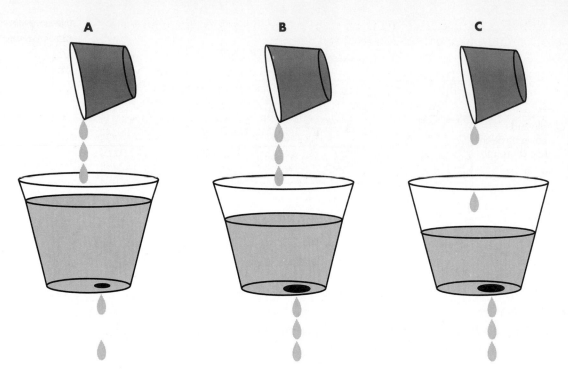

Fig. 3-2 The bucket analogy for understanding drug dosages and dosage intervals. **A,** If the rate at which water is poured into a bucket is greater than the rate at which it is leaving, the water level will rise. **B,** If the rate at which water is poured into a bucket is equal to the rate at which it is leaving, the water level will remain stable. **C,** If the rate at which water is poured into a bucket is less than the rate at which it is leaving, the water level will fall.

DOSAGE REGIMEN AND ROUTES OF ADMINISTRATION

The three components of therapeutic administration of drugs are as follows: the dose, the dosage interval, and the route of administration. Altering any component can result in drug concentrations that are too high or too low.

Drug Dose

A drug's dose is the amount of drug administered at one time. Because different drug manufacturers produce the same drug in various concentrations, the veterinary technician should always state the dose in units of mass, such as milligrams, grams, or grains, rather than the number of product units, such as tablets or capsules, or volume such as milliliters or "cc's." For example, the veterinary technician should avoid writing in the patient record that an animal received 1 tablet of amoxicillin because amoxicillin is available in tablet sizes ranging from 50 mg up to 400 mg. The same is true of the statement "Give 3 ml of xylazine" because 3 ml of a xylazine solution with a concentration of 20 mg/ml contains much less xylazine than 3 ml of a solution with a concentration of 100 mg/ml.

Some administration instructions differentiate between a **loading dose** and a **maintenance dose.** The loading dose is designed to raise the drug concentration to the therapeutic range in a short time. A loading dose is either a larger amount of drug administered one time, usually by intravenous (IV) or intramuscular (IM) route, or a rapid IV infusion rate, resulting in rapid achievement of therapeutic concentrations. Once therapeutic concentrations are achieved, periodic, small maintenance doses maintain the therapeutic concentrations. Therefore loading doses are used when the veterinarian wants drug concentrations to rapidly reach the therapeutic range.

Pharm Fact

A loading dose quickly attains therapeutic concentrations and is followed by smaller maintenance doses.

Dosage Interval

The time between administration of separate drug doses is referred to as the dosage interval. Dosage intervals are often expressed using Latin abbreviations (see Chapter 2). Veterinary technicians must understand these common abbreviations to administer the appropriate drug amount at the proper time.

Abbreviation	Dosage interval
SID	Once daily
BID	Twice daily
TID	Three times daily
QID	Four times daily
q4h	Every 4 hours
q6h	Every 6 hours
q8h	Every 8 hours
q12h	Every 12 hours
qd	Every day
q2d	Every 2 days ("every other" day)
prn	As needed

Pharmacists and medical professionals often refer to the dose (loading and maintenance) and the dosage interval together as the dosage regimen. The veterinary technician can determine the total daily dose, which is the total amount of drug delivered to an animal in 24 hours, by multiplying the dose by the frequency of administration (for example, 100 mg given 4 times daily results in a total daily dose of 400 mg). You can adjust the dosage interval and dose for medical reasons or to increase client compliance (the animal owner's willingness to administer the medication as directed) and still deliver approximately the same amount of drug each day. For example, the following dosage regimens are equivalent and provide a total daily dose of 480 mg:

480 mg SID
240 mg BID
160 mg q8h
120 mg q6h
80 mg q4h

Routes of Administration

Even if the correct dose is administered, the amount of drug that reaches the target tissues in the body can be significantly altered if the proper **route of administration** (the way a drug enters the body) is not used. Drugs given by injection are **parenterally administered,** which literally means "administered in the space between the enteric canal (the gastrointestinal tract) and the surface of the body." Drugs given by mouth, or per os (PO), are orally administered. Drugs that are applied to the surface of the skin such as lotions and liniments are topically administered. Aerosol administration usually means the drug is administered as a mist or gas via the respiratory tract.

Parenteral administration of drugs is further divided into specific routes. Intravenous (IV) administration means the drug is injected directly into a vein. Intravenous injections can be given as a single, large volume at one time, called an IV bolus, or slowly injected or dripped into a vein over several seconds, minutes, or even hours as an intravenous infusion. (Fig. 3-3 shows the differences in drug concentrations achieved by these variations of intravenous administration.) With a constant-rate IV infusion, drug levels eventually reach a plateau, or steady state, and remain there until the infusion is stopped.

Intravenous injection is not the same as intraarterial injection. Drugs given by this route are injected into an artery, not a vein, thus quickly producing high concentrations of drug in the tissues supplied by that artery. In contrast, after intravenous injection, blood containing the drug passes to the heart and is mixed and diluted with the remaining blood in circulation before it is delivered to body tissues. Inadvertent injection of drugs intraarterially (for example, injection into the carotid artery instead of the jugular

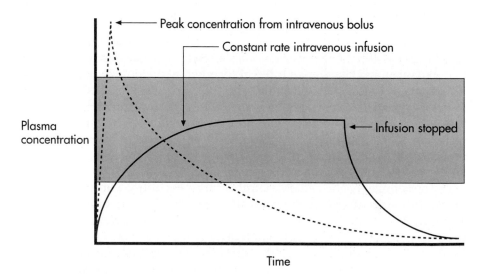

Fig. 3-3 Plasma concentrations of a drug after intravenous bolus injection and infusion. Color shows the therapeutic range.

vein) delivers a bolus (single, large amount) of drug directly to the tissues and can produce severe effects such as seizures or respiratory arrest. An accidental injection of a drug outside of the blood vessel (not within the vessel lumen) is extravascular or perivascular injection. Some drugs cause extreme local inflammation and tissue death if accidentally injected extravascularly.

Intramuscular (IM) administration involves injecting the drug into a muscle mass. Subcutaneous (SC or SQ) injections are administered deep beneath the skin into the subcutis. Intradermal (ID) injections are administered within, not beneath, the skin with very small needles. The intradermal route is usually reserved for skin testing procedures, such as testing for tuberculosis or reaction to allergenic substances. Intraperitoneal (IP) injections are administered into the abdominal body cavity and are frequently used when IV or IM injections are not practical (as in some laboratory animals) or large volumes of solution must be administered for rapid absorption. Each route of administration has its own pattern of drug absorption (speed and degree of absorption). The veterinary technician must know these patterns to identify the most advantageous route of administration for the patient or the clinical problem.

Pharm Fact

Accidental injection of a intravenous drug into an artery can produce severe adverse reactions.

MOVEMENT OF DRUG MOLECULES IN THE BODY

Part of the reason different routes of administration result in varied drug concentration curves is because of the way drug molecules move from one site to another by different mechanisms. There are four basic mechanisms: passive diffusion, facilitated diffusion, active transport, and pinocytosis and phagocytosis. The majority of drug movement through tissue fluid or membrane barriers is via passive diffusion.

Passive Diffusion

Passive diffusion is the random movement of drug molecules from an area of high concentration to an area of lower concentration. For example, when you pour a colored liquid into a glass of water, the color spreads, or diffuses, to all parts of the water. Similarly, when a drug is injected into the body, it passively diffuses from the injection site to areas of lower concentrations, eventually reaching a blood capillary and entering the systemic circulation. In this process no cellular energy is expended and no active transport process is performed by the body to direct the movement of drug molecules: hence the term *passive diffusion*.

Drug molecules move through body fluids by passive diffusion. Many drugs pass through biologic membranes such as cell membranes by passive diffusion. For a drug to diffuse from one side of a biologic membrane to the other, the drug must dissolve in the membrane, which is composed primarily of phospholipids, and diffuse down the concentration gradient from an area of high concentration on an area of lower concentration on the other side of the membrane. Thus if a drug can dissolve in a cell membrane, it readily passes through the membrane by passive diffusion without any energy expended by the cell to move the drug molecules. Passive diffusion continues until enough molecules have passed from an area of higher concentration to an area or areas of lower concentration to equalize the concentrations. At that point the concentration gradient is very small, and little difference exists in drug concentration in the areas of formerly high concentration and the areas of formerly low concentration. Drug molecules continue to move, however, such that an equal number move into and out of both areas. At that point the drug concentrations are in equilibrium. Theoretically, drug molecules move by diffusion from the site of administration to other areas throughout the body until equilibrium is attained among all compartments of the body.

Facilitated Diffusion

Facilitated diffusion is a passive transport mechanism across biologic membranes that involves a special "carrier molecule" in the membrane that facilitates the movement of certain drug molecules across the membrane. As in passive diffusion, facilitated diffusion involves no energy expended by the cell to move the drug molecules, and the direction of drug movement is determined by the concentration gradient (Fig. 3-4). In addition, once equilibrium is attained, the number of drug molecules crossing the membrane in either direction via the carrier remains the same.

Active Transport

Like facilitated diffusion, **active transport** of drug molecules involves a specialized carrier molecule. However, in active transport a drug molecule comes in contact with a specialized carrier molecule in the membrane, and the cell expends energy to move the drug molecule across or to "reset" the carrier molecule after transport so that it may transport again. Unlike diffusion, in which the direction of net drug movement is determined by the concentration gradient, active transport can move drug molecules against the concentration gradient from areas of low concentration to areas of higher concentration. Thus drugs can accumulate in high concentrations within a cell or body compartment via active transport.

Drugs actively transported may potentially reach such high concentrations within cells that they exert a toxic effect, such as that seen with aminoglycoside antibiotics. Because active transport requires cellular energy, anything that disrupts the cell's production of energy such as toxins or certain drugs prevents active transport of drug molecules across biologic membranes.

Physical Transport

Drug molecules may enter a cell by being physically engulfed by the cell, which involves one of two processes: pinocytosis ("cell drinking") or phagocytosis ("cell eating"). In both processes a portion of the cellular membrane surrounds the drug molecule and takes it within the cell. This is an active

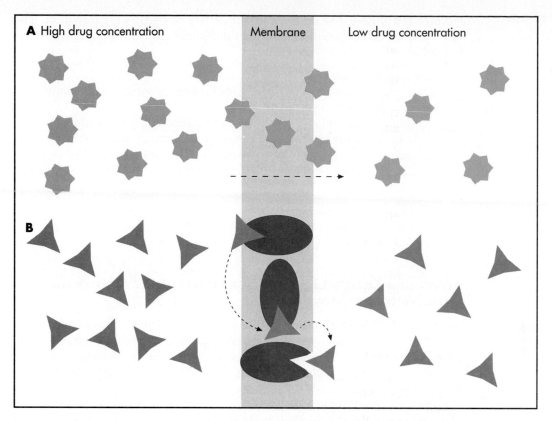

Fig. 3-4 Diffusion across a membrane. **A,** Passive diffusion. **B,** Facilitated diffusion.

process that requires the cell to expend energy. Pinocytosis and phagocytosis are especially important for movement of large drug molecules such as complex proteins or antibodies that would otherwise be unable to enter a cell or pass intact through a membrane barrier.

Effect of Transport Mechanisms on Drug Molecule Movement

Different drug transport mechanisms can determine not only the direction of drug molecule movement but also the rate at which the molecules move from one compartment to the next or through a membrane barrier. In facilitated diffusion and active transport, in which a carrier molecule is involved with drug molecule movement, the transport mechanism can only move a limited number of drug molecules at one time. If the transport system becomes overloaded or saturated, some drug molecules waiting to be transported begin accumulating. Thus the rate at which carrier-molecule transport mechanisms move drug molecules across the membrane has a maximum speed, sometimes called **t-max.**

In contrast to these carrier transport systems, the rate of passive diffusion is not limited because drug molecules simply diffuse through any part of the

Pharm Fact

Drugs that are actively transported across a membrane can accumulate in very high concentrations within cells or body compartments.

biologic membrane and do not rely on carrier molecules for transport. The rate at which molecules diffuse across the membrane is mostly related to the following:

- Concentration gradient
- Drug molecule size (with smaller molecules moving more rapidly than larger molecules)
- Lipophilic ("fat loving") nature of the molecule (with the ability to dissolve in fats, thus increasing the rate of movement across membranes)
- Temperature (the lower the temperature, the slower the diffusion)
- Thickness of the membrane (the thicker the membrane, the slower the diffusion)

Pinocytosis and phagocytosis are relatively slow mechanisms for drug transport because they involve a complex series of changes as the cell imbibes or ingests larger drug molecules.

Effect of a Drug's Lipophilic or Hydrophilic Nature on Drug Molecule Movement

As stated previously, drugs must dissolve, or be soluble, in a membrane to move across it by passive diffusion. Biologic membranes are largely composed of lipids (fats). Therefore to move across a membrane, drug molecules must be in a form that dissolves in fat or oil. This fat-loving form is known as the lipophilic form.

Some drug molecules dissolve more readily in water than in fat or oil. These "water-loving" forms are hydrophilic. When oil and water mix, they separate into two distinct layers. Hydrophilic drugs thus have difficulty dissolving in, and passing through, phospholipid (fat) cellular membranes. Conversely, lipophilic drugs tend to form into globules or balls when added to an aqueous (water-based) medium and therefore do not readily disperse throughout it.

Drug molecules that are polarized (contain charges at the ends of the molecule) or ionized (contain a net positive or negative charge such as HCO_3^-) readily dissolve in an aqueous medium and so are hydrophilic. Nonpolarized, nonionized drugs are less able to dissolve in water and can more readily pass through, lipid membranes and so are lipophilic. After administration of certain drugs, a specific percentage of the drug molecules go into a hydrophilic form and the remainder go into a lipophilic form. The degree to which a drug is predominantly in the hydrophilic or lipophilic form depends on the chemical nature of the drug and the environment in which it is placed.

PHARMACOKINETICS

Pharmacokinetics is the study (including mathematical descriptions) of how physiologic or drug characteristics affect drug concentrations within the body.

Movement of drugs into, through, and out of the body can be described in four basic steps: absorption, distribution, metabolism, and excretion (or elimination). Each step (sometimes described as ADME) may be altered by disease or physiologic conditions. The veterinarian and veterinary technician must recognize when these factors have been altered so that they can adjust the dosage to maintain drug concentrations within the therapeutic range. Failure to recognize or compensate for changing conditions can result in subtherapeutic responses in which the animal fails to respond or toxicity in which the animal experiences toxic side effects or dies.

Drug Absorption

After a drug has been ingested, injected, inhaled, or applied to the skin, it must be absorbed into the blood and travel to the body areas (target tissues) where it will have its intended effect. Movement of drug molecules from the site of administration into the systemic circulation is called **absorption.**

A drug is useless unless it is absorbed. Exceptions to this are drugs designed to work only where they are applied, such as local anesthetics, topical insecticides such as flea powders, and topical antibiotics and drugs that are intended to work within the lumen of the intestine and therefore need not be absorbed. With the exception of these locally acting medications, rapid, total absorption of the drug is desirable.

Effect of Route of Administration on Absorption

The route of administration (for example, PO and IM), directly affects the drug's **bioavailability,** which is the quantity of the drug administered that actually enters the systemic circulation. The IV route has no absorption phase because the drug is placed directly into the systemic circulation. Therefore 100% of a drug that is administered intravenously is absorbed, and these drugs have a bioavailability of 1. Drugs that are only partially absorbed have a bioavailability of less than 1. Drugs given by mouth or subcutaneously generally have the lowest bioavailability. Drugs given intramuscularly have only slightly less bioavailability than drugs given intravenously.

Not only the amount, but the rate at which drugs enter the body is also affected by the route of administration. Fig. 3-5 illustrates that drugs given intravenously almost instantly achieve their peak concentration (highest level) in the blood. Because drugs generally occupy the fluid component of blood and not the cells, blood concentrations of drugs are frequently (and more correctly) referred to as plasma, or serum, concentrations of drugs. As soon as the drug enters the blood (plasma), it begins to be excreted from the body. When a drug is injected as an IV bolus, the drug concentration immediately peaks and then gradually falls until all the drug has been excreted.

Drugs given intramuscularly take some time to diffuse from the injection site to the blood circulation. This is illustrated in Fig. 3-5 as a rapid increase of drug concentrations between the time of injection and attainment of the peak. Generally, drugs injected into muscle that is being exercised or used are absorbed rapidly; drugs injected into unused muscles are absorbed slowly because these muscles have less blood flow. Peak concentrations of

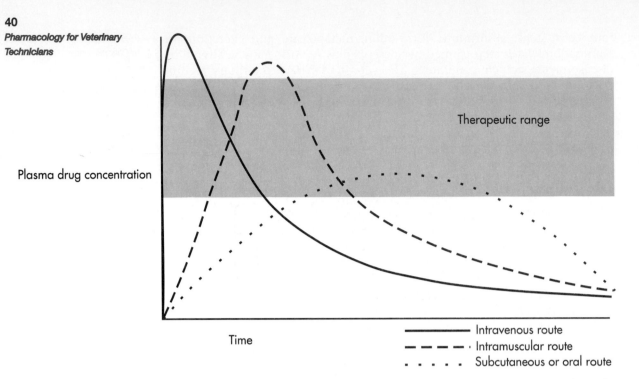

Plasma drug concentration

Time

Intravenous route
Intramuscular route
Subcutaneous or oral route

Fig. 3-5 Plasma drug concentrations attained after intravenous, intramuscular, subcutaneous, and oral administration.

drugs given intramuscularly are slightly lower than the peak from IV drug administration and occur within minutes of injection.

Drugs given by mouth or subcutaneously take longer to be absorbed because they must either diffuse farther to reach systemic circulation (SC injection) or they must pass through several barriers to be absorbed (PO administration). Because drugs given intramuscularly, subcutaneously, or by mouth attain therapeutic concentrations more slowly than drugs given intravenously, the IV route is preferred when the desired result is for a drug to have immediate effects on the body (as in emergency treatments). Unfortunately, many drugs are not formulated for IV administration and other routes must be used.

Because IV administration ensures that all the drug is immediately delivered into the systemic circulation, a short period (few minutes) often occurs during which serum concentrations of drugs are very high and in some cases may exceed the therapeutic range. Signs of toxicity could develop during this time unless drugs are given slowly by IV infusion. For example, injecting an animal with digoxin (a very widely used cardiac drug) as an IV bolus in loading-dose amounts might cause the animal to vomit or have serious cardiac arrhythmias (irregular heart beats) as a result of the high concentration in those first few minutes. Although some of these drugs can potentially be administered by IV bolus, the risk of short-term toxic concentrations may preclude their use. In those cases, slow IV infusion is recommended instead.

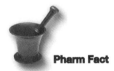

Pharm Fact

IV drugs that could cause toxicity if injected as an IV bolus may be safe if infused slowly.

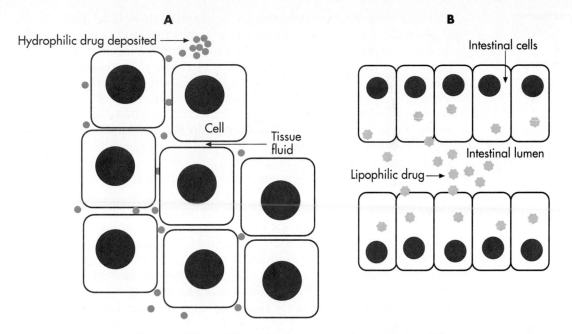

Fig. 3-6 Movement of hydrophilic and lipophilic drug molecules. **A,** Hydrophilic drug molecules at IM or SC injection site diffuse between cells. **B,** Lipophilic drug molecules in the intestinal lumen readily move through cell membranes.

Effect of Lipophilic and Hydrophilic Properties on Absorption

Drugs injected subcutaneously or intramuscularly are deposited in the fluid that surrounds the cells (extracellular fluid) and must diffuse through that fluid to reach the capillaries. Because extracellular fluid is an aqueous medium, hydrophilic drugs diffuse more readily than lipophilic drugs and hence are absorbed more quickly (Fig. 3-6). Some drugs that are injected intramuscularly or subcutaneously are formulated predominantly in a lipophilic form with the intent of slow absorption over hours to days. Such repository formulations are absorbed very slowly.

In contrast to drugs given subcutaneously and intramuscularly, drugs given by mouth must pass through cellular membranes to be absorbed from the lumen of the intestinal tract. Therefore drugs given by mouth must be in a lipophilic form to be readily absorbed from the gastrointestinal (GI) tract. Hydrophilic drugs, which are highly ionized or very polarized, are poorly absorbed from the gut. Some drugs (for example, some deworming agents and intestinal antibiotics) are chemically formulated to be hydrophilic to prevent absorption from the gut and maintain a high concentration within the intestinal lumen, where the drug exerts its effect.

Effect of pH of the Environment on Absorption

When you know the acidic or alkaline nature of a drug, the drug's pKa, and the pH of the drug's environment, you can determine whether the drug is in a predominantly ionized (hydrophilic) or nonionized (lipophilic) form. From that you should then be able to predict whether the drug will be well absorbed across a membrane barrier or will diffuse readily through tissue fluid.

Drugs given subcutaneously or intramuscularly are more readily absorbed in the hydrophilic form, and drugs given by mouth are more readily absorbed in the lipophilic form. The pH, which is the measure of acidity or alkalinity of the drug's environment, also affects drug absorption. After administration, some drugs are partially hydrophilic and partially lipophilic. The predominant form depends on the nature of the drug molecule and the pH of the drug's environment.

For example, after an aspirin tablet (acetylsalicylic acid) is swallowed and dissolves in the acidic environment of the stomach, which has a pH of 3, half the aspirin molecules are ionized and half are nonionized. However, as these molecules move out of the acidic environment of the stomach and into the more alkaline environment of the duodenum, which has a pH of about 5 near the stomach, the ratio of ionized to nonionized molecules changes dramatically. At this point most aspirin molecules are in an ionized form (about 100 ionized molecules for every 1 nonionized molecule).

This dramatic shift from fairly equal numbers of ionized and nonionized drug molecules in the stomach to a predominance of the ionized form in the duodenum would significantly reduce absorption of aspirin from the duodenum because most of the aspirin molecules are in a hydrophilic form, and orally administered drugs must be lipophilic to cross the membrane barriers of the gut. Because of its chemical characteristics, aspirin is more easily absorbed in the stomach than the intestine.

The chemical characteristics that determine the quantity of drug molecules converted into a lipophilic or hydrophilic form are determined by the drug's acidic or alkaline nature and pKa. The acidic or alkaline nature of a drug characterizes a drug molecule's ability to take up or release a hydrogen ion (H^+). A general rule is that as the environmental pH becomes more alkaline, weakly acidic compounds tend to shift more molecules into the ionized form. Conversely, as the environmental pH becomes more acidic, weakly alkaline compounds tend to shift more molecules into the ionized form. Sidebar 3-1 explains the differences between acidic and alkaline drugs.

In the previous example, aspirin is an acidic drug. In the more alkaline pH of the duodenum, the aspirin molecules are more in the ionized state than they were in the acidic environment of the stomach. In contrast, an alkaline drug such as the antiulcer medication cimetidine exists predominantly in the ionized form in the acidic environment of the stomach, with fewer molecules in the nonionized form. Thus the acidic or alkaline nature of a drug molecule influences which form (ionized or nonionized) will predominate as the pH of the environment changes (becomes more acidic or more alkaline).

Aspirin and sulfadimethoxine (an antibacterial agent) are both acidic drugs that become increasingly nonionized as the environmental pH becomes more acidic, and they become increasingly ionized as the pH becomes more alkaline. However, these two acidic drugs differ in the predominance of ionized or nonionized forms at a particular pH environment. For exam-

Sidebar 3-1

The Difference Between an Acidic Drug and an Alkaline Drug

An acid drug is a substance that, when in non-ionized form, can donate a hydrogen ion (H^+, or proton) and become ionized. Once in ionized form the drug molecule can acquire a hydrogen ion and revert to its nonionized form. In the following chemical equation the compounds act as acids. The R indicates the remainder of the drug molecule:

$$R—C{=}O \longleftrightarrow R—C{=}O + H^+$$
$$\text{OH (nonionized)} \quad \text{O}^- \text{ (now ionized)}$$

$$H_2SO_4 \longleftrightarrow HSO_4^- + H^+$$

An acidic solution such as an acid bath or gastric fluid contains many free H^+. The term *pH* is defined in reference to the number of free hydrogen ions. The more acidic the solution, the more free H^+ present in the solution. Thus any ionized molecules (hydrophilic forms) of an acidic drug present quickly encounter a free H^+, combine with it, and become nonionized (lipophilic). Therefore an acidic drug placed in an acidic environment exists primarily in the nonionized (lipophilic) form.

When a molecule of an alkaline drug accepts or combines with an H^+, it becomes ionized, which is the opposite of an acidic drug. Conversely, a molecule of an alkaline drug sheds that H^+ to become nonionized again. This is illustrated below in the equation for an alkaline drug:

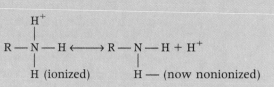

When a nonionized molecule of an alkaline drug is added to an acidic solution, which contains many free H^+, an H^+ combines with the nonionized molecule and converts it to a positively charged ionized molecule (hydrophilic form). Therefore the molecules of alkaline drugs placed in an acidic environment tend to become ionized, and more of the drug molecules are in the hydrophilic form. This is the opposite of what happens to a molecule of an acidic drug.

Weak acids and weak bases are acidic or alkaline compounds with a ratio of ionized to nonionized molecules that predictably changes as the drug encounters different pH ranges within the body (referred to as *physiologic pH*). In contrast, the molecules of strong acids such as hydrochloric acid (HCl) or strong bases such as sodium hydroxide (NaOH) usually do not shift between ionized and nonionized forms when encountering the pH range normally found within the body.

ple, in the stomach, which has a pH of 3, aspirin exists as approximately equal numbers of ionized and nonionized drug molecules (with a ratio of approximately 1:1). With sulfadimethoxine the ratio is approximately 1 ionized molecule to 1000 nonionized molecules in the same acidic stomach environment. Therefore sulfadimethoxine can more readily penetrate stomach cell membranes than can aspirin because more sulfadimethoxine molecules are in nonionized form. This difference can be attributed to the drug's *pKa*.

Each drug has a specific **pKa,** which is the pH at which all drug molecules are equally distributed between ionized and nonionized forms (ratio of 1:1). In the aspirin example, at a pH of 3, half the aspirin molecules are ionized and the other half nonionized. Therefore the pKa for aspirin is 3. For sulfa-

pH	Ionized:nonionized	pH	Ionized:nonionized
1	1 : 100	1	1 : 100,000
2	1 : 10	2	1 : 10,000
3	1 : 1	3	1 : 1,000
A 4	10 : 1	4	1 : 100 **B**
5	100 : 1	5	1 : 10
6	1,000 : 1	6	1 : 1
7	10,000 : 1	7	10 : 1
8	100,000 : 1	8	100 : 1

Fig. 3-7 Ratios of ionized to nonionized molecules of aspirin **(A)** and sulfadimethoxine **(B)** at various pH values. Color indicates pH at which the majority of drug molecules are in the ionized form.

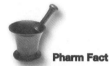

Pharm Fact

Acidic drugs exist mostly in the nonionized form in an acidic environment and mostly in the ionized form in an alkaline environment.

dimethoxine, half of the molecules are ionized and half are nonionized at a pH of 6; thus the pKa for sulfadimethoxine is 6.

The concept of pKa also applies to alkaline drugs. Acidic drugs exist predominantly in the nonionized form at any pH that is more acidic than that drug's pKa. In contrast, alkaline drugs exist predominantly in the ionized form at any pH that is more acidic than the drug's pKa. Figs. 3-7 and 3-8 show the way the ratio of ionized to nonionized molecules changes as the pH becomes more acidic or more alkaline. The ratio changes predictably for each increment of pH change. The ratio changes by a factor of 10 for each incremental change in pH. If the ratio is 1:100 at a particular pH, the ratio changes to 1:10 (1/10th of 100) and 1:1000 (10 × 100) at the next lower or higher pH.

In summary, acidic drugs exist predominantly in the nonionized form in an acidic environment and predominantly in the ionized form in an alkaline environment. Alkaline drugs exist predominantly in the nonionized form in an alkaline environment and predominantly in the ionized form in an acidic environment. The acidic or alkaline nature of a drug, its pKa, and the pH of the environment all determine the number of drug molecules that will be in the ionized or nonionized form.

Ion Trapping and Absorption of Drugs

Different compartments of the body have different pH environments. For example, the pH in the stomach is usually between 1 and 3, and in the duodenum the pH is 6 to 7. Within cells and most body fluids, the pH remains a fairly constant 7.4. A drug molecule could change from ionized form to nonionized form (or vice versa) as it passes from one compartment to another with a different pH. If a molecule enters a compartment whose pH causes a shift from nonionized to ionized (hydrophilic) form, the drug molecule may not be able to exit the compartment through the cellular membrane because it now exists in a hydrophilic form. This phenomenon is called **ion trapping.**

An example of ion trapping is seen when aspirin is taken by mouth. In the acidic environment of the stomach, the acidic aspirin exists predominantly in the nonionized form; these molecules readily penetrate the cells of the stomach wall (Fig. 3-9). However, the stomach cells' cytoplasm has a pH of 7.4,

pH	Ionized:nonionized
1	100 : 1
2	10 : 1
3	1 : 1
4	1 : 10
5	1 : 100
6	1 : 1,000
7	1 : 10,000
8	1 : 100,000

A

pH	Ionized:nonionized
1	10,000,000 : 1
2	1,000,000 : 1
3	100,000 : 1
4	10,000 : 1
5	1,000 : 1
6	100 : 1
7	10 : 1
8	1 : 1

B

Fig. 3-8 Ratios of ionized to nonionized molecules of diazepam **(A)** and lidocaine **(B)** at various pH values. Color indicates pH at which the majority of drug molecules are in the ionized form.

which is considerably more alkaline than the stomach environment. In an alkaline environment more of the acidic drug molecules shift to the ionized form, trapping them within the stomach cell membranes. As more lipophilic molecules enter, change into hydrophilic form, and become trapped within the aspirin molecules accumulate within the cells lining the stomach.

This does not mean that aspirin taken 3 weeks ago is still lodged in the cells of the stomach wall. The ratio of ionized to nonionized remains the same; some molecules remain in the nonionized form, even if the ratio is 1 nonionized to 10,000 ionized. As that single nonionized molecule passes out of the cell and into the blood, another ionized molecule is converted to the nonionized form to preserve the 1:10,000 ratio. This new nonionized molecule then moves out of the cell, and the cycle repeats until all the drug is absorbed and leaves the stomach cells. If the drug within the stomach wall cells had existed with most molecules in the nonionized form at a pH of 7.4, the drug would have been absorbed much more rapidly.

Ion trapping is used to treat animals that have received drugs or ingested poisons that are normally excreted by the kidney. As discussed in more detail later in this chapter, compounds in the lipophilic (nonionized) form in the kidney can passively diffuse through the renal tubular cells, enter an adjoining capillary, and be reabsorbed back into the systemic circulation. If these compounds are toxic, this reabsorption can cause additional damage because the agent is recirculated instead of excreted in the urine. However, if the pH of the urine can be changed so that the nonionized molecules become ionized, these hydrophilic molecules cannot passively diffuse through the renal tubular cell membranes and thus are trapped within the lumen of the renal tubule and excreted safely in the urine. Urinary acidifiers or alkalinizers are compounds that alter the pH of the urine and can be used to speed elimination of toxic agents such as strychnine.

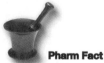

Pharm Fact

Urinary acidifiers or alkalinizers can be used to ion trap and hasten excretion of drugs or poisons.

Factors Affecting Absorption and Bioavailability of Orally Administered Drugs

Drugs given by mouth must be in the lipophilic form to penetrate the gastrointestinal (GI) mucosa and be absorbed. However, for a lipophilic drug to diffuse across the membrane barrier, it must be small enough to dissolve in

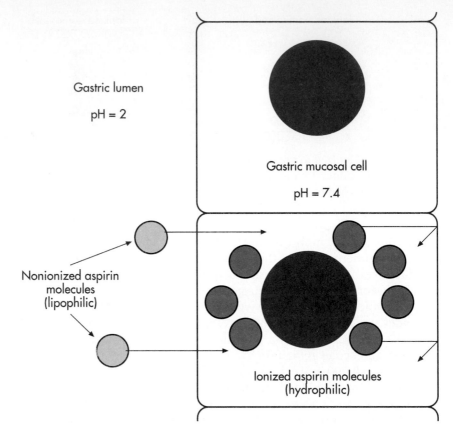

Gastric lumen

pH = 2

Gastric mucosal cell

pH = 7.4

Nonionized aspirin
molecules
(lipophilic)

Ionized aspirin molecules
(hydrophilic)

Fig. 3-9   Ion trapping of drug molecules in gastric mucosal cells.

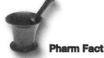

Pharm Fact

Drugs in liquid form usu-

ally have a faster onset of

action than drugs in solid

form.

the membrane. Large molecules such as antibodies and large proteins cannot readily diffuse through membranes because of their size. Tablets, granules, or powders cannot be absorbed until they break apart into much smaller particles. Thus dissolution, or dissolving, of the drug form (for example, tablet and powder) is a critical step in absorption of drugs given by mouth (Fig. 3-10).

Drugs in liquid form such as solutions and elixirs do not have a dissolution step and thus are usually more rapidly absorbed than solid dosage forms such as tablets. Thus liquid forms of a drug may have a quicker onset of action in the body than the same drug in solid form. For example, digoxin elixir is more rapidly absorbed because of the higher bioavailability and delivers more drug to the body than the tablet form.

Chapter 1 described sustained-release tablets and enteric-coated tablets as two special forms of oral drugs. Sustained-release medications dissolve slowly over minutes to hours while releasing small amounts of medication for absorption. The difference between systemic concentrations attained with a standard tablet and concentrations achieved with a sustained-release tablet are shown in Fig. 3-11. Enteric-coated tablets have a protective covering that prevents exposure of the drug to the harsh acidic envi-

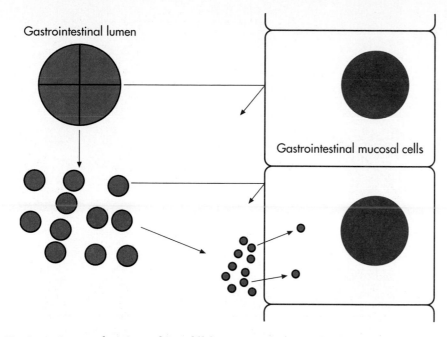

Fig. 3-10 Drugs administered in solid form must first completely dissolve to be absorbed.

ronment of the stomach. The enteric coating dissolves in the more alkaline environment of the duodenum, releasing the drug in this environment instead of in the stomach.

Gastric motility and intestinal motility can also affect absorption of an orally administered drug. *Gastric motility* refers to stomach contractions that move food and drugs from the stomach into the small intestine. Except for certain acidic drugs and other lipophilic compounds, most drugs are absorbed in the small intestine. The longer it takes for a drug to move into the small intestine, the longer it takes for the drug to be absorbed and exert an effect (Fig. 3-12). Thus conditions of decreased gastric motility or impaired gastric outflow can delay the onset of action of many orally administered drugs. For example, pyloric spasm delays gastric emptying, thereby causing a drug to be retained within the stomach for a prolonged period before it enters the intestine for absorption. Conversely, with increased gastric motility a drug may reach the intestine and begin to be absorbed sooner than normal.

The intestinal motility will determine if tablet dosage forms will have enough time to dissolve and be absorbed in the small intestine. If intestinal motility is increased, as in hypermotile diarrhea, the tablet may not remain in the small intestine long enough to be dissolved, and the drug may simply pass out of the body through the feces without being fully absorbed.

In contrast, decreased intestinal motility, as occurs with constipation or antidiarrheal treatment, can result in greater than normal absorption of the drug. Certain orally administered drugs such as neomycin exist primarily in the hydrophilic form and are designed to remain within the lumen of the

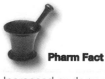

Pharm Fact

Increased or decreased GI motility can alter absorption of orally administered drugs.

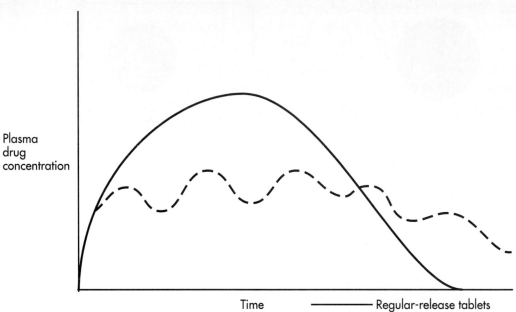

Fig. 3-11 Plasma drug concentrations attained after administration of standard tablets and sustained-release tablets.

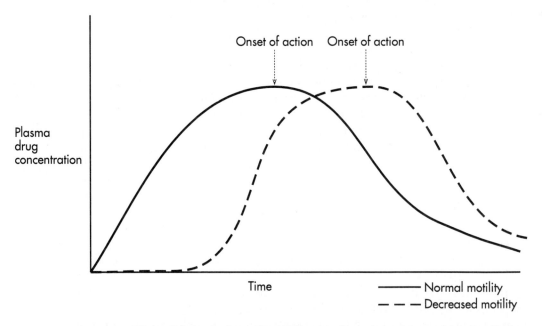

Fig. 3-12 Effect of decreased gastric motility on absorption of drugs from the duodenum.

intestine. They are not normally absorbed to any great extent. However, as illustrated earlier in the ion-trapping example, even if most drug molecules are in the hydrophilic form, a few molecules still exist in the lipophilic form and are absorbed. If the neomycin remains in the small intestine for an extended time, the few lipophilic molecules of neomycin continue to enter the body, eventually resulting in absorption of a significant amount of drug.

Even if a drug in solid form has dissolved into small particles, has remained in the intestine long enough to be absorbed, and is in the lipophilic form, one final barrier separates it from the systemic circulation. All blood that leaves the intestine travels by way of the hepatic portal system to the liver before it enters the systemic circulation. This allows the liver to screen and remove toxins absorbed from the GI tract before they can affect the rest of the body. Because drugs are viewed by the liver as foreign substances (xenobiotics), the liver may remove some drugs presented to it via the hepatic portal system. In some cases, such as with use of the tranquilizer diazepam in dogs, the liver removes so much of the drug that very little reaches the systemic circulation and hence has little effect on the body when given by mouth. Such extensive removal of the drug by the liver is called the **first-pass effect.**

Factors Affecting Absorption of Parenteral Drugs

Drugs injected subcutaneously or intramuscularly should be in the hydrophilic form so that they may readily diffuse through tissue fluid and reach a capillary to be absorbed. Anything that interferes with diffusion of the drug from the site of administration or alters blood flow to the injection site can delay absorption of the drug.

Tissue perfusion describes the extent of the blood supply to a tissue. If a tissue is well perfused by an extensive network of capillaries, the distance from the site of drug administration to a capillary is fairly short. Therefore a well-perfused tissue facilitates absorption of an injected drug. Because exercised skeletal muscle is well perfused, drugs injected intramuscularly are usually rapidly absorbed. In contrast, adipose (fat) tissue generally is poorly perfused, and drugs injected into a fat pad may remain there for an extended period without being absorbed. Subcutaneous tissues are not as well perfused as muscle but are better perfused than adipose tissue. Thus drugs given subcutaneously are not absorbed as quickly as those given intramuscularly, but the drug reaches systemic circulation much more quickly than any drug accidentally injected into a fatty deposit.

Tissue perfusion varies with physiologic conditions. An inactive muscle is not as well perfused as an active muscle; consequently, inactive muscles absorb drugs at a slower rate. Perfusion of subcutaneous tissue changes with the skin temperature. A body's exposure to cold temperatures causes the precapillary sphincters (circular rings of smooth muscle located at the entrance of the capillary) in the subcutaneous capillaries to contract (a process called *vasoconstriction*), thereby reducing blood flow to the area. This reduces loss of body heat, but it also reduces absorption of drugs injected subcutaneously. Thus drugs injected subcutaneously under these conditions must diffuse into deeper tissues to enter open capillaries, which delays absorption. Preparations of the local anesthetic lidocaine often contain epinephrine, a potent vasoconstrictor that slows the drug's absorption away from the site of administration, thus extending the duration of local anesthesia.

Vasodilation (dilation of blood vessels) enhances drug absorption. Vasodilation initiated by increased body temperature (such as from warm, ambient temperatures and exercise) or drugs (such as alcohol) increases perfusion to subcutaneous tissues, facilitating absorption of drugs injected subcutaneously.

DRUG DISTRIBUTION

Once absorbed, most drugs are not beneficial unless they reach target tissue such as certain cells, tissues, or organs. For example, the target tissue for the cardiac drug digoxin is the myocardium (heart muscle). If the drug cannot reach the myocardium for any reason, it will not benefit the patient. **Distribution** describes movement of a drug from the systemic circulation into tissues.

Barriers to Drug Distribution

In addition to barriers to drug absorption, barriers to distribution also exist. In most cases, drugs leave the bloodstream through capillaries. A common belief is that drugs have to be in a lipophilic form to move in and out of capillaries because they must pass through a membrane. In most cases this is not true.

The capillary walls are only as thick as one endothelial cell. With the exception of capillaries in the brain and a few other sites in the body, capillary walls are sufficiently permeable that drugs can move easily in and out by passing between rather than through the endothelial cells. These gaps, or **fenestrations** ("windows"), between cells allow small drug molecules to move readily back and forth while keeping larger molecules such as proteins like albumin and red blood cells within the capillary lumen (Fig. 3-13).

Capillaries in the brain are different from capillaries in other tissues because the endothelial cells abut closely with each other in what are called *tight junctions* instead of the usual open fenestrations (Fig. 3-14). Thus capillaries in the brain have no opening through which drug molecules can pass. Any drug molecules leaving or entering a brain capillary must be lipophilic because they have to traverse the capillary membrane. Cells surrounding the capillaries in the brain (for example, astrocytes and glial cells) provide an additional membrane for drugs to pass through. Hydrophilic drug forms encounter a significant blood:brain barrier; however, lipophilic drugs readily pass through this barrier.

Veterinary professionals often assume that in a pregnant animal, the placenta keeps drugs and toxins from reaching the fetus in much the same way as the blood:brain barrier protects the brain. This is not true, however, be-

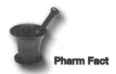

Pharm Fact

Lipophilic drugs readily pass through the blood:brain barrier, whereas hydrophilic drugs may be unable to penetrate this barrier.

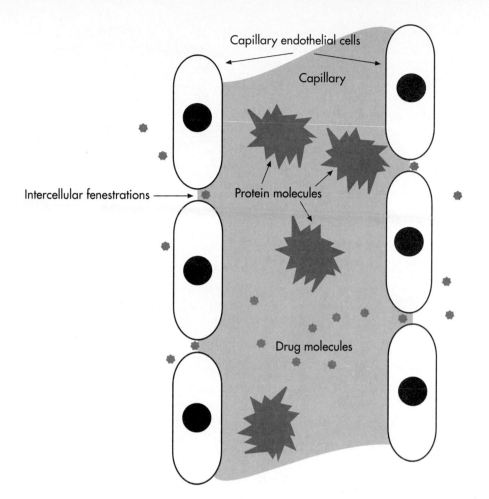

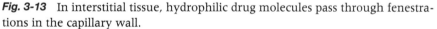

Fig. 3-13 In interstitial tissue, hydrophilic drug molecules pass through fenestrations in the capillary wall.

cause the capillaries in the placenta are permeable and allow most drugs to pass easily from maternal to fetal circulation. Therefore unless information exists to the contrary, the veterinary professional must assume that any drug given to a pregnant animal also reaches the developing fetus. Certain drugs administered at particular times in fetal development can result in spontaneous abortion, fetal malformation, or delivery of a weak neonate.

Effect of Tissue Perfusion on Drug Distribution

Drugs are usually distributed most rapidly and in greater concentrations to well-perfused tissues such as exercised skeletal muscle, the liver, kidneys, and the brain. In contrast, inactive skeletal muscle and adipose tissue are relatively poorly perfused, so drug delivery to these tissues is delayed. This

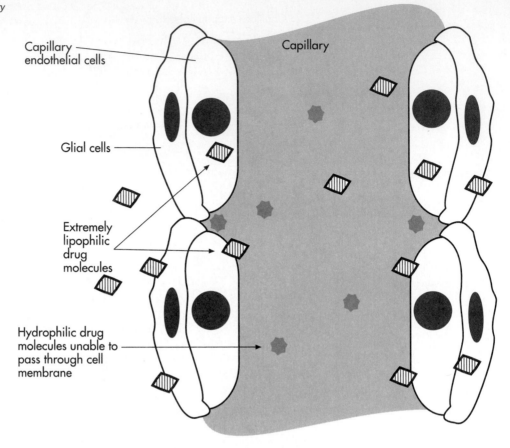

Capillary endothelial cells

Capillary

Glial cells

Extremely lipophilic drug molecules

Hydrophilic drug molecules unable to pass through cell membrane

Fig. 3-14 In CNS tissue, the blood:brain barrier allows only lipophilic drugs to enter the brain from the blood.

difference in perfusion explains the reason animals injected with short-acting barbiturates such as thiopental become anesthetized initially but quickly regain consciousness and require additional anesthetic.

Thiopental is a lipophilic drug; thus the blood:brain barrier poses no problem to its distribution. When thiopental is initially injected intravenously, it is first distributed to well-perfused tissues such as the brain. The drug accumulates rapidly and induces anesthesia. The thiopental remaining in the systemic circulation is slowly distributed into the less-perfused tissues such as fat and inactive muscle. While drug concentrations in the brain quickly reach equilibrium with the high blood concentrations, the drug continues to flow down a concentration gradient from the systemic circulation into the less-perfused adipose tissue.

As the drug leaves the blood and enters adipose tissue, drug concentrations in the blood decrease below concentrations in the brain. This reverses the concentration gradient, so the drug begins to flow from the brain back into the blood and eventually adipose tissue. This process of drug movement from one tissue, into blood, and into a second tissue is called **redistribution.** As the thiopental is redistributed from brain to blood to fat over a few minutes, the concentration of anesthetic drops in the brain and the animal wakes up (Fig. 3-15). Therefore, while perfusion generally determines which tissues receive the drug most quickly, eventually even the most poorly perfused tissues receive the drug, provided no physiologic barriers to the drug movement are present.

Effect of Plasma Protein Binding on Drug Distribution

Plasma contains circulating proteins that remain in systemic circulation because they are too large to pass through the capillary fenestrations. Some drugs bind to these proteins; these protein-bound drug molecules are not distributed to tissues (Fig. 3-16). Thus a significant proportion of a highly protein-bound drug remains in systemic circulation and acts as a reservoir of additional drug.

Because some molecules of a highly protein-bound drug exist in the free or unbound form (that is, they are not attached to the protein molecules), some drug is still delivered or distributed to the target tissue. The **protein-bound fraction** and the free fraction of the drug are in equilibrium. As free drug molecules move from the blood and into tissue along a concentration gradient, a roughly equivalent number of protein-bound drug molecules detach, or dissociate, from the protein molecules; these free drug molecules then move from the circulation and are distributed.

Recommended doses for highly protein-bound drugs are designed to compensate for the amount of protein-bound drug that remains in systemic circulation. Therefore reduction of the protein levels in the blood from any cause can greatly alter the pharmacologic effect of a "normal" dose of a highly protein-bound drug. For example, albumin is a plasma protein produced by the liver and is one of the principal proteins to which drugs bind. If an animal has liver disease and is unable to produce sufficient albumin or the animal has a protein-losing disease of the GI tract or kidney, less protein is available in the blood to bind to drugs. In this situation, a standard dose of a normally highly protein-bound drug results in a higher proportion of free drug molecules because less protein is available to bind the drug molecules. Therefore more drug molecules are distributed to the target tissue and have a greater pharmacologic effect. If the plasma protein level is sufficiently low, too much drug is available in the free form, which could result in toxic concentrations of drug in the target tissue.

The plasma protein level partially explains the reason animals with hypoalbuminemia (low plasma albumin level) require a smaller dose of barbiturates to be anesthetized. Barbiturates are normally highly protein bound. However, if the plasma albumin level is low, more barbiturate is free to diffuse into tissues (including the brain) and very high drug concentrations reach the brain, resulting in an anesthetic overdose from a "normal" dose of barbiturate. The dose of highly protein-bound drugs should be reduced in animals with liver disease, protein-losing enteropathy (intestinal disease), protein-losing nephropathy (kidney disease), or any other condition that alters protein-binding capacity.

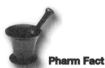

Pharm Fact

Standard doses of drugs that are highly protein bound may reach toxic concentrations in animals with low plasma protein levels.

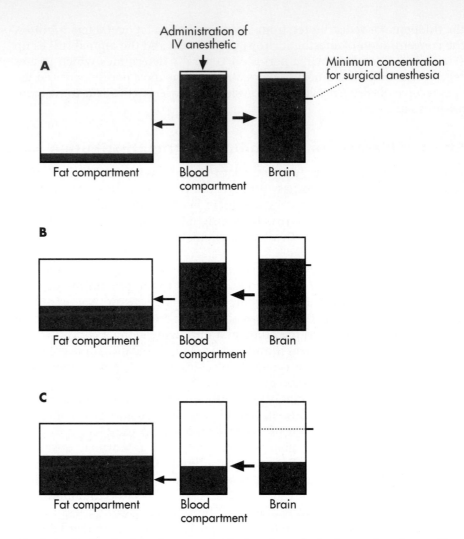

Fig. 3-15 Redistribution of an anesthetic drug from the brain to other tissues allows recovery from anesthesia. **A,** The drug moves quickly into the brain to cause surgical anesthesia. **B,** The concentration of anesthetic drug in the brain drops but is still sufficient to cause surgical anesthesia. **C,** The concentration of anesthetic drug in the brain drops below surgical anesthesia level, and the animal begins to awaken.

Volume of Distribution

The **volume of distribution (Vd)** is a pharmacokinetic value that approximates the degree to which a drug is distributed throughout the body. It assumes that the drug concentration in the blood is equivalent to the drug concentration equally dispersed throughout the rest of the body. Generally, the larger the volume of distribution for a drug, the more tissues the drug has penetrated and the lower the concentration in the blood.

For example, if you placed 100 mg of salt in a 1-L container of water (such as that shown in Fig. 3-17) and then placed 100 mg of salt in a second container of water with a volume of 10 L, which container would hold the more

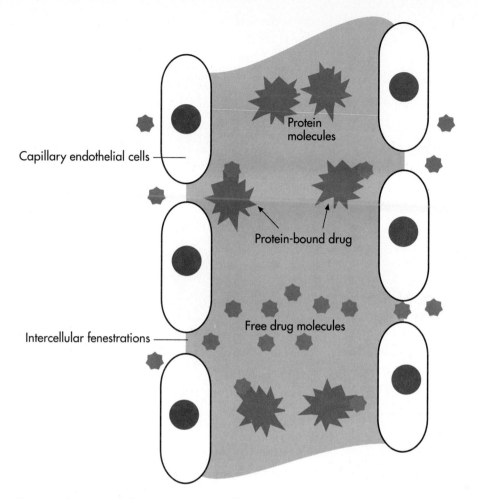

Capillary endothelial cells

Protein
molecules

Protein-bound drug

Free drug molecules

Intercellular fenestrations

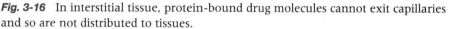

Fig. 3-16 In interstitial tissue, protein-bound drug molecules cannot exit capillaries and so are not distributed to tissues.

concentrated salt? The answer is that 100 mg of salt/1 L of water yields a salt concentration of 100 mg/1000 ml, or 0.1 mg/ml. In the 10-L container, 100 mg of salt/10 L of water is equivalent to 100 mg/10,000 ml, or 0.01 mg/ml. Thus the larger container holds the lower concentration of salt.

If the volume of distribution for a drug suddenly becomes larger (such as from accumulation of fluid within the abdomen, a condition called *ascites*), this might prevent a standard drug dose from achieving therapeutic concentrations because the drug amount is now diluted in a larger volume of body fluid. In this case the dose may have to be increased over the "normal" dose to attain concentrations in the therapeutic range. Conversely, in an animal that is severely dehydrated, the total body water is decreased and the volume of distribution for the drug is smaller, resulting in a higher concentration of drug in the remaining body fluids.

The apparent volume of distribution can be influenced by the protein binding of a drug. Volume of distribution is estimated by determining the

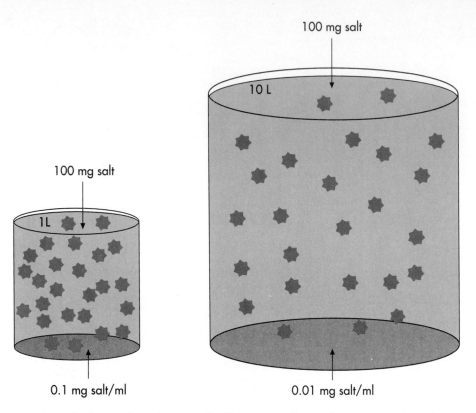

Fig. 3-17 The larger the volume of distribution, the lower the concentration of a drug.

drug concentration in the blood and then assuming the concentration is the same in all tissues of the body. However, in the case of drugs that are highly bound to plasma proteins, only the free drug molecules are readily distributed to tissues. Measurement of the plasma drug concentration (including both the free and the protein-bound drug molecules) shows that most of the original drug dose is still in the blood. The drug does not appear to penetrate tissues well because it is still mostly in the blood (high concentration, low volume of distribution, low penetration into the tissues). In reality, however, the few free drug molecules may be very lipophilic and readily penetrate tissues, but all the protein-bound drug still in the blood makes the apparent volume of distribution look small.

THE WAY DRUGS EXERT THEIR EFFECTS

Theoretically, if a drug is well absorbed and readily distributed in therapeutic concentrations to all tissues, it should have an effect on every tissue in the body. This is not always the case. For cells to respond to a drug molecule, usually the drug has to combine with a **receptor,** which is a specific protein molecule on or in the cell. A given receptor only combines with the molecule of certain drugs based on their shape or molecular structure. This con-

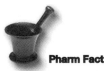

Pharm Fact

Cells can respond to a particular drug only if they possess a specific receptor for that drug.

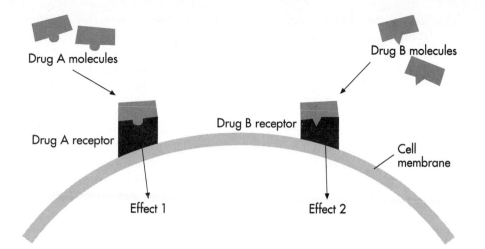

Fig. 3-18 Drug molecules have specific shapes that allow them to combine with specific receptors on the cell membrane surface and produce an effect. Drug A molecule combined with drug A receptor produces effect 1. Drug B molecule combined with drug B receptor produces effect 2.

cept may be compared with a key and lock: the receptor is the lock into which only the correct key (the drug) will fit (produce an effect). The effect of the correct drug molecule-receptor combination is some type of cellular change, such as the cell secreting substances, muscle cells contracting, or neuronal cells depolarizing (firing).

Cells do not have receptors for all drugs; only certain cells respond to certain drugs. For example, smooth muscle cells in the bronchioles of the lungs may have receptors to drug A, whereas smooth muscle cells in the uterus have no receptors to drug A. When drug A is administered, only the bronchiolar smooth muscle contracts, even though drug A is present at the uterus in therapeutic concentrations. The presence or absence of receptors and the number of receptors help determine whether a cell, a tissue, or an organ is sensitive to a particular drug.

As shown in Fig. 3-18, a cell surface (or sometimes cell organelles such as the nucleus and lysosomes) may have multiple types of receptors on it, each capable of combining with different specific drugs and each drug having a different effect on the cell. For example, when drug A combines with its receptor (see Fig. 3-18), the cell produces a response such as secretion of a protein. When drug B is present in therapeutic concentrations and combines with its specific receptor, the cell does not secrete protein but instead may be stimulated to divide. Hence, different drugs have different receptors and produce different effects.

Antagonists and Agonists

When drug A combines with its receptor, it produces a specific effect on the cell (see Fig. 3-18). We say that drug A has intrinsic activity when it combines with its receptor. A drug shaped similarly to drug A can combine with that

Injection of an antagonist drug may reverse the effects of an agonist drug.

same receptor but will produce no effect because of some characteristic about the second drug's shape or the way in which it combined with the receptor. The second drug has no intrinsic activity; it simply occupies the receptor site without producing a cellular effect. Drug A is an **agonist;** it produces an effect on the cell when it combines with its receptor. The second drug molecule is an **antagonist;** it is "antagonistic" to the effects of drug A (Fig. 3-19).

The effects of an agonist drug injection may be reversed by injection of an antagonist drug. This reversible antagonism is possible because for the most part, drug molecules do not just combine with the receptor and cease activity. Instead, they have a tendency to attach to and detach from the receptor and produce or maintain the cellular effect each time they recombine. If two drugs capable of combining with a particular receptor are present simultaneously at a receptor site, the drug with the greater number of molecules present is more likely to recombine with the receptor and produce an effect (agonist molecules) or prevent an effect (antagonist molecules).

One example is oxymorphone, a drug that combines with opioid receptors to produce analgesia (relief from pain), narcosis (induction of sleep from which the animal is not easily aroused), and respiratory depression. Because of the respiratory depression caused by oxymorphone, the effects of the drug are reversed using the narcotic antagonist naloxone. Naloxone has a structure similar to that of oxymorphone and thus can combine with the same opioid receptors. However, when it occupies these opioid receptors, naloxone produces no effect on the cell; no analgesia, narcosis, or respiratory depression occurs. Therefore naloxone is given in a sufficiently high dose that its molecules crowd out, or antagonize, the oxymorphone molecules at receptor sites and the animal begins to regain consciousness, feel pain, and breathe normally. At this point the effect of oxymorphone has been reversed by naloxone.

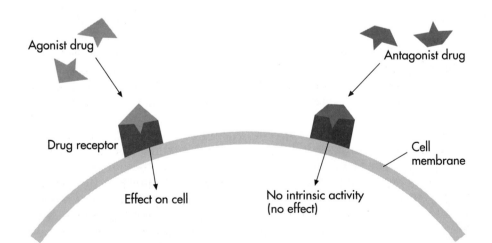

Fig. 3-19 An antagonist drug molecule occupies the cell's receptor sites, preventing the agonist drug from exerting its effect. The action of the antagonist drug combining with the receptor results in no effect.

In the previous example, oxymorphone and naloxone each had roughly an equal opportunity to occupy the same receptor. The number of drug molecules present at the receptor sites determined which drug had more of an effect (or noneffect) on the body. This form of competition between two drugs for receptors sites is called competitive antagonism. In the example, naloxone is a competitive antagonist to oxymorphone. Once the animal's narcosis reversed with naloxone, analgesia and narcosis could be produced again by simply giving more oxymorphone. This increases the number of oxymorphone molecules at the receptor sites and increases the chance for oxymorphone molecules to occupy more sites than naloxone. Because one drug's effect can be overcome by adding more of the other drug, and vice versa, this form of antagonism is sometimes also called *reversible, surmountable, antagonism.*

Some agonist drugs are less susceptible to the effects of an antagonist, and the agonist's effect is not readily reversed by giving more of the antagonist. The reason may be that the receptor has a greater affinity and combines more tightly with the agonist than with the antagonist. Sometimes an agonist physically alters the shape of the receptor, reducing the ability of an antagonist molecule to fit the receptor. These types of antagonism are shown in Fig. 3-20.

Agonist-antagonist interactions in which one drug seems to have an advantage over the other are called noncompetitive antagonism. This is also called *irreversible,* or *insurmountable, antagonism.* In most cases, if one of these noncompetitive agonist drugs attaches to the receptor, its effect declines over time, but the agonist's effect cannot be reversed simply by adding more antagonistic drug. Because the process of reversal is so slow, some reactions give the impression of being irreversible.

Up to this point drugs have been depicted as having an entirely agonistic or antagonistic effect on a cell. However, sometimes the purpose is to reverse just some effects of an agonist drug. For example, a veterinarian may give an animal oxymorphone to produce profound narcosis and analgesia for a moderately painful procedure. After the procedure is completed, the veterinarian may give an injection of butorphanol to reverse the effect. The animal partially recovers from the narcosis but retains some analgesia and still appears sleepy. This partial reversal phenomenon can be explained by examining butorphanol's interaction with the opioid receptor.

Butorphanol is a narcotic drug that combines with opioid receptors and therefore has the same basic configuration as oxymorphone and naloxone. Butorphanol produces analgesia and narcosis but not to the same extent as oxymorphone. Therefore when the animal receives butorphanol in concentrations high enough to antagonize the previously administered oxymorphone from the receptors, the animal loses the stronger degree of analgesia and narcosis produced by oxymorphone but retains the lesser degree produced by the butorphanol. The butorphanol partially reverses the oxymorphone effect; the butorphanol acts as a partial antagonist. Because it produced some analgesic and narcotic effect of its own, it is also a partial agonist. Drugs that behave in this manner are partial agonists/antagonists. Partial

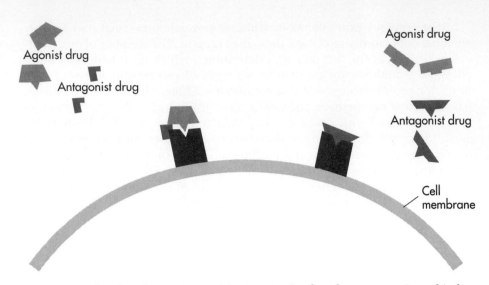

Fig. 3-20 Molecules of a noncompetitive antagonist alter the receptor site or bind more tightly to the receptor site than agonist drug molecules.

agonists/antagonists are very useful in reversing some potent effects of an agonist drug.

Nonreceptor-Mediated Reactions

Some drugs produce an effect without combining with receptors. For example, mannitol is classified as an osmotic diuretic. Mannitol molecules circulate in the blood and are excreted in the urine, where they "pull" water from the body and into the urine via osmosis. Mannitol does not accomplish this by combining with any receptor but by simply being present in the fluid environment.

Chelators are drugs that physically combine with ions or other selected compounds in the environment to produce their effects. For example, chelators are used to facilitate removal of lead from the body through chelation and excretion of the chelated product (combined chelator molecule and target molecule). Another common example of a chelator is the EDTA anticoagulant compound included in blood collection tubes that have lavender tops. The EDTA combines with calcium in the blood sample and prevents the clotting mechanism from turning the sample into a clot. No cellular receptor is involved in these examples; thus they are described as non–receptor-mediated reactions.

Another non–receptor-mediated reaction occurs when a person takes an antacid drug to combat heartburn or acid stomach. The calcium, aluminum, or magnesium in the antacid drug combines with the strong hydrochloric acid in the stomach to form a much weaker acid, thereby reducing stomach irritation. Again, the reaction involves a direct chemical change without a cellular receptor.

BIOTRANSFORMATION: THE WAY THE BODY ALTERS DRUGS

The body alters many drugs before they are eliminated. This process is referred to as **biotransformation,** or drug metabolism. The altered drug molecule is referred to as a *metabolite.* The liver is the primary organ involved in biotransformation. However, other tissues such as the lung, skin, and intestinal tract may also biotransform drug molecules. Biotransformation usually results in a molecule that is more hydrophilic and thus more readily eliminated by the kidney or liver.

Biotransformation is usually accomplished through enzyme action on the drug molecule and involves two steps. In phase I metabolism the original drug molecule is chemically transformed via oxidation, reduction, or hydrolysis of the molecule. In phase II metabolism, enzymes conjugate, or combine, the metabolite from phase I with another molecule such as glucuronic acid, sulfate, or glycine to produce a hydrophilic molecule.

After phase I is complete, the resulting metabolite usually has been rendered less biologically active. However, sometimes phase I biotransformation does not diminish the activity of the original compound or phase I biotransformation yields a compound with more activity than the original drug. Some drugs are formulated as prodrugs, which are inactive when administered but are activated by phase I biotransformation. A common example of this is the corticosteroid prednisone. Prednisone is converted by liver enzymes to prednisolone, which has antiinflammatory activity.

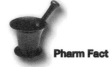

Pharm Fact

In some cases, biotransformation of a drug produces metabolites that are more potent than the original drug.

Drug Interactions Affecting Biotransformation

A veterinarian often administers several drugs to a patient at one time. Unfortunately, some drugs can interact with each other, altering their metabolism and producing higher or lower drug concentrations and adverse effects. In some cases, two drugs compete for the same limited number of biotransformation enzymes, saturating (overloading) the enzyme system and slowing metabolism of both drugs. This can result in accumulation of potentially toxic concentrations if the dose of each drug is not decreased.

Many drugs are normally metabolized by the mixed function oxidase (MFO) system, which is an enzyme system in the liver. This system is unique because the rate of metabolism can be increased, or induced, by continued exposure to that particular drug or class of drugs. In effect the body responds to repeated exposure to a particular set of drugs by increasing the rate of elimination. This **induced biotransformation** is one reason people and animals develop tolerance to the effects of certain drugs such as barbiturates and alcohol and must receive larger amounts to achieve the same effect.

When the MFO system has been induced by exposure to a particular drug, biotransformation of any other drug normally metabolized by the MFO system is also increased. Thus repeated use of phenobarbital, which is a barbiturate, for control of seizures also increases biotransformation of such drugs as phenylbutazone, digitoxin, estrogens, dipyrone, glucocorticoids, and others that use the MFO system. For this reason the dose of any other drugs affected by enzyme induction must be increased to compensate for more rapid biotransformation.

Species and Age Differences in Drug Biotransformation

A drug that is safe to use in one species may produce severe side effects in another. Cats metabolize some drugs poorly or not at all (Sidebar 3-2). Thus certain drugs that are safe for dogs, horses, or pigs may produce toxicity in cats.

Very young animals and (to a lesser extent) older animals also have a decreased ability to biotransform drugs (Sidebar 3-3). For this reason, veterinary professionals should always doublecheck the dose and precautions for a given drug before administering it to any animal less than 5 weeks old or older animals with reduced liver or kidney function. In older animals with reduced liver function it is necessary to reduce drug doses to prevent toxic accumulation of drugs.

Sidebar 3-2

The Reason Cats Cannot Tolerate Certain Drugs

Certain drugs must be used cautiously or not at all in cats to avoid toxic and potentially lethal side effects. The reason for intoleration of certain drugs can be compared with the bucket analogy. Consider what happens to the water level in the bucket if the rate of water addition remains the same but the hole in the bucket's bottom becomes smaller. The water accumulates in the bucket and the water level rises. Cats have a reduced ability to biotransform certain drugs and thus eliminate certain drugs slowly. Because of slower elimination, a drug dose proportional to that used in a dog could cause drug concentrations in a cat's body to rise to potentially toxic levels.

One of the most important drug conjugation pathways (phase II of biotransformation) in mammals involves combining a molecule of a phase I drug metabolite with a molecule of glucuronic acid. A cat's ability to synthesize the glucuronic acid is deficient in contrast to most other animals. Thus drugs that are normally metabolized using this conjugation pathway are shunted to other, less efficient metabolic pathways, requiring more time for the drug to be metabolized and subsequently eliminated.

Salicylate compounds (for example, aspirin, certain anticolitis drugs, and bismuth subsalicylate [found in Pepto-Bismol] are normally conjugated with glucuronic acid, but they are also excreted unchanged into the urine. Thus even though one of the major metabolic pathways for aspirin-like compounds is deficient (not absent) in cats, they can still tolerate careful use of these drugs.

Drugs that do not depend on extensive biotransformation by liver enzymes for elimination can usually be administered safely to cats. When in doubt, however, the veterinary technician should always read the drug package insert, consult a drug reference, or ask the doctor.

The Reasons Newborn or Young Animals Respond Differently to Drugs Than Adult Animals

Newborn and very young animals (less than 5 or 6 weeks old) tend to be less tolerant of certain drugs than mature animals. From birth to about 1 month of age, deficiencies in the neonatal liver slow the rate of drug biotransformation. Drugs that, in a mature animal, are normally oxidized, reduced, or conjugated with glucuronic acid as part of their biotransformation and excretion accumulate more readily in a young animals's liver because these metabolic pathways are more limited than in the adult liver, resulting in slower elimination of drugs.

Drugs that must be used very cautiously in neonates include ultra–short-acting barbiturates, some sulfonamide antibacterials, opioids, aspirin-like compounds (salicylates), some anticonvulsants, and local anesthetics (for example, procaine). By 5 weeks of age, the liver of most neonates functions near adult capacity. The exception is young foals, which appear to develop important enzymes in their liver within a few days of birth.

Drug distribution may also be different in young animals for several reasons. First, the blood:brain barrier in very young animals is more permeable to drugs than it is in adults. For this reason, drug doses that normally do not produce therapeutic concentrations in adults may produce significant concentrations in a young animal's brain. The same is true for some toxic agents. For example, significant accumulations of lead in the brain can lead to developmental problems in the central nervous system.

Because plasma albumin levels are comparatively low during the first 2 or 3 weeks of life, less protein is available to bind with drugs; thus more free drug molecules are available for distribution to tissues. Therefore doses of drugs that are normally highly protein bound must be reduced to compensate for a larger percentage of free drug molecules.

Water makes up a higher percentage of body weight in neonates and young animals than in adult animals. Therefore when a water-soluble (hydrophilic) drug is administered to a young animal and is distributed to the extracellular fluid throughout the body, it is diluted in a larger volume. Hence a given drug dose produces lower concentrations in a young animal than in an adult animal of the same weight.

Most drugs given by mouth to newborn ruminants (mammals with four-chambered stomachs) are absorbed in much the same way as in monogastric (single-stomach) animals. Therefore, in ruminants less than 4 to 6 weeks old, certain drugs may be more readily absorbed than after the rumen develops. Development of a functional rumen environment ("fermentation vat") may degrade some orally administered drugs, or the increasingly acidic pH in the ab-omasum (fourth compartment in the stomach) may alter the ratio of ionized to nonionized drug molecules, reducing drug absorption. Acidic drugs are less readily absorbed across the immature abomasum because of the more alkaline pH, whereas alkaline drugs may be more readily absorbed.

Because of these factors, veterinary professionals must review the package insert and other drug information closely before administering drugs to a neonate or young animal. The veterinary professional must remember that an adult dose adjusted for a young animal may be totally inappropriate because of differences in drug absorption, distribution, or biotransformation.

DRUG ELIMINATION

Drug **elimination,** or excretion (the removal of drug from the body), is greatly affected by dehydration; kidney, liver, or heart disease; age; and a variety of other physiologic and pathologic (disease) conditions. Failure to compensate for altered drug elimination is a common cause of inadvertent drug toxicity. By understanding the factors affecting drug elimination, the veterinary technician can help avoid problems with drug toxicity in patients.

Routes of Drug Elimination

The two major routes of elimination are via the kidney (into the urine) and via the liver (into the bile and subsequently the feces). Inhalant anesthetics and other volatile agents are mostly eliminated via the lungs, although some inhalant anesthetics (methoxyflurane and halothane) go through some hepatic biotransformation and **renal excretion.** Other less common routes of elimination include saliva, milk (in lactating animals), and sweat.

Renal Elimination of Drugs

In the kidney, circulating drugs are cleared from the blood through filtration and active secretion. Blood entering the kidney through the renal artery passes into smaller branches called the afferent arterioles and eventually moves through a tuft of capillaries called the glomerulus. Pressure within the glomerulus forces water and accompanying small molecules into the first part of the renal nephron called Bowman's capsule. The water and small molecules that have been filtered from the blood comprise the glomerular filtrate.

Most of the free (not protein-bound) drug molecules pass into the glomerular filtrate. Plasma proteins are too large to enter the glomerular filtrate; thus drugs bound to plasma proteins remain in circulation. If blood protein levels decrease, such as with hypoalbuminemia from chronic liver disease, more molecules will be in the free form and capable of passing into the glomerular filtrate and out the body in the urine.

The degree of renal perfusion (volume of blood flowing to the kidneys) also influences the amount of drug entering the glomerular filtrate. With hypotension (decreased systemic blood pressure), as from dehydration, blood loss, or shock, or with increased sympathetic nervous system stimulation, smooth muscle around the afferent arterioles constricts, decreasing blood flow into the kidney.

Reduced renal blood flow decreases filtration of drugs in the glomerulus, resulting in decreased elimination and increased concentrations of drugs primarily excreted by the kidney. This is the reason older animals with reduced renal function or animals with hypotension from any cause require reduced doses of renally excreted drugs. Conversely, if renal perfusion is increased by administration of medication that alters renal perfusion or infusion of intravenous fluids (causing an increase in blood volume and blood

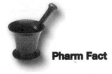

Pharm Fact

Drugs are primarily eliminated from the body through the kidneys and liver.

pressure), increased glomerular filtration results in more rapid removal of drug molecules from the systemic circulation.

After the glomerular filtrate has been formed in Bowman's capsule, it moves into the proximal convoluted tubule segment of the nephron. Here additional drug molecules, ions, and other small molecules may be added to the filtrate via a carrier-mediated transport process (usually active transport) that removes these molecules from the peritubular capillaries and secretes them into the renal tubule. In this way, concentrations of certain drugs such as penicillins and furosemide in the urine can increase significantly. Because penicillin is actively secreted into the proximal convoluted tubule, the resulting high concentrations of penicillin in the urine filtrate make it an ideal antibiotic for resolving urinary tract infections. Secretion of certain drug molecules into the proximal convoluted tubule requires significant energy; therefore anything that interferes with cellular energy production (for example, disease or toxicosis) reduces excretion of these drugs from the body.

The effect of plasma proteins on retention of drug molecules in the blood is more variable at the active secretion site than in the glomerulus. If the affinity, or attraction, between a protein-bound drug molecule in the peritubular capillaries and the carrier molecules involved in transporting it from the blood and into the urine is great, the drug molecule may separate from the plasma protein and combine with the carrier molecule. When the protein-bound drug molecule has a poor affinity for the carrier molecule, most drug molecules remain bound to the plasma proteins and thus remain in systemic circulation.

From the proximal convoluted tubule the filtrate moves into the loop of Henle, where some of the drug molecules may be reabsorbed from the filtrate into circulation. This occurs by passive diffusion; therefore drug molecules are reabsorbed to any significant extent only if they are in the lipophilic form (nonionized). Drug molecules that are hydrophilic (ionized) cannot pass through the cellular membrane of the renal tubule to reenter the circulation. As discussed earlier, drug molecules may shift from lipophilic to hydrophilic forms depending on the pH of the renal tubule filtrate. Any remaining drug molecules pass into the distal convoluted tubule and collecting ducts and out the body in the urine.

Hepatic Elimination of Drugs

Elimination of drugs via the liver is often called **biliary,** or **hepatic, excretion.** Hepatically excreted drugs usually move by passive diffusion from the blood into the hepatocyte (liver cell), at which point they are secreted into the bile or metabolized first and then secreted into the bile. The bile is then conveyed by the bile duct into the duodenum.

A drug that is excreted by the liver and arrives in the duodenum in lipophilic form could be reabsorbed across the intestinal wall and transported by the hepatic portal circulation back to the liver, where it is then excreted again by the liver or reenters the systemic circulation. This movement of drug from liver, to intestinal tract, and back to the liver is referred to as

enterohepatic circulation. Drugs that are reabsorbed intact (not metabolized) from the intestinal tract can exert a pharmacologic effect on the body; therefore some hepatically excreted drugs appear to have an extended duration of action in the body.

If the liver is compromised by acute disease or chronic degenerative processes such as cirrhosis (replacement of functional liver cells by nonfunctional fibrous tissue), the liver's ability to metabolize and/or eliminate drugs is reduced. Therefore the dose of drugs eliminated by biliary excretion must be reduced to prevent drug accumulation in toxic concentrations.

Half-life and Clearance: Measures of Drug Elimination Rates

Drug clearance is a term commonly used to describe the rate at which drug molecules are removed from the systemic circulation, presumably by elimination rather than distribution of the drug to tissues. A drug is rapidly **cleared** if it is quickly eliminated from the body. Reduced liver or kidney function reduces clearance of drugs eliminated by those organs.

The **half-life** of a drug is the time it takes to eliminate a certain proportion of a drug dose from the body. In Fig. 3-21, the drug concentration decreases over time in a predictable curve, not in a straight line. The drug concentrations drop by half at repeatable time intervals. In this example, drug concentrations drop by half every 2 hours until the drug is eliminated from the body. Therefore this particular drug has a half-life of 2 hours.

A drug's half-life reflects how quickly the drug is eliminated from the

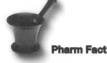

Pharm Fact

A drug's half-life reflects how quickly it is eliminated from the body.

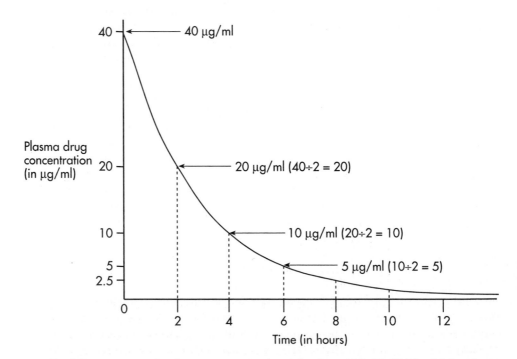

Fig. 3-21   Decrease in plasma concentrations of a drug with a half-life of 2 hours.

body and to some degree dictates how frequently the drug must be given to maintain concentrations within the therapeutic range. For example, most antibiotics used in veterinary medicine have a half-life of 2 to 3 hours. Therefore by 8 hours after administration, only about 6% of the original dose of an antibiotic with a half-life of 2 hours remains in the body (50% remains at 2 hours after administration, 25% at 4 hours, 12.5% at 6 hours, and 6.25% at 8 hours). In contrast, phenobarbital, a commonly used anticonvulsant (antiseizure) medication, has a half-life of approximately 2 days. Thus even within the span of 24 hours the drug concentration does not decrease even by half. Most antibiotics must be given every 6 to 8 hours, whereas phenobarbital is normally given only once daily.

A drug's half-life can also be used to estimate how efficiently the body is eliminating the drug. If the kidney is damaged or not well perfused, the half-life of a renally excreted drug increases. That is, it takes longer for the drug level to decrease by one half. The half-life of a drug excreted hepatically would not change if the kidneys were damaged because the hepatic elimination process has not been impaired. This example emphasizes the reason veterinary professionals must be aware of the way a drug is metabolized and excreted when selecting a drug or dosage regimen for animals with liver or kidney disease.

Relationship of Half-life to Steady-state Concentrations

Concentrations in the therapeutic range are quickly attained by administering large loading doses and then maintained with periodic maintenance doses. If only the maintenance dose is used (rather than first using a loading dose), the **peak** (highest) and trough (lowest) drug concentrations increase with each repeated dose because the next dose is given before all the drug administered with that dose has been eliminated. After a certain number of doses, peak concentrations plateau, or level out, and trough concentrations are about the same. At this point, concentrations of this drug for this dosage regimen have reached their **steady state** (Fig. 3-22).

The time it takes to reach steady-state concentrations is remarkably predictable for a particular drug. If the drug's half-life (in hours) is known, the time needed to achieve steady-state concentration can be determined by multiplying the drug's half-life by 5. Thus if amoxicillin has a half-life of approximately 2 hours, concentrations should reach steady state (all peak and trough concentrations the same thereafter) by 10 hours (5×2). In contrast, phenobarbital, which has a half-life of approximately 2 days, takes 10 days to reach steady-state concentrations. Therefore it may take days after initiating a dosage regimen of phenobarbital to attain the steady-state concentrations within the therapeutic range.

Drug Withdrawal Times

The presence of chemical or drug residues in beef, pork, lamb, chicken, and fish used for human consumption is a growing public health concern. Because of this, all drugs approved for use in food animals have mandated withdrawal times. The **withdrawal time** is the period after drug administration during which the animal cannot be sent to market for slaughter and the eggs

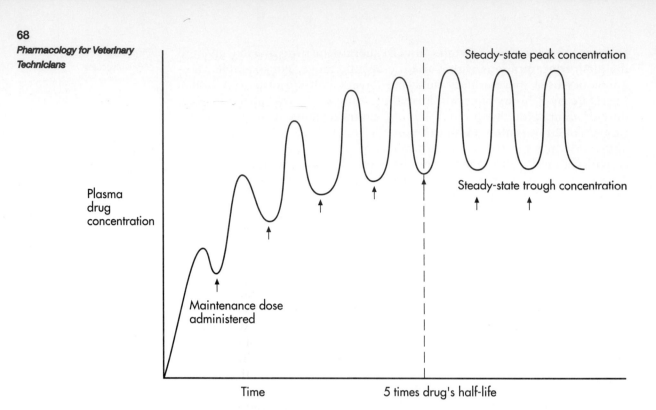

Fig. 3-22 After administration of each maintenance dose, plasma drug concentrations increase until they reach steady state.

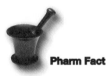

Pharm Fact

Although regulations pertaining to drug withdrawal times may cause added expense for producers, the regulations are necessary to prevent drug residues in food derived from animals.

or milk must be discarded. Withdrawal times cause additional expense to the food animal producer because the animal cannot be sent to market or the animal products (such as milk or eggs) cannot be sold.

The withdrawal time for drugs approved for use in food animals is calculated using the drug's half-life of elimination from the animal's body. The longer a drug's half-life, the longer the withdrawal time. Any factor that reduces the rate of elimination or clearance of a drug from the body prolongs the withdrawal time. As previously discussed, many factors can influence drug elimination. Veterinary professionals have a responsibility to public safety and food animal producers to know when a withdrawal time must be extended because of delayed elimination of drugs from the body. Veterinary technicians play an important role in helping to educate and reinforce the intent of withdrawal times so that food animal producers view regulations pertaining to withdrawal times as directly related to public health and not as arbitrary government interference.

USING CONCEPTS OF PHARMACOKINETICS

This chapter discussed the factors that influence movement of drugs into, through, and out the body. By remembering the "leaky bucket" analogy and the fact that the amount of drug entering the body must balance the amount of drug leaving the body, you should be able to understand the way these factors affect the daily care and treatment of veterinary patients. As you become more familiar with the principles underlying good veterinary care, you will begin to recognize situations in which the "normal" dose of a drug may not be safe or effective for a particular patient. A vigilant veterinary technician can help the veterinarian prevent animal illness or death from inappropriate administration of a drug.

Recommended Reading

Boothe DM: Principles of drug therapy for the practicing veterinarian. In Bonagura JD: *Kirk's current veterinary therapy XII,* Philadelphia, 1995, WB Saunders.

Brown SA et al: *Small animal medical therapeutics,* New York, 1992, JB Lippincott.

Rowland M, Tozer TN: *Clinical pharmacokinetics: concepts and applications,* Philadelphia, 1989, Lea & Febiger.

Review Questions

1. The veterinarian asks you to administer four drugs. Each has a different route of administration. Drug A must be given PO, drug B must be given IV, drug C must be given SC, and drug D must be given IM. Where are each of these drugs going to be placed in the body? Which drug will reach its peak plasma concentration the fastest?

2. The veterinarian is reviewing a brochure for a new drug that says "Our drug reaches concentrations of 40 μg/ml within 2 hours after administration." The doctor comments that the drug concentration by itself does not indicate how effective the drug is. What is the reason for this and what information is necessary to better assess the usefulness of this new drug?

3. A dosage regimen specifies 15 mg/kg IV and then 5 mg/kg q8h. Which is the maintenance dosage and which is the loading dose? What is the advantage of using a loading dose?

4. The veterinarian wants to "lengthen the dosage interval" for a drug now being given at 50 mg q6h PO for 3 days. Which component of this dosage regimen must be altered?

5. The recommended total daily dose for a drug is 480 mg. What are the equivalent total daily doses for the following dosage intervals? Which dosage schedule is the client most likely to follow?

     _____ mg q12h   _____ mg q8h   _____ mg q4h

     _____ mg TID   _____ mg q24h   _____ mg QID

6. A drug's package insert states that the drug can be given as an IV bolus or by IV infusion. What is the difference in these methods of administration?

7. You place a jugular catheter in a horse. The drug you are to administer must be given intraarterially. Is it appropriate to administer the drug into the jugular catheter?

8. A drug's package insert has a caution statement that says "Do not give this drug extravascularly." What does this mean? How would you be able to tell if you had injected it extravascularly?

9. If a drug is given in aerosol form, where would you expect the largest drug concentration to be immediately after administration?

10. Why is it that an animal might respond to injection of a drug directly into the carotid artery with severe central nervous system signs, whereas an intravenous injection of the same drug into the jugular vein in the same general area in the neck results in no adverse effects?

11. Rank the following injection routes in order of most superficial to most deep injection site:

    _____ intramuscular _____ intradermal _____ subcutaneous.

12. If you were injecting a drug IP, in what body area would you inject it?

13. Drugs move through the body by a variety of mechanisms, including diffusion and active transport. Which mechanism of drug movement is described in the following?
    a. A local anesthetic injected SC produces a spreading feeling of numbness in the skin.
    b. Large drug molecules are taken up by macrophage "scavenger" cells in the alveoli of the lungs.
    c. The cells of the renal tubules accumulate concentrations of aminoglycoside antibiotic that greatly exceed drug concentrations in the plasma.
    d. A hydrophilic drug moves along a concentration gradient into a cell.

14. If an animal ingests a poison that impairs cellular metabolic processes, could an antidote drug cross the cell membrane and move into the cell even though the cell cannot expend energy? Which drug transport processes would be disrupted and which would not?

15. Why do facilitated diffusion and active transport have maximum rates at which they can transport drug molecules across a membrane and passive diffusion does not?

16. Which drug would attain higher concentrations within the body after absorption: 100 mg of drug A with a PO bioavailability of 0.25 or 100 mg of drug B with a PO bioavailability of 0.40?

17. Digoxin is a cardiac drug with a narrow therapeutic index. (Highest concentrations in the therapeutic range are very close to the lowest effective concentrations.) Considering the plasma drug concentration curves for various routes of administration, why is IV administration not recommended for drugs with a narrow therapeutic range such as digoxin?

18. Why is a drug absorbed well if given subcutaneously but the same drug is not absorbed well when given by mouth?

19. If a drug is in hydrophilic form when given subcutaneously, how is it able to enter the capillaries?

20. Which would be more readily absorbed from the stomach (pH of 2 to 3): an acidic drug or an alkaline drug, both with a similar pKa?

21. Why do some drug molecules move readily out of the stomach lumen but then become trapped within the cells of the stomach wall?

22. Indicate which of the following hypothetical drugs is most likely to have a predominance of drug molecules in the ionized form and which in the nonionized form:

Acidic drug	pKa of 3	Placed in medium with pH of 6
Acidic drug	pKa of 2	Placed in medium with pH of 9
Acidic drug	pKa of 5	Placed in medium with pH of 2
Acidic drug	pKa of 7	Placed in medium with pH of 5
Acidic drug	pKa of 7	Placed in medium with pH of 7
Alkaline drug	pKa of 6	Placed in medium with pH of 9
Alkaline drug	pKa of 9	Placed in medium with pH of 8
Alkaline drug	pKa of 5	Placed in medium with pH of 2
Alkaline drug	pKa of 5	Placed in medium with pH of 8

23. Which drug is most rapidly absorbed from an SC injection site where the pH of the extracellular fluid is 7.4? Why is this drug most quickly absorbed?

Drug A	Acidic drug	pKa of 3.4
Drug B	Acidic drug	pKa of 5.4
Drug C	Alkaline drug	pKa of 6.4
Drug D	Alkaline drug	pKa of 8.4

24. You are working with a renally excreted drug that is primarily an acidic drug with a pKa of 6. To increase the rate of elimination of this drug, should the urine be acidified or alkalinized?

25. The manufacturer of an antibiotic claims that the enteric coating on the product enhances the drug's effectiveness. How could this be possible?

26. A cat with pylorospasm (contraction of the muscles surrounding the outflow tract from the stomach, which delays passage of stomach contents into the intestine) is given an alkaline drug with a pKa of 6. What effect would pylorospasm have on the rate of drug absorption or the amount of drug absorbed?

27. Why would an orally administered antibiotic tablet not be well absorbed in an animal with diarrhea?

28. Why are some toxic materials not very toxic when ingested but are extremely lethal if accidentally injected?

29. Why are drugs injected subcutaneously absorbed more slowly on a cold day than those injected on a hot day?

30. Diabetic animals are often overweight. Why should you be careful not to accidentally inject insulin (given for control of diabetes mellitus) into the fat?

31. Why are many antibiotics effective for infections at other body sites often not effective against bacterial infections involving the brain?

32. You inject an appropriate dose of thiopental IV into a thin dog and the animal stops breathing, reacting as though it received an overdose. The veterinarian looks over your shoulder and says, "Don't worry, the redistribution will take care of it." What is the significance of that comment?

33. A very thin dog with chronic liver disease has low plasma protein levels. The dog requires treatment with a drug that is highly protein bound. Considering the dog's poor body condition and low plasma protein levels, should the standard drug dose be increased or decreased?

34. Which drug would probably better penetrate tissues: drug A with a volume of distribution of 1 L or drug B with a volume of distribution of 3 L? If equal amounts of drug A and drug B were given to an animal, which would be present in greater concentrations in the plasma?

35. Digoxin is a cardiac drug with an apparent volume of distribution that seems to exceed the total volume of water possible within an animal's body. For example, in an animal with a body water volume of 3 L, the volume of distribution for digoxin may be 4 L. How is this possible? (Remember that digoxin selectively binds to sites in skeletal and cardiac muscle in high concentrations.)

36. In an animal with an increased volume of distribution as a result of ascites, would drug concentrations in the body likely be higher or lower than normal?

37. A dog is hospitalized because of insecticide poisoning. The veterinarian is concerned and says, "We can't use an antidote to reverse the effect because the insecticide is a noncompetitive agonist." What is the significance of that comment?

38. Pentazocine (Talwin-V™) is a partial narcotic agonist/antagonist. What effect would pentazocine have on an animal if it was given after a strong narcotic such as oxymorphone? How would this effect be different than that of a true narcotic antagonist such as naloxone?

39. Explain how a chelator drug can produce its effect when placed in a cell-free test tube of serum or within the lumen of the intestine, where there are no cells and hence no cellular receptors to which the drug can attach.

40. Why must veterinary professionals be concerned about using hepatically biotransformed drugs in young animals and cats? Should we have similar concerns about administering drugs that are excreted unchanged through the kidneys?

41. A dog is being treated with phenobarbital to control epileptic seizures. Why must the dosage be adjusted 2 to 3 weeks after therapy begins? Is the dose likely to be increased or decreased at that time and why?

42. What effect would decreased renal perfusion have on blood concentrations of a drug excreted through the kidneys?

43. A particular dose of penicillin is effective against a specific bacterium in the urine. When the same bacterial strain is found in other tissues in the body, however, the same dose of penicillin is not nearly as effective. Explain how this is possible.

44. An animal has ingested a poison and the doctor gives it activated charcoal repeatedly for several hours via a stomach tube because of enterohepatic circulation. Why must the charcoal be given repeatedly rather than only once or twice?

45. The doctor comments, "These fluids will increase drug clearance." What is the significance of that comment?

46. A horse is given an IV bolus injection of a new antibiotic. Concentrations of the drug in the blood are as follows (drug injected at hour 0):

Hour 0	0 μg/ml
Hour 1 postinjection	24 μg/ml
Hour 2 postinjection	19 μg/ml
Hour 3 postinjection	12 μg/ml
Hour 4 postinjection	9.5 μg/ml

What is the half-life of this drug in the horse? If the normal therapeutic concentration for this drug is 7 to 30 μg/ml, how many hours after the drug was administered should the next dose be given to maintain concentrations within the therapeutic range? What would be the concentration at 7 hours?

47. Why is a loading dose more necessary with a drug that has a long half-life than with a drug that has a short half-life?

48. Which food animal drug would require a longer withdrawal time: drug A with a half-life of 30 minutes or drug B with a half-life of 5 hours?

Drugs Affecting the Gastrointestinal Tract

Key Terms

acetylcholine
acetylcholinesterase
adsorb
α receptor
antacid
anticholinergic drug
antiemetic
antispasmodic
cathartics
chemoreceptor trigger
   zone (CRTZ)
colonic
dopaminergic antagonist
emesis
emetic (vomiting) center
enteric
gastric
gastric acid rebound
   syndrome
H_2 antagonists
hypermotility
hypersecretion
hypomotility
malabsorption
maldigestion
melena
oxyntic (parietal) cells
parasympatholytic drug
peristaltic contractions
protectant
purgative
segmental contractions
tenesmus
vagal stimulation

Function and Control of the
   Gastrointestinal Tract
Emetics
   The Vomiting Reflex
   Induction of Vomiting
   Types of Emetics
Antiemetics
Antidiarrheals
   Antidiarrheals that Modify Intestinal
      Motility
   Antidiarrheals that Block
      Hypersecretion

Adsorbents and Protectants
Laxatives, Lubricants, and Stool
   Softeners
Antacids and Antiulcer Drugs
Ruminatorics and Antibloat
   Medications
Other Drugs Used for Gastrointestinal
   Problems
   Antimicrobials
   Oral Electrolyte Replacements
   Pancreatic Enzyme Supplements
   Corticosteroids

Learning Objectives

*After studying this chapter,
the veterinary technician should know the following:*

Ways gastrointestinal function can be altered by drugs

Mechanics of vomiting and the way it can be induced

Types of diarrhea and the ways they can be controlled

Drugs that modify the stool

Drugs used to treat ulcers

Drugs used to modulate rumen motility

Various diseases affect the gastrointestinal (GI) tract of animals and may cause vomiting, colic (abdominal pain), bloat, diarrhea, and constipation. A variety of medications available as prescription and over-the-counter (OTC) drugs treat these conditions. Because these drugs are readily available and widely used, technicians should be aware of their side effects and adverse reactions and be able to answer clients' questions about medications used to treat GI ailments. (A box listing GI drugs can be found at the end of this chapter.)

FUNCTION AND CONTROL OF THE GASTROINTESTINAL TRACT

The diversity of anatomic differences between species is more pronounced with the GI tract than with any other organ system. Although the GI tracts of various domestic species appear different, they have many similarities in function and control. To simplify, the monogastric (single stomach) animal has three functional segments of GI tract: the stomach, intestines, and cecum and colon. Drugs and functions related to the stomach are defined as **gastric** (for example, gastric ulcers, gastric blood flow, or gastric emptying). Drugs and functions related to the duodenum, jejunum, or ileum are usually referred to as **enteric,** and those related to the colon are referred to as **colonic.**

Ruminants (four stomach mammals) have a unique GI configuration: they have a more elaborate "prestomach" group of compartments. The rumen, reticulum, omasum, and abomasum (the "true" stomach) aid in breakdown and processing of a ruminant's herbivorous (plant) diet. Generally, the reticulum receives food from the esophagus (except in nursing animals), acts as a "mixing stomach," and passes the mixed ingesta into the rumen. The rumen acts as a large mixing and fermenting vat for breakdown of foodstuffs. Coarse materials are regurgitated from the rumen into the mouth for further mastication, a process known as "chewing cud". The omasum and abomasum are concerned primarily with further mixing, some digestion, and absorption.

The nervous system, endocrine system, and a variety of compounds released by cells and intestinal microbes all influence normal and abnormal functioning of the GI tract. The parasympathetic nervous system and drugs that mimic its effects increase digestive secretions, blood flow to the GI tract, gut (GI) motility, and smooth muscle tone. All these processes help digest food and absorb nutrients, which is the reason that the parasympathetic nervous system is sometimes referred to as the *"rest and restore"* system.

In contrast, the sympathetic nervous system, which triggers the fight or flight mechanism, decreases blood flow to the GI tract and redirects the blood toward skeletal muscle and other organs and tissues needed for an emergency response. This decreased blood supply decreases intestinal secretions, intestinal motility, and absorption of food. Drugs that mimic the effects of the sympathetic nervous system have similar effects

Prostaglandins are compounds produced by the body that usually have local effects. In the intestinal tract, prostaglandin E (PgE) is produced by the intestinal smooth muscle and mucosa. Its effect is mostly protective, it in-

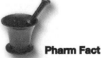

Pharm Fact

Drugs that decrease prostaglandins also decrease the self-protective mechanisms of the stomach.

creases intestinal mucus and fluid production, decreases gastric hydrochloric acid secretion, increases intestinal motility, and improves blood flow to areas in which PgE is active. Drugs that inhibit the effects of prostaglandins reverse these protective responses, and drugs that mimic prostaglandins produce similar effects as prostaglandins.

Histamine, which is released by basophils and mast cells during inflammation or allergic reactions, binds to H_2 receptors located on the gastric **oxyntic (parietal) cells** that produce hydrochloric acid in the stomach. Stimulation of these H_2 receptors, which are slightly different from the H_1 receptors associated with the respiratory tract (see Chapter 6), results in additional secretions of hydrochloric acid and increased gastric acidity (Fig. 4-1). Mast cell tumors have a known potential to cause gastric or duodenal ulcers by releasing massive amounts of histamine into the body.

Oxyntic cells also contain receptors for **acetylcholine** and gastrin. Gastrin is released from the stomach wall (antral area) in response to the presence of proteins in the stomach, distention of the stomach, or increased stimulation by the parasympathetic nervous system. Although histamine, gastrin, and acetylcholine each can stimulate gastric hydrochloric acid production, the receptor sites on the oxyntic cells for all three agents must be occupied for maximum acid production.

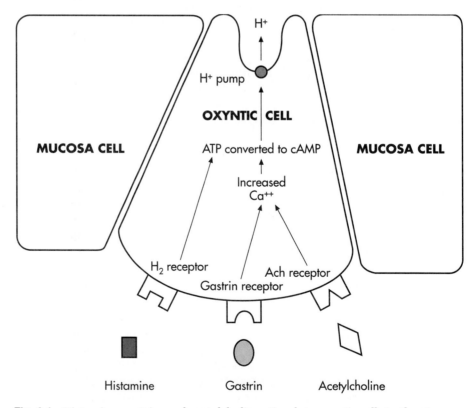

Fig. 4-1 Histamine, gastrin, and acetylcholine stimulate oxyntic cells in the stomach to produce hydrochloric acid.

Bacterial toxins, released by some types of bacteria, can stimulate secretion of fluids by intestinal cells, resulting in profuse diarrhea and dehydration. *Salmonella enteriditis* and other enteric bacteria often produce characteristic intestinal signs through this mechanism.

The veterinary technician should know the role of the autonomic nervous system and the effects of PgE, histamine, and bacterial toxins to understand the mechanism by which intestinal disease occurs and the ways intestinal drugs can reverse clinical signs.

EMETICS

Emetics are drugs that induce vomiting. **Emesis** (vomiting) is induced to remove an ingested toxic substance before it can be absorbed into the body. For this reason, emetics must be reliable and rapid acting.

The Vomiting Reflex

The complex process of emesis is controlled by a group of neurons in the medulla of the brainstem, known as the vomiting, or emetic, center (Fig. 4-2). The vomiting reflex may be triggered by input from four types of stimuli:

- Stimulation of the vagus nerve caused by irritation of tissues or organs innervated by the vagus nerve (for example, GI tract organs, peritoneum, and kidney capsule)
- Direct stimulation of the chemoreceptor trigger zone, located near the emetic center in the medulla
- Stimulation of nerves of the inner ear involved with balance (motion sickness)
- Stimulation of higher centers of the brain by emotional stimuli

The emetic center coordinates the muscle groups and autonomic functions that produce vomiting (in species capable of vomiting). The neurons of the vomiting center have **α receptors** (a type of adrenergic receptor involved with the sympathetic nervous system) and serotonin receptors. Stimulation of these receptors on the emetic center neurons evokes the vomiting reflex. Cats seem to be especially sensitive to sympathetic nervous system stimulation of the emetic center induced by natural stress or administration of drugs that stimulate the α receptors. Blocking the serotonin receptors or α receptors with antagonistic drugs can help control emesis.

The **chemoreceptor trigger zone (CRTZ)** is a specialized area of receptors in the central nervous system (CNS) that detects toxic substances in the blood and cerebrospinal fluid (CSF) and subsequently stimulates the emetic center to produce vomiting. The CRTZ can be stimulated by drugs, either as a desired effect or an undesirable side effect, from toxins associated with renal failure, excessive ketones associated with diabetes mellitus, bacterial toxins, and other metabolic toxins.

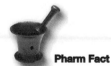

Pharm Fact

The vomiting center of cats is very sensitive to drugs that stimulate α receptors.

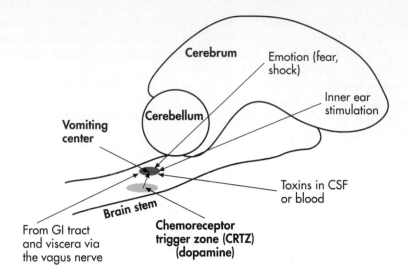

Fig. 4-2 The vomiting center in the brainstem receives impulses from the chemoreceptor trigger zone, GI tract, and cerebrum.

Sensitivity of the CRTZ to different drugs or chemicals varies among species and explains the reason some drugs produce emesis in one species but not another. For example, because the CRTZ of dogs contains more dopamine receptors than the CRTZ of cats, drugs or toxins that normally stimulate dopamine receptors or drugs that normally stimulate release of dopamine more readily produce emesis in dogs than cats. Conversely, **dopaminergic antagonists,** or antidopaminergic drugs, tend to decrease vomiting in dogs but have much less antiemetic effect in cats.

The CRTZ of dogs also contains more receptors to histamine than the CRTZ of cats. This correlates with histamine being a potent emetic agent in dogs but not cats. In contrast, the CRTZ of cats is much more sensitive to drugs that stimulate α_2 receptors, which explains why xylazine, a sedative and anesthetic agent that stimulates α_2 receptors, produces a strong emetic effect in cats and a much lesser emetic effect in dogs. Because of these differences in CRTZ sensitivities, dogs and cats often require different antiemetic drugs to counteract toxins or compounds that have stimulated vomiting through the CRTZ.

The vestibular apparatus in the inner ear is responsible for balance and also connects to the CRTZ and the vomiting center via cranial nerve VIII (vestibulocochlear). Excessive inner ear stimulation such as from irregular circular motion (for example, from car travel) generates impulses to the CRTZ in dogs and the emetic center in cats and dogs, stimulating these centers and producing emesis. Again, because of the different pathways from the vestibular apparatus to the emetic center, drugs that control motion sickness in cats may not be as effective in dogs, and vice versa.

In people the cerebral cortex (a higher brain center) can stimulate vomiting under circumstances of extreme emotional shock, such as viewing a tragic or painful situation. It is uncertain to what extent higher brain centers initiate vomiting in animals, although some animals tend to vomit when stressed or excited, possibly as a result of release of sympathetic neurotransmitters and stimulation of α receptors on the CRTZ and emetic center.

Of the methods described above for initiation of vomiting, the most common (in animals) are probably irritation of the intestinal tract and direct stimulation of the CRTZ. When the GI tract becomes irritated by viral or bacterial infection, a foreign body, overdistention, or chemicals, impulses travel via the vagus nerve (a parasympathetic nerve) to the emetic center where the vomiting reflex is initiated. This mechanism can be protective by preventing absorption and facilitating removal of an irritating or a harmful ingested substance.

Induction of Vomiting

Emetics are most often used to induce vomiting in animals that have ingested toxic substances. They should not be used in all cases of poisoning, however. The veterinarian or a Poison Control Center should be consulted before inducing emesis because the risk of aspiration (inhalation) of stomach contents into the lungs and subsequent death from aspiration pneumonia may outweigh the benefit of induced vomiting. Vomiting also should not be induced if a corrosive substance, such as alkali cleaning agents, acids, or oxalate products, was ingested because corrosives can extensively damage the oral and esophageal mucosa. If burns on the oral mucosa are observed in an animal that has ingested an unknown substance, it must be assumed that the compound was corrosive unless proven otherwise.

Pharm Fact

Induction of vomiting in an animal that has ingested a corrosive substance is contraindicated because vomiting corrosive poisons can further damage the esophagus and oral cavity.

Emesis should not be induced in animals that have ingested volatile (easily evaporated) liquids such as gasoline, light petroleum products, and most oils. Volatile liquids usually do not stimulate the normal gag reflexes and may be easily aspirated into the lungs during vomiting.

The veterinary professional should not induce emesis in an animal that is comatose, extremely depressed, unconscious, or lacking a functional gag reflex. If you have to heavily sedate an animal that is vomiting or induce emesis in a semiconscious or tranquilized animal, you should place a cuffed endotracheal tube and inflate the cuff to reduce the risk of aspiration pneumonia. Some anesthetic agents such as barbiturates, or tranquilizers such as acepromazine, decrease the vomiting reflex, counteracting the effect of some emetic agents.

The veterinary professional should not induce emesis in an animal that is convulsing or showing preictal (preseizure) signs (for example, after ingestion of strychnine or other CNS stimulants). Vomiting can trigger seizure activity in these animals. You should not induce emesis in an animal with bloat, gastric torsion, or esophageal damage because the weakened stomach or esophageal wall can perforate or rupture during vomiting. Finally, you should not attempt to induce emesis in horses, rabbits, or many rodent species because these species either cannot vomit or the act of vomiting may result in complications such as rupture of the stomach.

When weighing the risks and benefits of inducing vomiting in an animal that has ingested poison, the veterinary professional must also consider whether the toxic substance is still in the stomach and proximal duodenum because these areas are the most likely to be evacuated by vomiting. Most liquid toxins pass beyond this area or are absorbed into the systemic circulation within 2 hours after ingestion. Solid poisons such as rat bait blocks and pelleted rodenticides may still be in the stomach up to 4 hours after ingestion depending on the speed of gastric emptying. If an animal has been vomiting for some time after ingestion of a toxic material, giving an emetic to induce additional vomiting has no clear benefit.

Types of Emetics

There are two general categories of emetics: centrally acting and locally acting. Centrally acting emetics include drugs such as apomorphine, which directly stimulates dopamine receptors in the CRTZ to produce emesis. When given by IV or IM injection, apomorphine quickly causes emesis in dogs. Because of the lesser role of dopamine receptors in emesis in cats, apomorphine is a less effective emetic in cats.

Another method of apomorphine administration consists of placing the apomorphine tablet directly into the conjunctival sac of the eye. The apomorphine is quickly absorbed through the mucous membranes of the conjunctiva and rapidly induces vomiting. After the desired effect is achieved, the tablet is removed and the remaining residue is flushed from the eye to prevent further absorption.

Apomorphine is a morphine derivative. When it combines with the opioid receptors in the medullary respiratory centers of the brainstem, respiration may be depressed if a large dose is given. Although the respiratory depressant effects of apomorphine can be reversed with a narcotic antagonist such as naloxone, its emetic effects, which are mediated by dopamine receptors, are not affected by naloxone. Dopaminergic antagonists such as phenothiazine tranquilizers (for example, acepromazine and droperidol) may combat the vomiting caused by apomorphine. If an animal is tranquilized with a drug like acepromazine, subsequent administration of acepromazine will not produce the desired rapid and complete vomiting because the dopaminergic receptors on which apomorphine works are blocked by the acepromazine.

Another effective centrally acting emetic for cats is xylazine (Rompun, Anased). This sedative and anesthetic agent stimulates α_2 receptors in both the CRTZ and the emetic center in cats, producing emesis within minutes of injection. This emetic effect can be reversed using α_2 antagonists such as yohimbine (Yobine).

In contrast to the rapidly acting, centrally acting emetics such as apomorphine and xylazine, locally acting emetics such as syrup of ipecac do not produce an immediate effect. Syrup of ipecac, available at most local drugstores, produces its emetic effect by irritating the GI tract and causing parasympathetic stimulation of the emetic center. When absorbed from the intestine into the systemic circulation, syrup of ipecac also stimulates the CRTZ. Syrup of ipecac does not produce vomiting until 10 to 30 minutes after administration; the ipecac must pass from the stomach into the intestine to produce the required local irritation and to be absorbed.

The 10- to 30-minute lag between ipecac administration and onset of vomiting can lead uninformed clients or veterinary professionals to believe the initial dose was ineffective, causing them to administer multiple doses of the drug before vomiting begins. Multiple doses can result in serious complications because high concentrations of ipecac are cardiotoxic (toxic to the heart muscle). Animals with ipecac overdose may exhibit arrhythmias, hypotension, and myocarditis (inflammation of the heart muscle). If multiple doses of ipecac have not induced vomiting, the animal may require gastric lavage (flushing of the stomach) to remove the excess ipecac. Under normal conditions a standard dose of ipecac does not produce significant cardiac abnormalities.

Syrup of ipecac and extract of ipecac are not the same. Extract of ipecac is 14 times more potent than the syrup. Cardiotoxicity and death can result if extract of ipecac is given at doses normally given for syrup of ipecac.

Another common mistake is to administer activated charcoal and syrup of ipecac at the same time. Also known as "the universal antidote," activated charcoal **adsorbs** the syrup of ipecac to its surface, preventing it from contacting the GI lumen wall and causing the GI irritation needed for induction of emesis. In addition, coating of the charcoal by the ipecac prevents the charcoal from adsorbing the toxin for which it was given. Thus these compounds should not be given simultaneously. However, it is common to first give syrup of ipecac to induce vomiting and then, after the vomiting, to give the charcoal to adsorb any toxin remaining in the GI tract.

Outdated syrup of ipecac is often ineffective for inducing vomiting, but it still can cause cardiotoxicity. Therefore, outdated syrup of ipecac should not be used unless absolutely necessary.

Other local emetics include hydrogen peroxide, a warm concentrated solution of salt and water, and a solution of powdered mustard and water. These emetics do not work consistently. In addition, warm concentrated salt water may cause salt toxicity. Inducing vomiting by forcing a finger to the back of an animal's throat usually results in a struggle and bitten fingers but seldom any vomiting.

ANTIEMETICS

Antiemetics prevent or decrease vomiting. The veterinary professional must remember that vomiting and diarrhea are naturally protective mechanisms that remove irritating or toxic substances from the intestinal tract. Prevention of vomiting by use of antiemetics may allow the offending substance to remain in the GI tract longer or may mask clinical signs that would help determine disease progression and recovery. Therefore antiemetics should only be used when the vomiting reflex is no longer beneficial to the animal.

Phenothiazine tranquilizers such as acepromazine (PromAce), chlorpromazine (Thorazine), and prochlorperazine (Compazine, Darbazine) are commonly used to control vomiting caused by motion sickness. Some veterinary gastroenterologists also advocate chlorpromazine for controlling vomiting associated with acute gastroenteritis.

Pharm Fact

Antiemetics should only be used when vomiting is no longer providing a benefit to the animal.

Phenothiazine drugs block dopamine receptors in the CRTZ and the emetic center, thereby reducing vomiting. These drugs also have an antihistamine effect, which is the reason they are effective in preventing or controlling motion sickness. (Histamine is involved in vomiting stimulated by the vestibular apparatus.) Although phenothiazine drugs do have some anticholinergic activity (that is, they block activity of the parasympathetic nervous system), this antiemetic effect is not very potent and thus does not prevent vomiting caused by parasympathetic impulses entering the vomiting center from GI, peritoneal, pharyngeal, or other visceral stimulation.

As discussed in Chapter 8, phenothiazines have α-adrenergic receptor antagonist activity and therefore block the vasoconstrictive effect of α-1 receptors. The net effect is peripheral vasodilation and a subsequent drop in blood pressure. For this reason, animals that are hypovolemic (have reduced blood volume) from dehydration associated with prolonged vomiting and diarrhea should be rehydrated before phenothiazine antiemetic therapy is initiated.

In normal animals phenothiazine drugs produce little tranquilization at the doses usually used for antiemetic effect. However, in depressed animals or those that have received other CNS depressant drugs, a tranquilizing effect may be evident. Phenothiazines should not be used in animals with a history of seizures or those prone to seizure activity (such as animals that have ingested strychnine).

Antihistamines are the main ingredient in drugs used to control motion sickness in people. Veterinarians occasionally use dimenhydrinate (Dramamine) and diphenhydramine (Benadryl) for prevention of motion sickness. These drugs decrease impulses sent from the vestibular apparatus to the emetic center during continuous motion. Like phenothiazines, antihistamines are less effective in blocking the vomiting stimulus caused by **vagal stimulation** (parasympathetic nervous system stimulation) from the intestinal tract and so are less effective in blocking vomiting associated with gastroenteritis.

Antihistamines have a sedative effect on animals, similar to that observed in people, and thus may adversely affect the performance of working animals. These drugs can also decrease the wheal and flare reaction used to gauge the body's reaction to antigens in intradermal allergy testing. Antihistamines should not be used for at least 4 days before allergy testing.

Atropine, aminopentamide (Centrine), and isopropamide (combined with prochlorperazine in Darbazine) are **parasympatholytic,** or **anticholinergic, drugs** that block the effect of the parasympathetic nervous system. Anticholinergic drugs theoretically prevent vomiting by blocking the impulses traveling to the CNS via the vagus nerve and the motor impulses traveling to the muscles involved with the vomiting reflex via the vagus nerve. Anticholinergic drugs also decrease secretions by the intestinal tract and overall gut motility.

Anticholinergic drugs usually do not completely block the vomiting response and may actually increase vomiting associated with gastric atony (lack of tone) and decreased intestinal motility. Many veterinarians still use anticholinergics, but most gastroenterologists do not recommend anticholinergics for use as antiemetics except for vomiting associated with irritable bowel syndrome or excessive stimulation of the parasympathetic nervous system.

Metoclopramide (Reglan) is a centrally acting antiemetic that also has local antiemetic activity. Its central-acting effect is through the antidopaminergic action on the CRTZ. Metoclopramide acts locally by increasing lower esophageal muscle tone, relaxing the pyloric outflow tract of the stomach, increasing gastric motility without increasing secretions, and increasing motility of the duodenum and jejunum. These local effects increase stomach tone and are useful in certain syndromes that produce vomiting associated with gastric stasis (relaxed stomach tone).

Metoclopramide has also been useful for a particular condition in which otherwise healthy dogs intermittently vomit small amounts of bile-tinged fluid, usually in the morning. Although this condition is not life threatening, it is annoying to the pet owner because of the yellow stains from the bile pigments. A dose of metoclopramide given to these dogs in the evening usually helps correct this situation.

Metoclopramide has other CNS effects in addition to its antiemetic effect. It can produce sedation and should not be used in conjunction with phenothiazine tranquilizers because of the potential for an added sedative effect. Occasionally, cats given a dose of metoclopramide show frenzied behavior. Because metoclopramide relies on vagal stimulation for much of its local antiemetic activity, use of atropine or narcotic analgesics in conjunction with metoclopramide can negate the local antiemetic effect.

Veterinarians are beginning to use cisapride (Propulsid), a newer drug for humans, to control vomiting associated with gastric stasis (lack of motility). Like metoclopramide, cisapride increases lower esophageal tone and peristalsis while accelerating gastric emptying. It has been used in dogs to reduce regurgitation associated with megaesophagus (dilated esophagus) and to treat cats with chronic constipation or frequent vomiting from hairballs. (Vomiting of hairballs is usually preceded by a phase of gastric stasis). As with metoclopramide, simultaneous use of anticholinergic agents may negate the activity of cisapride.

ANTIDIARRHEALS

Antidiarrheals combat various types of diarrhea. Like vomiting, diarrhea is normally a protective mechanism that helps remove irritating or toxic substances from the intestinal tract. Knowing the general type and cause of diarrhea helps in selection of the proper treatment:

- Maldigestion or malabsorption of food, which creates an osmotic force from undigested food that retains water within the bowel lumen, increasing the volume and fluid content of the feces
- Hypersecretion of intestinal fluids into the bowel lumen, as caused by bacterial enterotoxins (toxins in the bowel lumen) or general inflammation of the bowel
- Increased permeability of the intestinal mucosa, resulting in loss of protein, fluid, serum, or even blood cells into the bowel lumen
- Altered intestinal motility, resulting in increased movement of liquid feces

Pharm Fact

The veterinarian should use an antidiarrheal drug that counteracts the specific underlying cause of the diarrhea.

Intestinal motility involves two types of contractions: **segmental contractions,** which mix the contents of the bowel, and **peristaltic contractions,** which propel the food along the tract (Fig. 4-3). Increased segmental contractions slow movement of feces along the tract, and inhibition of segmental contractions or increased peristaltic movement results in more rapid movement of ingesta along the tract.

In many GI diseases a short period of **hypermotility** (increased movement of bowel contents by rapid peristalsis) is followed by a longer period of **hypomotility** (decreased peristalsis) and atony (few or no segmental contractions). The straining to defecate that occurs with spastic contractions of the colon, such as found in colonic or rectal inflammation and irritation, is called **tenesmus.** Each of these intestinal movements can be affected by different types of antidiarrheal drugs.

Antidiarrheals That Modify Intestinal Motility

Antidiarrheals that affect gut motility slow the movement of bowel contents by decreasing peristaltic movements or increasing segmental contractions in the small intestine. Narcotic or opioid analgesics are C-V or C-III controlled drugs that increase segmental contractions and reduce peristaltic movements. Over-the-counter (OTC) versions of these drugs contain the same ingredients but at lower concentrations. These drugs are thought to have an antisecretory effect, which reduces the hypersecretory diarrheal effects of certain bacterial toxins and prostaglandins.

Narcotics commonly used to combat diarrhea include diphenoxylate (Lomotil), paregoric (tincture of opium), and loperamide (Imodium and Imodium A-D, the latter of which is the OTC version). These compounds often

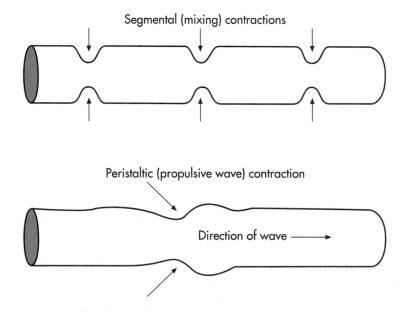

Fig. 4-3 Segmental and peristaltic contractions of the intestines.

contain a subtherapeutic dose of atropine designed to produce a slightly uncomfortable dryness in the mouth to dissuade abuse of the opioid.

A disadvantage of narcotics (when used as antidiarrheals) is that their analgesic effect can mask pain that is used to monitor progression or resolution of disease. Another disadvantage is that narcotics can cause excitement ("morphine mania") in cats. Because these drugs decrease gut motility and slow the transit time of intestinal contents, they also prolong the contact time between the bowel mucosa and pathogenic bacteria such as *Salmonella enteriditis* and enterotoxins, which could increase the damage caused by these agents. This is a major concern in horses with bacterial enteritis. Therefore these compounds should not be given until the infectious agent or enterotoxin has been cleared from the bowel. Narcotics should not be given to animals with head trauma because these drugs tend to increase cerebrospinal fluid pressure or intracranial pressure, which can exacerbate cranial hemorrhage or swelling.

Anticholinergics are parasympatholytic drugs that decrease the effect of the acetylcholine neurotransmitter on the GI tract. These drugs are used as **antispasmodics** because they decrease spastic colonic contractions and control diarrhea associated with these contractions. Atropine is used less often than isopropamide or aminopentamide because of its wider range of side effects and its short duration of activity.

These drugs are not particularly effective for most small bowel diarrheal problems because most small bowel diarrhea is associated with flaccid, or atonic, bowels (that is, "limp," with little or no tone, few segmental contractions, and weak peristaltic movement). Decreased segmental contractions result in loss of resistance to the flow of bowel contents so that even weak peristaltic movement produces rapid passage of liquid contents through the bowel.

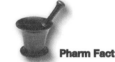

Pharm Fact

Parasympatholytic drugs block the parasympathetic effect and allow the sympathetic effect to dominate; therefore any condition in which sympathetic tone is already high is a contraindication for use of these drugs. For example, animals with cardiac arrhythmias, tachycardia (such as in cats with hyperthyroidism), or ileus (lack of intestinal motility) should not be treated with parasympatholytics. Decreased GI motility also prolongs contact of toxins or irritant substances with the bowel mucosa, prolonging their damaging effect on the bowel or increasing the degree of absorption into the body.

Parasympatholytic drugs should not be given to animals with cardiac arrhythmias, tachycardia, or ileus associated with increased sympathetic activity.

Antidiarrheals That Block Hypersecretion

Enterotoxins such as the toxins produced by *Escherichia coli* in the gut directly stimulate the secretory cells of the intestinal tract to secrete more fluid into the intestinal lumen. In addition, inflammation of the bowel results in the production of PgE, which further stimulates intestinal mucosal cells to secrete fluid and mucus into the lumen. Bowel inflammation also damages the "tight junctions" between cells lining the intestinal tract, which allows small–molecular-weight sugars, fluid, and larger protein molecules to be lost into the intestinal lumen.

If inflammation or cellular destruction continues, the intestinal tract may become so porous that red blood cells escape into the intestinal lumen, resulting in bloody diarrhea. Secretory diarrhea can be dangerous to animals because rapid loss of fluids from the body can produce life-threatening dehydration. Antidiarrheal-antisecretory drugs block intestinal fluid loss by preventing contact of enterotoxins with the intestinal mucosa or decreasing the inflammatory response of the intestinal tract wall.

Bismuth subsalicylate, the active ingredient in Pepto-Bismol, breaks down in the gut to bismuth carbonate and salicylate. The bismuth coats the intestinal mucosa, possibly protecting it from enterotoxins, and has some antibacterial activity. The major antisecretory effect, however, is probably from the salicylate (an aspirin-like compound), which decreases inflammation and blocks formation of prostaglandins that would normally stimulate fluid secretion.

Although the bismuth is not well absorbed into the systemic circulation, the salicylate is absorbed; therefore these compounds should be used with caution in cats because of their limited ability to metabolize and excrete salicylates. Some clinical investigaters recommend limiting use of bismuth subsalicylate in cats to no more than 24 hours.

The bismuth that remains in the bowel can cause a dark, tarry appearance in the stool, resembling **melena** (stools darkened by digested blood). This color change should not be interpreted as an indication of gastric or small intestinal hemorrhage. Bismuth is radiopaque and may be evident on abdominal radiographs.

Veterinary patients commonly reject Pepto-Bismol because of its taste. Refrigerating the liquid form reduces the peppermint flavor, which may make it easier to administer. The tablet form greatly facilitates administration of the drug.

A potent antiprostaglandin that has been used in animals with GI problems is flunixin meglumine (Banamine). Unfortunately, this antiprostaglandin effect also increases the risk of gastric or intestinal ulceration and even perforation in dogs. Although it is used for relief of colic in horses and to some degree for calf scours, flunixin is not the drug of choice for treatment of diarrhea in other animals (see Chapter 12).

Chlorpromazine, the phenothiazine tranquilizer that is sometimes used as an antiemetic, has some antisecretory effects. It inhibits the intracellular mechanism for secretion of fluids. In treatment of secretory diarrhea, chlorpromazine may have some benefit in addition to its antiemetic effect.

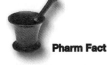

Pharm Fact

Orally administered bismuth can cause a tarry appearance in the stool.

Adsorbents and Protectants

Bacterial enterotoxins cause hypersecretion and irritating compounds produce acute diarrhea by direct contact with intestinal mucosal cells. Any drug that prevents these agents from contacting the intestinal mucosa could theoretically reduce the diarrheal response, which is the underlying principle of adsorbents and **protectants.** An adsorbent causes another substance to adhere to its outer surface, thus reducing contact of that substance with the intestinal tract wall. Although not usually used as an antidiarrheal agent, activated charcoal adsorbs enterotoxins to its surface, preventing them from contacting the bowel wall. The charcoal and adsorbed enterotoxin are then excreted in the feces.

Kaolin and pectin (Kaopectate) are often used together for symptomatic relief of vomiting or diarrhea in people and animals. The kaolin-pectin combination may adsorb enterotoxins. Whether kaolin-pectin has any significant effect in controlling diarrhea in veterinary patients is questionable. Because of their adsorbent qualities, kaolin-pectin combinations can decrease absorption of some antimicrobials and possibly digoxin. Therefore if kaolin-pectin compounds are used with other oral medications, the kaolin-pectin should be given at least 2 hours before or 3 hours after the other drugs.

LAXATIVES, LUBRICANTS, AND STOOL SOFTENERS

Laxatives, lubricants, and stool softeners are used to increase the fluid content of and/or soften the feces to facilitate defecation. These types of drugs are used to control chronic constipation (for example, in older cats), facilitate passage of trichobezoars (hairballs), evacuate the colon before radiographic procedures, and ease passage of stool after perianal surgery or in animals with severe pelvic fractures.

Laxatives, **cathartics,** and **purgatives** facilitate evacuation of the bowels. Laxatives are considered the most gentle of this class of drugs, whereas cathartics are more marked in their evacuating effect, and purgatives are potent in their actions. Irritant laxatives, including castor oil and phenolphthalein, work by irritating the bowel, resulting in increased peristaltic motility. Castor oil is converted in the duodenum to ricinoleic acid, which is a very irritating compound. Because of their stimulant activity, these compounds should not be used in animals with suspected obstructed bowel or impacted feces or those with tenesmus resulting from colonic irritation or rectal/anal surgery.

Bulk laxatives are much more gentle than irritant laxatives. These drugs osmotically pull water into the bowel lumen or retain water in the feces. Hydrophilic colloids or indigestible fiber (bran, methylcellulose, Metamucil) are not digested or absorbed to any degree and therefore create an osmotic force to produce their laxative effect. Psyllium is a hydrophilic compound that has gained popularity for its purported health benefits. It produces a laxative effect but also increases flatulence.

Hypertonic salts such as magnesium (Milk of Magnesia, Epsom salts) and phosphate salts (Fleet Enema) are also bulk laxatives that are poorly absorbed and create a strong osmotic force to attract water into the bowel lumen. Large doses of hypertonic salts should be avoided because they can severely dehydrate an animal.

Although these salts are poorly absorbed, if they are given in large doses or remain in the bowel for an extended period, they may be absorbed in sufficient amounts to cause electrolyte imbalances. For example, absorption of excessive magnesium salt can cause muscle weakness and CNS alterations. Absorption of phosphate from phosphate and sodium phosphate salt laxa-

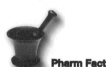

Pharm Fact

Irritant laxatives and
purgatives should not be
used in animals with
bowel obstruction or fecal
impaction.

tives or enemas can cause hypocalcemia to the extent of producing hypocalcemic tetany. Because cats are especially susceptible to these electrolyte imbalances, phosphate laxatives and sodium phosphate enemas, including soaps with a high phosphate content, should not be used in feline patients.

Lubricants (for example, mineral oil, cod liver oil, white petrolatum, and glycerin) are given to facilitate stool passage through the bowel. Mineral oil is most commonly used for horses with impactions and is administered by stomach tube. The greatest danger associated with use of this oil is aspiration into the lungs with subsequent pneumonia. Because mineral oil has no distinct taste and does not readily stimulate swallowing, aspiration is a risk in all species if the oil is not given by stomach tube.

Cod liver oil and white petrolatum are common ingredients of laxatives used in cats and dogs. As with mineral oil, these oils dissolve lipid-soluble toxins and therefore are sometimes used to decrease absorption of certain ingested toxic substances. Controversy exists because some toxicologists believe that these oils may increase absorption of lipid-soluble toxins. Long-term use of nonabsorbable oils can decrease absorption of lipid-soluble vitamins such as A, D, E, and K from the bowel.

Glycerin is most commonly used as a suppository, and therefore does not carry the risk of aspiration. Glycerin suppositories facilitate stool passing through the colon of animals with severe pelvic fractures or compression of the pelvic canal, through which the colon and rectum pass.

Docusate sodium succinate (Colace) is a stool softener that acts as a "wetting agent" by reducing the surface tension of feces and allowing water to penetrate the dry stool. Docusate sodium succinate and related calcium and phosphate compounds may also stimulate colonic secretions, resulting in increased fluid content of feces. This compound is commonly used after anal surgery (for example, anal sacculectomy and perianal fistula surgery), when passage of a firm stool may be painful.

ANTACIDS AND ANTIULCER DRUGS

Inflammation of and damage to the gastric and duodenal mucosa, with possible ulceration, can result from hyperacidity, reflux of bile from the duodenum into the stomach, accumulation of metabolic toxins (as in renal failure), stress from surgery or disease, or conditions that inhibit PgE formation. In ruminants, increased carbohydrate intake such as with grain overload can result in production of significant amounts of acidic byproducts by the rumen microflora (that is, bacteria and protozoa), causing the rumen pH to become very acidic. Rumen acidosis kills the normal rumen flora and causes irritation or ulceration of the rumen and adjoining compartments of the intestinal tract.

Several drugs commonly used in veterinary medicine can also contribute to GI irritation and ulcer formation. Nonsteroidal antiinflammatory drugs such as aspirin, phenylbutazone, flunixin meglumine (Banamine), and indomethacin (Indocin) inhibit formation of PgE, which normally helps maintain mucus production and regenerative processes of the intestinal tract. Because of its lipophilic state in an acidic pH, aspirin can diffuse directly into stomach cells and may accumulate to significant concentrations within these cells, causing cellular damage. Corticosteroids increase the risk of gastritis and ulceration by decreasing mucus production and increasing gastric acid production.

Antacids and antiulcer drugs are commonly used to prevent, control, or reverse damage to the intestinal tract related to various conditions. Gastric acid is normally produced by oxyntic (parietal) cells in the stomach when stimulated by acetylcholine (from the parasympathetic nervous system), histamine, and gastrin. Antacids are given to increase the stomach or rumen pH; the increased alkalinity reduces gastric irritation from hyperacidity or maintains the proper pH for rumen microbes to function.

Antacids are classified as systemic and nonsystemic antacids. Nonsystemic antacids, which come in either liquid or tablet form, are composed of calcium, magnesium, or aluminum. These antacids are administered by mouth to directly neutralize acid molecules in the stomach or rumen. Such OTC products as Tums and Rolaids are nonsystemic antacids made primarily of calcium. Other nonsystemic antacids include magnesium products such as Riopan and Carmilax, aluminum products such as Amphojel, and combinations of magnesium and aluminum products such as Maalox.

Calcium and aluminum antacids often cause constipation as a side effect, whereas magnesium products often produce diarrhea. Products containing both aluminum and magnesium attempt to balance these constipating and diarrheal effects. Repeated use or large doses of nonsystemic antacids may cause electrolyte imbalances because of absorption of these electrolytes.

Calcium antacids are a factor in **gastric acid rebound syndrome.** In this situation the calcium carbonate in the antacid triggers release of gastrin, with a subsequent increase in hydrochloric acid production after the calcium carbonate antacid has moved beyond the stomach. The result can be a rebound of gastric acid production and a subsequent drop in gastric PH because the antacid is no longer present in the stomach to compensate for the increased acidity.

These nonsystemic antacids also may interfere with absorption of other drugs from the bowel. The increased pH of the GI lumen may convert some drugs to a predominantly hydrophilic form that is less able to penetrate the intestinal mucosa (see Chapter 2). Drugs also may become adsorbed to or chelated with antacids, for example, tetracyclines with calcium antacids. Absorption of digoxin, acepromazine, and corticosteroids given by mouth may be decreased by concurrent use of antacids. When these drugs must be used concurrently, antacids should be given 2 to 3 hours before or after these other drugs.

In contrast to the local neutralizing effect of nonsystemic antacids, systemic antacids decrease acid production in the stomach. Systemic antacids include cimetidine (Tagamet), ranitidine (Zantac), and famotidine (Pepcid) and are often referred to as **H$_2$ antagonists** because they block the H$_2$ histamine receptor located on oxyntic (parietal) cells in the stomach. Blocking this receptor markedly decreases the stimulus for gastric acid production. These drugs are

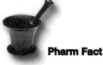

Pharm Fact

Electrolyte imbalances
may occur with repeated
use of certain antacids.

available in injectable and oral forms; cimetidine and famotidine are also available in OTC forms as Tagamet-HB and Pepcid-CD, respectively. Of these three drugs, only cimetidine and ranitidine inhibit the hepatic enzymes responsible for metabolism and breakdown of some cardiac drugs (beta blockers, calcium channel blockers, and quinidine), theophylline, and anticonvulsant drugs such as diazepam and phenytoin. Simultaneous use of systemic antacids with these drugs results in slowed metabolism, increased plasma drug concentrations, and toxic drug concentrations unless the dose is reduced. Surprisingly, barbiturate metabolic interactions with cimetidine are not clinically significant.

Omeprazole is described as an *acid blocker.* Unlike systemic antacids that block stimulation of acid production, omeprazole binds to the luminal surface of the stomach's oxyntic cells and inhibits the pump that normally transports hydrogen ions into the stomach lumen. Fewer hydrogen ions in the stomach result in a less acidic environment. Omeprazole comes in a capsule that contains too much drug for most patients that weigh less than 40 lb. In those cases the powdered drug is removed from the capsule and the appropriate amount is repacked in a smaller gelatin capsule or (as has been suggested by one gastroenterologist) mixed with liquefied soft margarine, which is then refrigerated to solidify and later cut into smaller pieces for administration.

Sucralfate (Carafate) is an antiulcer drug used to treat ulcers of the stomach and upper small intestine. The drug has been called a "gastric Band-Aid" because it forms a sticky paste in the stomach that binds with the proteins found in open, active ulcers. In effect the drug selectively adheres to the ulcer site, protecting it from the acidic environment of the stomach. In addition, it stimulates prostaglandin release, promoting protective mechanisms such as increased mucus production.

Sucralfate requires the presence of an acidic environment to bind most effectively to the ulcer site. The full clinical significance of antacid use with sucralfate has not been resolved in veterinary medicine; however, the veterinarian should avoid administering sucralfate simultaneously with antacids or other drugs that alkalinize the stomach environment because of the need for an acidic pH for maximum binding of sucralfate to the ulcer site. In spite of the required acidic environment, clinical investigators have used sucralfate to treat esophageal ulcers by crushing the tablets and mixing then with warm water to form a slurry that is administered by mouth.

Misoprostol (Cytotec) is a synthetic PgE_1 drug. As do natural prostaglandins in the stomach, this drug increases mucus production, decreases acid production, and facilitates the stomach's protective mechanisms for defense and healing. Although this drug has been used with mixed results as an ulcer preventive (for example, in animals receiving large doses of nonsteroidal antiinflammatory drugs), it is more effective in healing existing ulcerations. Because it is a prostaglandin, it stimulates the remainder of the intestinal tract and may produce diarrhea or abdominal discomfort such as cramping and colic as side effects. The drug is fairly expensive but is extremely effective in the treatment of animals that have accidental overdose of nonsteroidal antiinflammatory drugs or severely stressed animals (for example, animals with neurologic injuries or those that have undergone extensive surgery), who have an increased risk of ulcer formation.

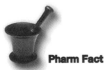

Pharm Fact

Most modern antibloat medications work by reducing the surface tension of foam in the rumen.

RUMINATORICS AND ANTIBLOAT MEDICATIONS

Ruminatorics stimulate an atonic or a flaccid rumen. In the past, compounds containing strychnine, tartar, and barium chloride were used to stimulate rumen motility in ruminants recovering from disease or severe distress in which the rumen function had ceased. These compounds are occasionally still used by livestock producers, but the ruminatorics used by veterinarians work more predictably and without as many side effects.

Neostigmine, marketed as the veterinary product Stiglyn, combines with the enzyme **acetylcholinesterase** and prevents it from breaking down acetylcholine. This increases parasympathetic stimulation, resulting in increased GI stimulation, increased bronchial secretions, bronchoconstriction, decreased heart rate, miosis (constricted pupils), and urination. Because of these effects, neostigmine should not be used in animals with GI obstruction, asthma, or bradycardia or with other drugs such as organophosphates that increase parasympathetic tone. Neostigmine has also been used in dogs to diagnose and treat myasthenia gravis, a neuromuscular disease.

Bloat, or ruminal tympany, occurs in ruminants as a result of gas accumulation in the rumen. The gas may be present either as free gas or within a froth of very small bubbles, which is known as "frothy bloat." Antibloat medications act by reducing numbers of rumen microorganisms that produce the gas or by breaking up the bubbles formed in the rumen with frothy bloat. In past years, compounds such as oil of turpentine, pine oil, gasoline, creolin, and even formaldehyde have been used to kill rumen microorganisms and reduce distention. Use of these compounds carried the risk of tissue irritation, tainting of milk, and other potentially toxic side effects.

Most modern veterinary bloat medications act by decreasing the surface tension of foam in the rumen, causing the small bubbles to rupture and form much larger gas pockets that can be eructated (belched) from the rumen. Mineral oil or ordinary household detergents mixed with mineral oil are often used to decrease the viscosity of the rumen contents, decrease the stability of the bubbles, and remove the froth. Some commercial antibloat preparations contain vegetable oils and emulsifiers, and other products contain poloxalene. Dioctyl sodium succinate (DSS) also reduces the viscosity of rumen contents, which allows the foam to dissipate. The optimal use for these products is via oral administration or by direct injection (into the rumen through the flank using a large-bore needle) in the early stages of bloat.

OTHER DRUGS USED FOR GASTROINTESTINAL PROBLEMS

Antimicrobials

Although antimicrobials usually are not needed or indicated for most common GI problems, a few can be useful in certain circumstances. Sulfasalazine (Azulfidine) is a combination antimicrobial that is broken down by GI bacteria into the sulfonamide sulfapyridine, and the aspirin-like prostaglandin-blocking agent aminosalicylic acid. Most of the antiinflammatory effect of sulfasalazine occurs in the colon, where it combats inflammatory bowel disease. As with many other sulfonamides, animals treated with sulfasalazine may develop keratoconjunctivitis sicca ("dry eye"). Clients should be instructed to examine the corneas for dryness or haziness while their animal is receiving sulfasalazine.

Tylosin (Tylan) is an antibiotic very similar to erythromycin. Tylosin is used in cattle and swine to treat susceptible gram-negative and gram-positive bacteria as well as *Chlamydia* and *Mycoplasma* infections. Veterinarians should not use it in horses because the drug may cause severe diarrhea that sometimes leads to death. Use of tylosin for enteritis and colitis in dogs and cats, which is an example of an unapproved, extra-label use, has produced variable results.

Metronidazole (Flagyl) is an antimicrobial that is effective against anaerobic bacteria such as those found in the colon and the protozoan *Giardia*. It may be used to treat chronic diarrhea if giardiasis is suspected but no *Giardia* organisms have been identified on repeated fecal examinations. Toxic side effects, including CNS signs such as head tilt, staggering, disorientation, proprioceptive deficits (inability to sense the position of the limbs), and seizures, have been observed in animals receiving this drug for long periods. Drug use should be stopped immediately if CNS signs develop. Usually these neurologic signs disappear after several days.

Oral Electrolyte Replacements

Various liquid and powder products containing electrolyte salts (Enterolyte, Resorb, Pedialyte) are used to replace ions lost with diarrhea or vomiting. These products generally are recommended for calves, lambs, and foals with scours or diarrhea. However, they are also used in small companion animals.

Electrolyte replacers work best with conditions of secretory diarrhea in which no significant dehydration is present and the animal is not vomiting. Animals with significant dehydration or vomiting should be rehydrated with suitable fluids given via the IV route. If this is not possible or economically feasible, these electrolyte solutions can be given by mouth. Absorption of electrolytes may be impaired in animals with severe intestinal damage.

Pancreatic Enzyme Supplements

Dogs and cats may be affected by a syndrome referred to as *exocrine pancreatic insufficiency,* in which the pancreas fails to produce sufficient amounts of the digestive enzymes lipase, which breaks down lipids; amylase, which breaks down starches; and various proteinases, which break down proteins. Failure

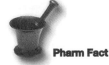

Pharm Fact

Metronidazole is often used in chronic diarrhea cases where giardiasis is suspected but no *Giardia* organisms have been found.

to digest these food components results in **maldigestion** and subsequent **malabsorption** of nutrients. The osmotic effect of these undigested nutrients produces a voluminous, pale, malodorous type of diarrhea with weight loss.

In animals with exocrine pancreatic insufficiency, pancreatic enzyme supplements such as Viokase and Pancrezyme are added to the animal's food before feeding. Unfortunately, commercially available enzyme supplements vary in their enzyme content. In addition, the supplemental enzymes are denatured by the acidic environment of the stomach, rendering the lipase and proteinases (to a lesser degree) largely ineffective.

These enzyme products may be mixed with the food at least 15 to 20 minutes before the food is offered; however, the effectiveness of lipase in breaking down fats is minimal because it depends on the proper temperature and pH. Because gastric acid inactivates these enzymes, it has been suggested that H_2 blockers such as cimetidine may decrease the breakdown of the enzyme supplement. Unfortunately, no significant improvement in fat digestion is observed when cimetidine is also used, and the cost of the H_2 blocker does not justify its limited benefit.

Most enzyme supplements are in powder form but are also available as tablets. The tablet form has been fairly ineffective in dogs. However, digestion is significantly increased when the tablets are crushed before administration. Enteric-coated enzyme tablets apparently have no advantage, even though the enteric coating protects the enzymes from the acidic environment of the stomach. The lack of efficacy with the enteric-coated enzymes may be related to insufficient dissolution of the coating or the relatively fast intestinal transit time in veterinary patients. Thus despite attempts to improve the effectiveness of enzyme supplements, animals with pancreatic exocrine insufficiency are likely to have subnormal digestion of fats and may not regain the weight that was lost before enzyme treatment.

Corticosteroids

Corticosteroid use in GI disease is controversial because the beneficial anti-inflammatory effect is offset by immunosuppression (decreased immune function), increased gastric acidity, suppression of normal gastric protective and healing mechanisms, and increased risk of infection. Some chronic inflammatory bowel problems such as eosinophilic gastroenteritis may respond very well to corticosteroids. Important precautions in using corticosteroids include using the smallest dose necessary to control clinical signs, then as soon as possible decreasing the dose to minimize side effects, and monitoring the animal's progress closely for signs of gastric problems or other adverse systemic effects. (Corticosteroids are discussed in greater detail in Chapter 10.)

Gastrointestinal Drug Categories and Names*

Emetics

Apomorphine
Extract of ipecac
Syrup of ipecac
Xylazine (Rompun, Anased)

Antiemetics

Phenothiazine tranquilizers
  Acepromazine (PromAce)
  Chlorpromazine (Thorazine)
  Prochlorperazine (Compazine, Darbazine)
Activated charcoal
Aminopentamide (Centrine)
Atropine
Cisapride (Propulsid)
Isopropamide
Metoclopramide (Reglan)
Yohimbine (Yobine)

Antidiarrheals

Anticholinergics
  Aminopentamide (Centrine)
  Atropine
  Isopropamide (Darbazine)
Opioid analgesics
  Diphenoxylate (Lomotil)
  Loperamide (Imodium)
  Paregoric
Blockers of hypersecretion
  Bismuth subsalicylate
  Chlorpromazine
  Flunixin meglumine (Banamine)
Adsorbents/protectants
  Activated charcoal
  Kaolin/pectin

Laxatives and stool softeners

Castor oil
Docusate sodium succinate (Colace)

Hydrophilic colloids/fiber
Hypertonic salts
  Magnesium
  Phosphate
Lubricants
  Mineral oil
  Cod liver oil
  Glycerin
  White petrolatum
Phenolphthalein

Antacid/antiulcer drugs

Nonsystemic antacids
  Magnesium products (Riopan, Carmilax)
  Aluminum products (Amphojel)
  Calcium products (Tums, Rolaids)
Systemic antacids
  Cimetidine (Tagamet)
  Famotidine (Pepcid)
  Ranitidine (Zantac)
Misoprostol (Cytotec)
Omeprazole
Sucralfate (Carafate)

Ruminatorics and antibloat medications

Dioctyl sodium succinate
Neostigmine (Stiglyn)
Poloxalene

Other GI drugs

Antibiotics
  Metronidazole (Flagyl)
  Sulfasalazine (Azulfidine)
  Tylosin (Tylan)
Oral electrolyte replacements
Pancreatic enzyme replacements
Corticosteroids

*Brand names are in parentheses.

Recommended Reading

Boothe DM: GI pharmacology update, *Vet Previews Purina Pub Vet* 1(2):2, 1994.

Clark SE: Pharmacologic management of colic. In Auer L, editor: *Equine surgery,* Philadelphia, 1992, WB Saunders.

Constable PD: Introduction to the ruminant forestomach. In Howard J, editor: *Current veterinary therapy 3—food animal practice,* Philadelphia, 1993, WB Saunders.

Davis LE: Drugs affecting the digestive system. In Howard J, editor: *Current veterinary therapy 3—food animal practice,* Philadelphia, 1993, WB Saunders.

Hoefer HL: *Gastrointestinal diseases of ferrets,* Proceedings of the North American Veterinary Conference, Orlando, Fla, Jan 1995.

Jergens AE: Acute diarrhea. In Bonagura JD, editor: *Kirk's current veterinary therapy XII,* Philadelphia, 1995, WB Saunders.

Jergens AE: Diagnosis and symptomatic therapy of acute gastroenteritis, *Compend Cont Educ* 16(12):1555, 1994.

Jones BD: *Therapy for acute vomiting,* Proceedings of the North American Veterinary Conference, Orlando, Fla, Jan 1996.

Jones BD: *Therapy for acute secretory diarrhea,* Proceedings of the North American Veterinary Conference, Orlando, Fla, Jan 1996.

Matz ME: Gastrointestinal ulcer therapy. In Bonagura JD, editor: *Kirk's current veterinary therapy XII,* Philadelphia, 1995, WB Saunders.

Murray MJ: Gastrointestinal ulceration. In Auer L, editor: *Equine surgery,* Philadelphia, 1992, WB Saunders.

Papich MG: Antiulcer therapy, *Vet Clin North Am Small Anim Pract* 23(3):497, 1993.

Rings DM: Diseases of the ruminant forestomach. In Howard J, editor: *Current veterinary therapy 3—food animal practice,* Philadelphia, 1993, WB Saunders.

Tams TR: *Use of cisapride to control vomiting in cats,* Proceedings of the North American Veterinary Conference, Orlando, Fla, Jan 1995.

Tams TR: *Drug therapy of GI disease,* Proceedings of the North American Veterinary Conference, Orlando, Fla, Jan 1996.

Twedt DC: *Controlling chronic colitis,* Proceedings of the North American Veterinary Conference, Orlando, Fla, Jan 1996.

Washabau RJ, Elie MS: Antiemetic therapy. In Bonagura JD, editor: *Kirk's current veterinary therapy XII,* Philadelphia, 1995, WB Saunders.

Review Questions

1. The package insert for drug A states that its site of action is enteric, and the insert for drug B states that its site of action is gastric. In what part of the body does each of these drugs work?

2. What effects do the sympathetic nervous system and the parasympathetic nervous system have on the GI tract and its function?

3. After answering Question 2, explain what effect acetylcholine and epinephrine (or drugs that imitate their effects) have on the GI tract.

4. The doctor comments that in many diseases, treatment is focused on reducing the effects of prostaglandins but prostaglandins are often beneficial to the intestinal tract. What is the significance of this comment?

5. What three factors work together to stimulate oxyntic (parietal) cells to produce hydrochloric acid?

6. Explain the mechanism that causes a dog to vomit soon after eating a decomposing animal carcass.

7. Explain the mechanisms that cause a dog to vomit during a car ride, a cat to vomit from stress, and a dog to vomit from an overdose of digoxin.

8. By what mechanism do antihistamines prevent motion sickness? Are antihistamines more effective in dogs or cats? Why?

9. Why is xylazine (Rompun, Anased) more likely to cause vomiting in cats than in dogs?

10. A pharmaceutical sales representative is touting a "brand new" drug that is primarily antidopaminergic. "It's a great drug for those cats that continually vomit hairballs," he explains. Considering what you know about vomiting mechanisms in cats, is this new drug likely to be effective for cats vomiting hairballs?

11. A client presents his dog for emergency treatment, saying the dog lapped up some antifreeze (ethylene glycol) 10 minutes ago. You remember that antifreeze can damage the animal's kidneys and cause death. Because antifreeze is a liquid, it will be absorbed very quickly. Which drug is most appropriate to induce vomiting: syrup of ipecac, hydrogen peroxide, or apomorphine?

12. In which cases is it inappropriate to induce emesis?
    a. A dog that ingested 2 ounces of corrosive drain opener 5 minutes previously
    b. A cat that lapped up a small puddle of strong alkali cleanser 1 hour previously
    c. A horse that ingested rat poison 15 minutes previously
    d. A dog that ate baking chocolate 1 hour previously and has been vomiting ever since
    e. A dog that ate strychnine mole bait 3 hours previously and is having seizures
    f. A cat that ate five Tylenol (acetaminophen) tablets 12 hours previously

13. Apomorphine is not very effective in inducing vomiting in cats. What other veterinary drug is an effective emetic as well as an analgesic and sedative in cats?

14. The new associate veterinarian in your practice is trying to induce vomiting in a dog that ingested rat poison 15 minutes ago. He administered syrup of ipecac 10 minutes ago, but the dog has not yet vomited. He assumes the emetic has failed and is about to administer a second dose. What has the new doctor failed to consider?

15. While arranging drug containers in the pharmacy, you find an old bottle labeled *Ipecac Extract.* Is this the same drug as syrup of ipecac?

16. A client presents a small puppy that ate some granular fertilizer an hour previously. He has already given the puppy some syrup of ipecac at home, plus some activated charcoal (universal antidote). He asks why the puppy has not yet vomited the fertilizer. How would you answer this question?

17. Why are phenothiazine tranquilizers such as acepromazine effective in preventing motion sickness?

18. Why should very dehydrated animals not receive phenothiazine tranquilizers as antiemetics before they are rehydrated?

19. A client says, "I thought Benadryl was used for colds and allergies! Why are you giving it to my dog to prevent motion sickness?" How would you answer this question?

20. What is an anticholinergic drug? What is a parasympatholytic drug? What effect do these drugs have on the GI tract?

21. Metoclopramide (Reglan) is said to have an advantage over other antiemetics because it has centrally acting and locally acting antiemetic effects. What is meant by this?

22. What other antiemetic drugs should not be given simultaneously with metoclopramide? Why?

23. What drug, similar to Reglan, is effective in reducing hairball vomiting in cats?

24. Why is one antidiarrheal agent effective in one animal but not in another?

25. What are four general physiologic causes of diarrhea?

26. Do motility-modifying antidiarrheal drugs increase or decrease segmental or peristaltic contractions?

27. How does hypomotility cause diarrhea?

28. What is tenesmus?

29. Which antidiarrheals increase segmental contractions and reduce peristaltic contractions?

30. What are the side effects of opioid antidiarrheals?

31. Why are atropine, isopropamide, and aminopentamide more effective in controlling large bowel diarrhea than small bowel diarrhea?

32. Why are hypersecretory diarrheas generally more dangerous than diarrhea associated with changes in intestinal motility?

33. Why is Pepto-Bismol fairly effective in controlling hypersecretory diarrhea? Does it really "coat and soothe" the intestinal tract?

34. A client is concerned because for the past 2 days her dog's stools have been a dark color and she thinks the discoloration is caused by digested blood. She mentions that she has been giving the dog bismuth subsalicylate (generic) for the past 2 days. The doctor is unavailable to speak with the client. What reasonable explanation can you give the client to explain the stool discoloration?

35. A client telephones to ask about giving Pepto-Bismol to his cat. What is an appropriate response?

36. Activated charcoal and kaolin and pectin compounds are sometimes effective in controlling diarrhea. What is their mechanism of action?

37. Why should a drug like Kaopectate *not* be given simultaneously with other oral medications?

38. Under what circumstances should such laxatives as castor oil or phenolphthalein *not* be given?

39. Which type of enema compounds should *not* be used in cats?

40. Why might a patient require supplemental vitamins if it is receiving long-term therapy with laxatives?

41. Docusate sodium succinate is given to animals with severe pelvic fractures and to cattle with bloat. What is the drug's action in each case?

42. How can nonsteroidal antiinflammatory drugs cause damage to the intestinal tract?

43. Systemic antacids are much more expensive than nonsystemic antacids. Is the higher expense justified by greater efficacy?

44. Do antihistamine cold medications also block stomach acid production as Tagamet does?

45. A client calls and says she received a free sample of Pepcid-CD (famotidine) in the mail. She asks whether giving it to her dog after it vomits is appropriate to help settle the dog's stomach. What is an appropriate response?

46. What is the difference between an H_2 blocker and the drug known as the "acid blocker"?

47. Which drug functions as a band-aid in treatment of gastric ulcers? Is this drug usually given with antacids?

48. Prostaglandins can cause undesirable intestinal effects, yet misoprostol is a prostaglandin used to treat gastric ulcers. Explain this.

49. What do strychnine and neostigmine have in common?

50. What type of common household product is a common ingredient of antibloat medications? How does it work?

51. What antimicrobial is used in treating inflammatory bowel disease? Where is its site of action?

52. In what animals should the antibiotic tylosin *not* be used? Why?

53. What antimicrobial is indicated for treatment of giardiasis in dogs? What side effects are commonly observed with use of large doses or with standard doses given for long periods?

54. What are some indications for use of oral electrolyte supplements?

55. Why are the signs of pancreatic exocrine insufficiency not completely alleviated by oral supplementation with pancreatic enzymes?

Chapter **5**

Drugs Affecting the Cardiovascular System

Normal Cardiac Function
    Cardiac anatomy and dynamics of
        blood flow
    Electrical conduction through the
        heart
    Depolarization, repolarization, and
        refractory periods
    Role of the autonomic nervous
        system in cardiovascular function
Antiarrhythmic Drugs
    Antiarrhythmic drugs that inhibit
        sodium influx
    β-Blocker antiarrhythmic drugs
    Calcium channel blocker
        antiarrhythmic drugs
Positive Inotropic Agents
Vasodilators
    Vasoconstriction in heart disease

Vasodilator drugs
    Hydralazine
    Nitroglycerin
    Angiotensin-converting enzyme
        inhibitors
    Prazosin
Diuretics
    Loop diuretics
    Thiazide diuretics
    Potassium-sparing diuretics
    Osmotic diuretics
    Carbonic anhydrase inhibitors
Other Drugs Used in Treating
    Cardiovascular Disease
    Aspirin
    Bronchodilators
    Sedatives and tranquilizers

Key Terms

absolute refractory
   period
adrenergic drug
aldosterone
α_1 *receptor*
α_2 *receptor*
angiotensin I and II
angiotensin-converting
   enzyme (ACE)
arrhythmia
atrioventricular (AV) block
atrioventricular (AV) node
automaticity
β_1 *receptor*
β_2 *receptor*
bradycardia
cholinergic receptors
depolarization
diuresis
down-regulation
ectopic focus
hypokalemia
mitral insufficiency
negative inotropic drug
positive inotropic drug
PR interval
premature ventricular
   contraction (PVC)
relative refractory period
renin-angiotensin system
repolarization
sinoatrial (SA) node
supraventricular
   arrhythmia
tachycardia
up-regulation
vasoconstriction
vasodilation
ventricular arrhythmia

Normal heart anatomy

Dynamics of blood flow through the heart

Types of antiarrhythmics and the way they exert their effects

Types of positive inotropes and the way they exert their effects

Types of vasodilators and the way they exert their effects

Types of diuretics and the way they exert their effects

Treatment of cardiovascular problems is challenging for several reasons: cardiac drugs have complex mechanisms of action that can be difficult to understand; several cardiac drugs may be used simultaneously, so drug interactions must be considered; and many cardiac drugs have serious side effects that must be anticipated. In addition, impaired cardiovascular function may alter the normal absorption, distribution, metabolism, and elimination of these drugs. (A box listing cardiovascular drugs can be found at the end of this chapter.)

The veterinary professional must have knowledge of normal and abnormal cardiac physiology to understand the intended effect of a cardiac drug, determine whether the goals of the therapy are being met, and detect toxic side effects early enough to prevent serious consequences. Veterinary technicians often monitor hospitalized cardiac patients and listen to client descriptions of the animal's status at home and therefore must have a working knowledge of the effects of cardiac drugs and early signs of complications.

This chapter presents principles of cardiac drug use. Many specifics of individual cardiac drug mechanisms have been excluded for brevity and to focus on the key elements of each drug. Veterinary professionals should review the package insert or published information for any cardiac drug before administering it to a veterinary patient.

NORMAL CARDIAC FUNCTION

Many complex feedback mechanisms regulate function of the cardiovascular system. This chapter contains a brief review of cardiovascular physiology and pathology. More detailed information is contained in veterinary cardiology, physiology, and internal medicine textbooks.

Cardiac Anatomy and Dynamics of Blood Flow

The mammalian heart acts like a two-pump system. A fairly small pump on the right side pumps blood to the lungs and back to the heart, and a larger, stronger pump on the left pumps blood throughout the remainder of the body and back to the heart. The vessels returning blood to the right side of the heart are the vena cavae. Blood flows from the vena cavae into the right atrium, through the tricuspid, or right atrioventricular (AV), valve, and into the right ventricle. From the right ventricle, blood is pumped through the pulmonic valve (pulmonary refers to the lungs) into the pulmonary arteries, to the lungs, and back to the heart via the pulmonary veins.

With few exceptions, arteries carry blood away from the heart and veins carry blood toward the heart. Blood from the pulmonary veins enters the left atrium, passes through the mitral, or left atrioventricular (AV), valve, and into the left ventricle. Finally, blood is pumped out of the left ventricle, through the aortic valve, and into the aorta for distribution throughout the body.

The valves in the heart allow only one-way flow of blood and open and close passively. They swing like a one-way door in response to pressure changes between the atria and ventricles or between the ventricles and pulmonary arteries or aorta. The valves do not "force" blood from one part of the heart to another; they prevent reversal of blood flow.

Electrical Conduction Through the Heart

The heart beats in a very specific, coordinated manner. Special "wiring," or a conduction system, in the heart muscle ensures that the electrical impulses, or waves of depolarization, that control heart contraction move through the heart in a very specific sequence. These waves of depolarization are recorded on an electrocardiogram (ECG).

Each heart muscle cell has the potential to depolarize ("fire") spontaneously and independently, a property called **automaticity.** If a cardiac muscle cell were removed and placed in a special physiologic solution to keep it alive, the cell would spontaneously contract at a rate determined by that cell's physical and biochemical makeup. A specialized group of cardiac cells in the right atrium depolarizes more rapidly than any other cells in the heart. This group of cells is called the **sinoatrial (SA) node** (Fig. 5-1). Cells in the SA node depolarize 50 to 150 times per minute depending on the species. (Larger species generally have slower rates.) The rate at which cells in the SA node depolarize determines the heart rate. For this reason the SA node is often referred to as the heart's pacemaker.

When cells in the SA node depolarize, a wave of depolarization spreads in all directions through first the right and then the left atrium. As this wave of depolarization passes from one cardiac muscle cell to another, each cell contracts. This wave passes so quickly that both atria contract almost simultaneously, pushing blood through the AV valves into the ventricles. On the ECG strip this atrial depolarization (and subsequent contraction of atrial muscle cells) is reflected as a small bump called the *P wave*. The wave components of the ECG shown in Fig. 5-2 proceed in alphabetical order, from *P* through *T* as you view the strip from left to right.

The wave of depolarization spreads around the atria and is prevented from entering the ventricles by a cellular barrier to electrical impulses that acts like an electrical insulator. In normal animals the depolarization wave

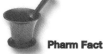

Pharm Fact

Cardiac muscle cells can depolarize spontaneously, a property called *automaticity.*

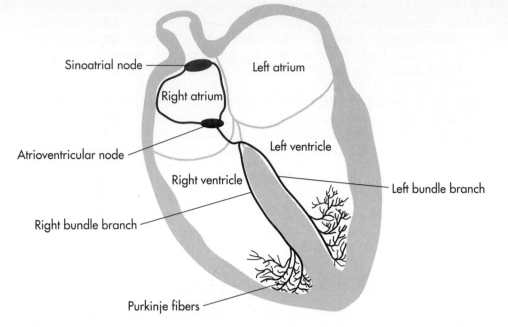

Fig. 5-1 Pathway of depolarization conduction from the SA node to the ventricles.

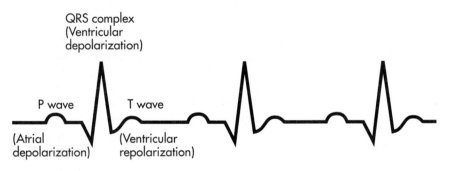

Fig. 5-2 Components of a normal ECG tracing.

can reach the ventricles only through a specialized cluster of conducting cells called the **atrioventricular (AV) node.** The wave of depolarization enters the AV node and is delayed there for a fraction of a second before entering the ventricles. This short delay allows the atria to complete their contraction before the ventricles begin contracting, and provides enough time for blood to move from the atria into the ventricles. Without this slight delay the atria and ventricles would contract at the same time and blood would not be pumped efficiently. On the ECG this period of conduction delay in the AV node shows up as a flat line after the P wave and is referred to as the P-R interval or the P-QRS interval.

After the depolarization wave passes through the AV node, it travels rapidly in the interventricular septum (wall between the right and left ventricles) along a specialized conduction pathway known as the bundle branches. The bundle branches conduct the electrical impulse to the Purkinje fibers, located at the apex (conical end) of the heart. The depolarization wave emerges from the Purkinje fibers at the apex and spreads rapidly throughout the ventricular muscle cells, causing them to contract from the apex toward the heart valves and push blood through the pulmonic and aortic valves and to the lungs and body.

Depolarization (and contraction) of the ventricles is reflected as a large wave on the ECG called the QRS complex. The QRS complex is composed of a small Q wave, a large R wave, and a small S wave, all clumped together. After the ventricles contract, the ventricular muscle cells relax and repolarize (reset) in preparation for the next depolarization wave. This period of ventricular cell repolarization is displayed as the T wave on the ECG strip.

An ECG pattern shows the way electrical impulses are traveling through the heart. Any deviation from the normal pattern of cardiac depolarization or repolarization is apparent as abnormal P waves, bizarre QRS complexes, or skewed T waves.

Depolarization, Repolarization, and Refractory Periods

Many cardiac drugs affect depolarization or repolarization, either as an intended effect or as a side effect; therefore the veterinary technician must have a basic understanding of the processes that take place within cardiac cells during depolarization and repolarization.

Depolarization and repolarization may be compared with the mechanics of a mousetrap. The mousetrap is set by moving the spring-loaded wire loop in place. After the trap snaps shut, it cannot "fire" again until it is reset. Cardiac cells act in a similar manner. In its resting state a cardiac cell is much like the mousetrap, ready to snap shut. When the cardiac cell is stimulated, it fires, or depolarizes. Like the tripped (depolarized) mousetrap, the cardiac cell cannot depolarize again until it is repolarized (reset). Thus repolarization of the cardiac cell is like resetting the mousetrap, preparing it to fire again.

Depolarization and repolarization primarily involve movement of ions, specifically sodium (Na^+) and potassium (K^+), across the cardiac cell membrane. Although other ions such as chloride (Cl^-) and calcium (Ca^{++}) are involved, for simplicity this discussion focuses only on sodium and potassium. In its resting state the cardiac cell is polarized; that is, it has two distinct "poles," or segregated areas, of electrical charge. In resting cardiac cells the polarization is between sodium ions, which are found in high concentrations outside the cell membrane, and potassium ions, which are found in high concentrations inside the cell membrane (Fig. 5-3). Although this polarized state is referred to as the *resting state,* the cell is actually expending energy to pump the Na^+ out and the K^+ in and maintain polarization even if a stray ion leaks across the membrane. The pump itself is a specialized protein within the cell membrane called the sodium-potassium-ATPase pump. The enzyme ATPase is used to supply the sodium-potassium pump with energy stored in the cell's adenosine triphosphate (ATP). The pump can maintain polarization of these ions in the resting state

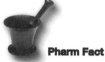

Pharm Fact

Depolarization and repolarization of heart muscle cells can be compared with tripping and resetting a mousetrap.

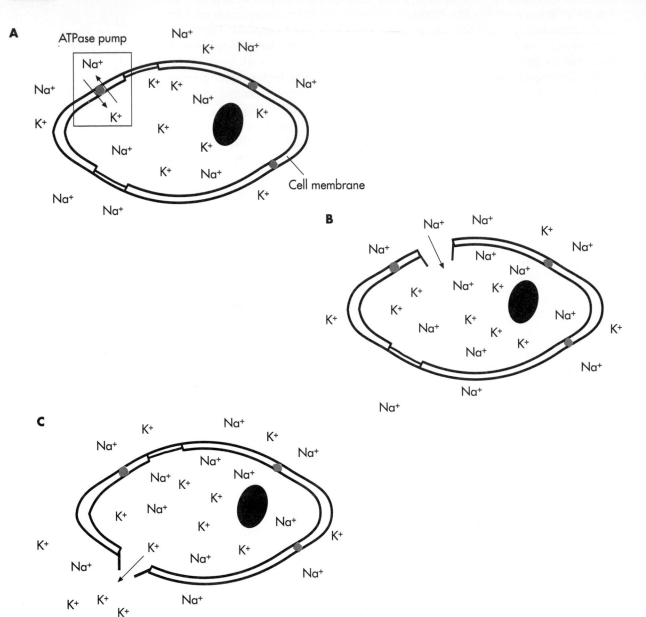

Fig. 5-3 Changes in sodium *(Na+)* and potassium *(K+)* ion concentrations during depolarization and repolarization. **A**, In the resting state, the Na^+/K^+ ATPase pump increases intracellular K^+ concentrations while pumping Na^+ out of the cell. **B,** During depolarization, the Na^+ channels open, allowing Na^+ to move into the cell along the concentration gradient. **C,** During repolarization, the Na^+ channels close, the K^+ channels open, and K^+ moves out of the cell.

because the Na$^+$ and K$^+$ have difficulty crossing the cellular membrane except through specialized Na$^+$ and K$^+$ channels that are closed during the
resting state.

The cardiac cell remains in this polarized resting state until the appropriate stimulus occurs. This stimulus is either the depolarization of adjoining
cardiac cells or a change in electrical charge within the cardiac cell itself.
When the stimulus occurs, the Na$^+$ channels (sometimes called "gates")
open, allowing Na$^+$ to move into the cell. The concentration gradient of Na$^+$
(high outside the membrane, low inside) and the slightly negative charge
within the cell from negatively charged intracellular proteins cause the Na$^+$
to move readily through the open channels into the cardiac cell. This influx
of Na$^+$ is known as **depolarization** because the two ion populations are no
longer kept apart, or polarized.

As the positively charged Na$^+$ flood into the cell, the net charge within
the cardiac cell becomes positive (*phase 0* in Fig. 5-4). When the charge within
the cell becomes positive, the Na$^+$ channels close and the K$^+$ channels open.
The concentration gradient of K$^+$ (high inside the membrane, low outside) and
the increasingly positive charge within the cell cause the K$^+$ to quickly leave
the cell through the open K$^+$ channels, taking with them their positive charges
and causing the inside of the cardiac cell to become more negative (*phases 1, 2,
and 3* in Fig. 5-4). This movement of K$^+$ out of the cell is called **repolarization**
because the ion populations are separated and the cell is polarized again.

Neurons tend to have a rapid succession of depolarization and repolarization phases, whereas cardiac muscle cells tend to have a plateau phase
(*phase 2* in Fig. 5-4) between the influx of Na$^+$ during depolarization and the
efflux (outflow) of K$^+$ during repolarization. During this plateau phase,

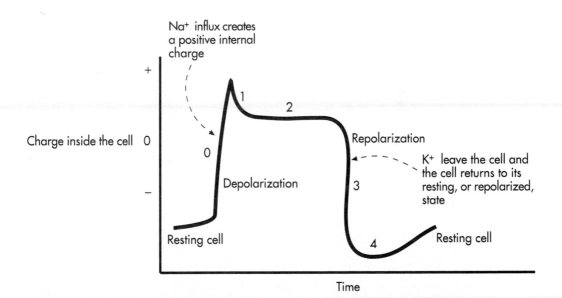

Fig. 5-4 Relative changes in electrical charge within a cardiac muscle cell during
depolarization and repolarization.

Ca^{++} and Na^+ continue to move into the cell through "slow channels," thus maintaining the positive charge of the plateau phase. Repolarization rapidly occurs when these slow channels close.

At the completion of K^+ efflux and repolarization, the Na^+ and K^+ are located on the "wrong" sides of the cellular membrane, having passed through their respective channels during depolarization and repolarization. At this point the sodium-potassium pump begins to reestablish the "proper" location of the Na^+ and K^+ by pumping the Na^+ out of the cell and pumping the K^+ into the cell.

The line in *phase 4* in Fig. 5-4 moves gradually upward. This is because most cardiac cells are somewhat permeable to Na^+. As the Na^+ leak in (faster than they can be pumped out), the charge within the cell becomes more positive until it reaches a threshold, at which point depolarization takes place. This phenomenon of Na^+ leaking helps explain the reason cardiac cells depolarize spontaneously without stimulation (automaticity).

As mentioned earlier, after a cardiac cell has depolarized, it cannot depolarize again until it has repolarized. The time during which the cardiac cell cannot depolarize is called the *refractory period*. This is divided into the **absolute refractory period** and the **relative refractory period.** A cardiac cell (or nerve) is absolutely refractory in phase 0 of the depolarization and repolarization cycle because no matter how strong the stimulus applied to the cell, the cell cannot depolarize again with the Na^+ channels already open and Na^+ already entering the cell. As the cell begins to repolarize in phases 2 and 3, a sufficiently strong stimulus may be able to elicit a weak depolarization response. In this relative refractory period the cell may be depolarized again if the stimulus is sufficiently strong. The cell becomes relatively less refractory to depolarization stimuli as it progresses from phases 1 through 3.

The refractory period is essential to prevent a wave of depolarization from traveling throughout the heart (such as from the right atrium to the left atrium and back again) in a continuous sequence. For example, when the wave of depolarization travels around the atria, it stops when it returns to the areas that are in the refractory period of the cycle. If the refractory period were shortened for some reason and the cells were able to fire again when the wave of depolarization returned, the wave would be propagated and the coordinated contraction of the heart would quickly turn into a series of rapid, uncoordinated contractions termed atrial or ventricular flutter or fibrillation.

Role of the Autonomic Nervous System in Cardiovascular Function

The autonomic nervous system, which is composed of the sympathetic and parasympathetic branches, regulates many organ and system functions at an unconscious level. The sympathetic nervous system (also known as the "fight or flight" response system) increases the heart rate and force of contraction, elevates blood pressure, causes constriction of peripheral blood vessels, decreases perfusion and activity of the GI tract, and dilates the bronchioles. All these functions improve the body's ability to survive a crisis. The

Pharm Fact

Sympathetic stimulation predominates as the body prepares for emergency action, and parasympathetic stimulation predominates as the body rests.

increased heart rate delivers more blood to the muscles for movement, and vasoconstriction of peripheral vessels shunts blood away from the skin (resulting in less bleeding in the event of injury) and GI tract (negating the need to digest food during an emergency) and directs it to critical areas of the body. Bronchodilation allows more oxygen to reach the lungs and reduces accumulation of carbon dioxide.

Neurons of the sympathetic nervous system release the neurotransmitters epinephrine (adrenaline) and norepinephrine. These compounds bind to specific types of receptors called adrenergic receptors to produce the fight or flight changes. Drugs that bind to these receptors and have intrinsic activity can mimic the effects of epinephrine and norepinephrine and are called *adrenergic agonists*. In contrast, drugs that block these receptors, called *adrenergic antagonists*, inhibit the sympathetic influence on an organ or tissue.

Epinephrine, norepinephrine, and adrenergic agonists can bind to several different types of adrenergic receptors. These receptors, α_1, α_2, β_1, and β_2 adrenergic **receptors,** are located on cells in different tissues. When stimulated, these receptors help carry out the sympathetic nervous system response. β_1 receptors are located in the heart. They increase the rate and strength of contraction and speed of conduction of the depolarization wave. Stimulation of β_1-adrenergic receptors by norepinephrine or adrenergic agonist drugs is responsible for the "racing heart" (tachycardia) experienced during exercise, fear, or excitement.

β_2 Receptors are found in smooth muscle surrounding blood vessels of the heart and skeletal muscles and surrounding the terminal bronchioles in the lungs. When stimulated, β_2-adrenergic receptors cause smooth muscle to relax, dilating blood vessels in the skeletal muscle and heart (vasodilation) and dilating airways in the lungs (bronchodilation). In contrast to the vasodilating effect of β_2 receptors, stimulated α_1 receptors cause smooth muscle surrounding blood vessels in the skin and intestinal tract to contract, decreasing blood flow (vasoconstriction). Thus in fight or flight situations, blood is shunted away from the skin and digestive tract (α_1 effect) and toward the heart and skeletal muscles (β_2 effect). α_2 Receptors are located on the ends of neurons that release norepinephrine (see Chapter 8).

Although α_1, β_1, and β_2 receptors are all stimulated by sympathetic neurotransmitters and adrenergic agonist drugs, they are not necessarily stimulated equally. For example, epinephrine has a very strong α_1 effect (vasoconstriction of peripheral blood vessels) and a weaker β_2 effect (vasodilation of cardiac and skeletal muscle blood vessels). When epinephrine is released by the body or injected as a drug, blood pressure increases because blood is shunted away from the skin without increased flow to skeletal muscles. This "selective" stimulation of receptors is a common characteristic of drugs used in cardiovascular and respiratory therapeutics. Use of a drug that focuses on a single adrenergic receptor helps prevent undesirable side effects.

The parasympathetic nervous system (sometimes referred to as the "rest and restore" system) causes many effects opposite those of the sympathetic nervous system. The parasympathetic system slows the heart rate (opposite of β_1-adrenergic effect), increases blood flow to the intestinal tract (opposite of α_1-adrenergic effect), and decreases the diameter of the bronchioles (opposite of β_2-adrenergic effect). The parasympathetic nervous system has little effect on peripheral blood vessels and thus does not antagonize the vasoconstriction of skin vessels caused by the sympathetic nervous system.

Neurons of the parasympathetic nervous system secrete acetylcholine as the principal neurotransmitter. Acetylcholine combines with **cholinergic receptors** to produce parasympathetic effects. As with adrenergic receptors, different types of cholinergic receptors exist. For simplicity, these differences will be mentioned only when they play a significant role in specific drug actions or physiologic phenomena.

The parasympathetic and sympathetic nervous systems are always producing some effect on the body, often simultaneously on the same organ or tissues. The system producing the stronger effect at any particular moment determines whether the body shows sympathetic or parasympathetic signs. This is the reason adrenergic antagonists tend to cause parasympathetic nervous system signs, whereas cholinergic antagonists cause sympathetic nervous system signs.

ANTIARRHYTHMIC DRUGS

An **arrhythmia** is any abnormal pattern of electrical activity in the heart. As discussed earlier, the waves of depolarization follow a specific sequence, starting in the SA node and ending with contraction of the ventricles. Sometimes, however, another area of the myocardium (heart muscle) or conducting system begins to depolarize out of sequence or more rapidly than the SA node, disrupting the normal electrical pattern. This abnormal site of depolarization is called an **ectopic focus.** Ectopic foci are often areas of damaged myocardial cells with membranes that allow leakage of Na^+ into the cell more rapidly than normal, resulting in quicker attainment of the threshold for depolarization.

ECGs detect arrhythmias caused by ectopic foci or other abnormalities. An ectopic focus in the ventricles may be indicated on the ECG as a single, large, bizarre wave. This single wave is referred to as a **premature ventricular contraction (PVC)** because it represents depolarization of the ventricles out of the normal sequence, causing the ventricles to contract prematurely (Fig. 5-5). Single, intermittent PVCs on the ECG do not significantly affect the heart's ability to pump blood and sometimes occur in healthy animals under general anesthesia. However, multiple PVCs may result in a series of rapid contractions, referred to as *flutter.* If the conduction disturbance is severe, the heart simply quivers and has no coordinated contractions, a rapidly fatal condition termed *ventricular fibrillation.* Antiarrhythmic drugs are used to control ectopic foci or reverse disorganized conduction of electrical impulses through the heart to prevent fibrillation.

Various types of antiarrhythmic drugs help control different arrhythmias. Therefore the veterinary professional must know the type of arrhythmia present before choosing the appropriate antiarrhythmic drug. Arrhythmias are divided into two general groups: those that result in an increased heart rate **(tachycardia)** and those that cause a decreased heart rate **(bradycar-**

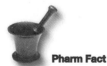

Pharm Fact

The type of arrhythmia must be identified before the correct antiarrhythmic drug can be chosen.

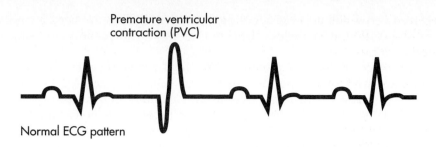

Fig. 5-5   Abnormal QRS complex indicating a PVC produced by an ectopic focus.

dia). These arrhythmias are further subdivided according to location of the ectopic foci or lesion causing the arrhythmia. A **supraventricular arrhythmia** indicates that the cause of the problem is "above" the ventricles and thus originates in the SA node, atria, or AV node. A **ventricular arrhythmia** indicates that the problem originates in the ventricles. For example, an animal with an accelerated heart rate caused by atrial fibrillation has a supraventricular tachycardia. Once the type of arrhythmia has been determined, an effective antiarrhythmic drug is used to reestablish a normal conduction sequence, or sinus rhythm.

Antiarrhythmic Drugs That Inhibit Sodium Influx

Lidocaine, quinidine, and procainamide reverse arrhythmias primarily by decreasing the rate of Na^+ movement into the cell. Without normal Na^+ influx at depolarization, the steep phase 0 is retarded, resulting in less effective depolarization. The phase 4 leaking of Na^+ into the cell is also slowed, decreasing automaticity in the bundle branches and Purkinje fibers as well as in any abnormal ectopic foci in damaged tissue. Because depolarization of an ectopic focus is slowed but the SA node is unaffected by these antiarrhythmic drugs, the SA node can regain control of the heart rate.

Lidocaine, which is also used as a local anesthetic under the name of Xylocaine, is only available in injectable form. The extensive biotransformation by the liver (first-pass effect) and gastrointestinal irritation it causes if given by mouth preclude its use as an oral medication. The preferred route of administration of lidocaine for treatment of arrhythmias is intravenously because absorption after intramuscular injection is erratic. For animals that have a lidocaine-responsive arrhythmia but require an oral drug for long-term maintenance, tocainide (another lidocaine-like compound) can be used. This drug has less of a first-pass effect and is much more effective than lidocaine when given by mouth.

Lidocaine is one of the drugs of choice for controlling PVCs and ventricular arrhythmias in cardiac patients or animals under anesthesia. Although lidocaine works well in controlling PVCs and ventricular ectopic foci, it has little efficacy against atrial ectopic foci, atrial fibrillation, or atrial flutter. For these arrhythmias, procainamide and quinidine are more effective.

Cats appear to be somewhat more sensitive to the effects of lidocaine than other species. Conduction disturbances have been observed in cats that have received very small doses of lidocaine; however, this has not been a consistent observation. Nonetheless, these reports do warrant caution in using lidocaine in cats.

Toxic effects of lidocaine produce signs ranging from sedation, ataxia, and drowsiness with slight overdoses to central nervous system (CNS) excitement and seizures with larger overdoses. Generally, seizure activity stops soon after lidocaine administration is halted because the body rapidly metabolizes the lidocaine. Cardiovascular depression caused by toxic doses is much less common with lidocaine than with quinidine or procainamide.

Veterinary technicians must realize that lidocaine is sometimes packaged in vials with epinephrine. Lidocaine with epinephrine is designed for use as a local anesthetic, *not* as an antiarrhythmic drug. Epinephrine causes vasoconstriction in the area of injection and reduces movement of lidocaine away from the site of administration (see Chapter 3). If an animal with an arrhythmia is accidentally injected intravenously with lidocaine that contains epinephrine, the animal will experience sympathetic stimulation of the heart by epinephrine, causing tachycardia, greater consumption of oxygen by the myocardium, and increasingly unstable conduction of impulses through the heart. This could cause death in an animal with cardiac disease. For this reason the technician should always closely examine the label on the bottle of lidocaine before using it to treat arrhythmias.

Procainamide and quinidine are drugs that belong to the same general class as lidocaine. However, theoretically they are effective against both ventricular ectopic foci and supraventricular tachycardia caused by atrial flutter or fibrillation. Although these drugs have been used for supraventricular arrhythmias in horses, they are not very effective against atrial fibrillation in dogs or cats. Hence they are more commonly used for their ventricular antiarrhythmic effects. Quinidine and procainamide are available in oral forms and therefore are used for long-term maintenance of patients with ventricular arrhythmias.

Quinidine frequently causes vomiting, diarrhea, and anorexia. In contrast, procainamide appears to be well tolerated and causes fewer GI problems. When given too rapidly intravenously, quinidine can cause severe hypotension and potentiate (make greater) the effect of other hypotensive drugs such as acepromazine.

Veterinary professionals must be aware of the interaction between quinidine and digoxin because these cardiac drugs may be used together. Quinidine displaces digoxin from its binding sites in cardiac and skeletal muscle cells while simultaneously decreasing digoxin elimination. These actions can double plasma digoxin concentrations and produce digoxin toxicity. Digoxin doses should be decreased by half for animals being treated simultaneously with quinidine.

Procainamide is available in two forms of tablets. The standard tablet is usually given 4 times per day, whereas the sustained-release form (Procan-SR) is given only 3 times per day. The veterinary technician should not break sustained-release tablets in half to achieve a proper dose. Instead the technician should use a slightly smaller dose or the standard procainamide tablets. Because of the rapid GI transit time of dogs as compared with that of people, owners should check the dog's stool to make sure that intact sustained-release tablets are not passing through the intestines and out the body with the feces.

β-Blocker Antiarrhythmic Drugs

β_1 Receptors are located primarily in the heart. When stimulated by the sympathetic nervous system or by sympathomimetic drugs, β_1 receptors cause the heart to beat more rapidly and with greater strength. However, sympathetic stimulation, which normally increases as the body attempts to compensate for a weakened, diseased heart, can also make the heart more electrically unstable, allowing ectopic foci to appear and arrhythmias to develop. Thus decreasing β_1 sympathetic stimulation may help reduce generation of ectopic foci and arrhythmias. Drugs that block β receptors are known as *beta blockers*.

Propranolol (Inderal) is a prime example of this group of antiarrhythmics. It blocks stimulation of β_1 receptors by epinephrine, norepinephrine, and other β-stimulating drugs. It decreases the heart rate and prevents tachycardia in response to stress, fear, or excitement by depressing the automaticity of the SA node and slowing conduction of the depolarization wave through the AV node. Automaticity of cardiac muscle cells and cells of the bundle branches is also decreased, reducing the chance of ventricular ectopic foci developing.

Because beta blockers decrease sympathetic stimulation, they cause the heart to contract with less force. Drugs that decrease the strength of contraction are referred to as **negative inotropic drugs** (negative inotropes). In animals with congestive heart failure, the increased contractile force from sympathetic tone normally helps compensate for the weakened condition of the heart. Therefore while treatment with a beta blocker decreases arrhythmias, its negative inotropic effect could also cause a marginally functional heart to become worse, leading to congestive heart failure. For this reason, beta-blockers must be used with caution in animals with myocardial failure.

Another problem with many beta blockers is that they may not be specific for β_1 receptors but may also block β_2 receptors. Stimulation of β_2-adrenergic receptors of the sympathetic nervous system normally causes bronchodilation as well as vasodilation in cardiac and skeletal muscle. Blocking the β_2 receptors in the lungs allows the parasympathetic nervous system to dominate, resulting in reflex bronchoconstriction. The newer beta blocker antiarrhythmic drugs such as nadolol, timolol, and atenolol are selective for β_1 receptors, thus reducing the β_2 antagonist side effects.

β_1 receptor stimulation increases the speed of the depolarization waves through the cardiac conduction system. Therefore blocking these β_1 receptors should allow parasympathetic dominance on the SA and AV nodes, slowing conduction of impulses through the heart and decreasing the heart rate. These effects are evident on the ECG as a slowed heart rate (from decreased SA node depolarization) and as a prolonged interval between the P wave (atrial depolarization) and the QRS complex (ventricular depolarization) because of slower conduction through the AV node. If conduction through the AV node is delayed long enough, the depolarization wave may "die out" and not reach the ventricles. This phenomenon shows up on the ECG as a P wave without a corresponding QRS complex and is referred to as *heart block,* or **atrioventricular (AV) block.** This might be detected on auscultation or pulse palpation as an intermittent "missed beat."

Because slowing of the heart rate and conduction speed results from parasympathetic stimulation, AV block and bradycardia can be reversed with atropine, which is a parasympathetic antagonist. As a general rule, when treating bradycardia or early heart block associated with use of β_1-blocking antiarrhythmics, it is better to decrease the beta-blocker dose than to use an additional drug to combat the heart block. In cases of beta-blocker overdose, atropine may be necessary to maintain cardiovascular function.

Animals that have been receiving a β_1 blocking drug for some time may appear to become tolerant of the beta blocker. The slower heart rate associated with the antiarrhythmic effect of the drug may begin to reverse itself. In this case the "resistance" is not necessarily caused by induction of liver enzymes but is more likely a result of **up-regulation** of the β-adrenergic receptors. With up-regulation, cardiac muscle (and other tissues containing β receptors) begins to produce more β receptors to counteract the blocking activity of the beta-blocking antiarrhythmics. These additional receptors make the tissues more sensitive to compounds such as epinephrine and norepinephrine that stimulate β receptors and less responsive to beta blocking. Without an additional increase in the β-blocker dose, this up-regulation, or proliferation of additional β receptors, increases the heart rate and risk of arrhythmias.

In animals that have up-regulated their β receptors in response to beta-blocker drugs, administration of the beta blocker must not be stopped suddenly. With all the additional receptors on the surface of cardiac cells induced by beta-blocker administration, the heart is very sensitive to β_1-stimulating drugs or endogenous compounds such as epinephrine. If β-blocker administration is suddenly stopped, even a normal release of epinephrine by the body may result in extreme tachycardia and possibly severe arrhythmias. Thus if a beta blocker has been used for a long time, it should be gradually discontinued to allow the body to "down-regulate" the additional receptors and the decreased sensitivity of the cardiac tissue to normalize.

Calcium Channel Blocker Antiarrhythmic Drugs

Calcium channel blockers include verapamil, nifedipine, and diltiazem. Although calcium channel blockers are not used very frequently to treat arrhythmias in veterinary patients, verapamil and diltiazem have been used successfully for treatment of supraventricular tachycardia, atrial fibrillation, and atrial flutter. All these drugs combat arrhythmias by blocking Ca^{++} channels of cardiac muscle cells, resulting in decreased conduction of depolarization waves and decreased automaticity of parts of the conduction system. Unfortunately, blocking the Ca^{++} channels can also decrease the

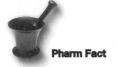

Pharm Fact

Patients receiving β_1 blockers for some time may develop tolerance to the drugs.

strength of contraction and cardiac output. Therefore calcium channel blockers should be used with caution or not at all in animals with congestive heart failure because of their negative inotropic effect.

A more common use of diltiazem is in cats with hypertrophic cardiomyopathy, in which the heart becomes very thickened and enlarged such that it cannot contract efficiently. Calcium channel blockers help decrease the size of the heart in some affected cats.

POSITIVE INOTROPIC AGENTS

Positive inotropic drugs (positive inotropes) increase the strength of contraction of a weakened heart. Most positive inotropic agents work by directly or indirectly making more Ca^{++} available to the contractile proteins in the muscle cell or by increasing the affinity between Ca^{++} and contractile proteins.

Catecholamines (norepinephrine, epinephrine, and dobutamine) are the body's natural positive inotropic agents and are released in response to sympathetic nervous system stimulation. **Adrenergic drugs** (sometimes called sympathomimetics) are usually synthesized catecholamines or other compounds with essentially the same chemical structure of endogenous catecholamines.

Adrenergic drugs and catecholamines produce a positive inotropic effect by stimulating β_1 receptors in the cardiac muscle. They improve contractility of a weakened heart for short periods only because repeated use reduces the number of catecholamine receptors on cell surfaces, decreasing the cells' ability to respond to stimuli. This phenomenon, called **down-regulation,** is the reason adrenergic drugs lose their ability to produce significant positive inotropic effects within hours to days after initiation of therapy.

Catecholamines are used for short-term treatment, whereas digoxin is the drug of choice for maintaining long-term positive inotropic effects. Digoxin exerts its positive inotropic effect primarily by making more Ca^{++} available for the contractile elements within cardiac muscle cells. It does this indirectly by inhibiting the cell's sodium-potassium-ATPase pump, which allows Na^+ to accumulate within the cardiac cell. This relatively small increase of Na^+ displaces Ca^{++} from its "holding area" in the cell, making more Ca^{++} available to contractile elements and resulting in an increased force of contraction. However, increased Na^+ inside the cardiac muscle cell also increases the risk of spontaneous depolarization and ectopic foci.

Digoxin improves myocardial cell contraction but has a very different effect on the SA and AV nodes. Digoxin enhances the parasympathetic effect on these nodes, slowing the heart rate (SA node effect) and delaying conduction of impulses from the atria to the ventricles through the AV node. Therefore digoxin is often used to control supraventricular tachycardia caused by atrial fibrillation. An animal can live with atrial fibrillation, but it cannot live with the ventricles beating so rapidly that they inefficiently pump blood. Because digoxin delays conduction through the AV node to the ventricles, the rate of ventricular contraction is slowed. Thus the tachycardia is controlled even though the atrial fibrillation is not eliminated.

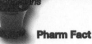

Some diuretics used in heart patients can predispose the patient to digoxin toxicity.

Digoxin has a small therapeutic index; that is, the dosages that achieve therapeutic concentrations are very close to the dosages that produce toxic concentrations. Early signs of digoxin toxicity include anorexia, vomiting, and diarrhea, reflecting the drug's stimulatory effects on the chemoreceptor trigger zone (see Chapter 4). Owners of animals receiving digoxin should be instructed to contact the veterinarian immediately if these early signs of toxicity occur.

As toxic concentrations of digoxin accumulate further, the heart rate slows (SA node effect) and the PR interval on the ECG lengthens (first-degree AV block). As toxicity increases, bradycardia (slow heart rate) becomes more pronounced and the PR interval lengthens until occasional atrial impulses fade out in the AV node (second-degree AV block), resulting in a P wave without a QRS complex.

If the toxicity progresses, theoretically the AV node could become completely blocked. This third-degree, or complete, AV block is characterized by the ventricles' beating independently of the atria. This type of block is usually associated with severe myocardial disease and not usually produced by the digoxin toxicity itself. Because digoxin's slowing of SA and AV node conduction is mostly through enhancement of the parasympathetic effect on these nodes, some of the AV block and SA bradycardia can be reversed with atropine, which blocks acetylcholine, the neurotransmitter primarily associated with parasympathetic effects on the body.

Because the cardiac cells are destabilized by increased intracellular Na^+, animals with digoxin toxicity also often show increased PVCs (evidence of ectopic foci) or bigeminy (see Chapter 8). Digoxin toxicity is made worse by **hypokalemia** (low blood potassium level) or hypomagnesemia (low blood magnesium level). Some of the diuretics commonly used in cardiac therapy also cause loss of K^+, and the resulting hypokalemia can predispose an animal to digoxin toxicity.

Digoxin has a long half-life, so once toxicity develops, signs may persist for hours or days until drug concentrations fall below the toxic range. Generally, if an animal receiving digoxin suddenly shows anorexia or vomiting, digoxin therapy should be stopped and the animal examined by a veterinarian. If an ECG suggests digoxin toxicity (that is, shows bradycardia, increased PR interval, or AV block), digoxin use should be halted for at least 24 hours. In uncomplicated cases of digoxin toxicity, digoxin can usually be resumed after skipping only one or two doses and resuming with a slightly smaller dose.

Digoxin is primarily excreted by the kidneys; therefore animals with impaired kidney function, such as older animals with chronic renal failure, will have decreased elimination of digoxin resulting in markedly elevated concentrations in the blood. Plasma concentrations of digoxin should be regularly monitored in animals with impaired renal function so that the dosage regimen can be adjusted to avoid toxicity but maintain effectiveness.

Cats tolerate digoxin less well and require much smaller doses than dogs. Some clinicians calculate digoxin doses by the animal's body surface area in square meters (mg/m^2) on the premise that small dogs and very large dogs tend to be overdosed and underdosed, respectively, if their dose is calculated by body weight (mg/kg).

Digoxin is available as elixir and tablets. As discussed in Chapter 3, elixirs are more rapidly and efficiently absorbed from the GI tract than tablets. The bioavailability of digoxin in tablets is only 60% versus about 75% for the elixir. If the dosage form is switched from tablets to elixir or vice versa, the dose must be adjusted to prevent overdosing or underdosing. The following equation can help approximate a new calculated dose:

$$\text{Dose in tablet form (mg)} \times 0.6 = \text{Dose in elixir form (mg)} \times 0.75$$

For example, a dog is being treated with 0.1 mg tablets. The equivalent dose of elixir is determined as follows:

$$0.1 \text{ mg in tablet} \times 0.6 = X \text{ mg of elixir} \times 0.75$$
$$0.06 \text{ mg} = X \text{ mg of elixir} \times 0.75$$
$$0.06/0.75 = X \text{ mg of elixir}$$
$$X = 0.08 \text{ mg of elixir}$$

Because more of each elixir dose is absorbed than each tablet dose, a smaller elixir dose is required (0.08 mg rather than 0.1 mg) to attain concentrations equivalent to those attained with tablets.

VASODILATORS

Vasoconstriction of peripheral blood vessels is a normal physiologic response to the drop in blood pressure caused by congestive heart failure, hemorrhage, dehydration, and any other condition that decreases blood volume or the amount of blood pumped by the heart. This protective mechanism increases arterial blood pressure but also the heart's workload by increasing the resistance to blood flow through the vessels. Vasodilator drugs are used to relieve some of the workload by opening the constricted sphincters, decreasing resistance to flow, and making it easier for the heart to pump blood through these vessels.

Vasoconstriction in Heart Disease

Vasoconstriction associated with congestive heart failure is caused by several different mechanisms; therefore different types of vasodilators must be used to counteract it. When blood pressure begins to fall, the body attempts to compensate with sympathetic stimulation, which causes the heart rate to increase (β_1 receptors) and the precapillary arterioles to constrict (α_1 receptors) (Fig. 5-6).

Another effect of increased sympathetic tone is vasoconstriction of the renal artery, which decreases renal perfusion and consequently reduces formation of urine and water loss. Although vasoconstriction of the renal artery does not directly increase blood pressure, it further reduces the loss of blood volume and initiates a secondary vasoconstriction and fluid conservation mechanism called the **renin-angiotensin system** (Fig. 5-7).

back) through the mitral valve and back into the left atrium. Hydralazine causes arteriolar vasodilation, which decreases arterial blood pressure and reduces resistance to blood flow from the ventricle into the aorta. This allows more blood to flow into the aorta and less to flow back into the left atrium. Although the valve itself remains poorly functional, at least some of the normal direction of blood flow through the left heart is restored.

Theoretically, an arterial vasodilator such as hydralazine should increase blood flow through pulmonary arteries clogged with canine heartworms. However, hydralazine is not very effective in such animals because the drug works "downstream" from where most adult heartworms are causing occlusion and the arteriolar vessels in the pulmonary tree are often sufficiently damaged or altered (by the heartworms) such that they do not dilate in response to the drug.

Hydralazine's arteriolar vasodilative effect often reduces blood pressure below normal; therefore sympathetic tone increases, resulting in vasoconstriction of the kidney's afferent arterioles (which carry blood into the glomeruli) and reducing perfusion of the kidneys. Decreased urine formation stimulates the renin-angiotensin system, which causes Na^+ and water retention. Therefore hydralazine is often used with a diuretic to prevent an increased blood volume in these cases.

Nitroglycerin

Unlike hydralazine, which causes dilation of the small arterioles, nitroglycerin relaxes the blood vessels on the venous side of the circulation. In addition to venodilation (dilation of veins), nitroglycerin may also help dilate coronary arterioles by relaxing the vascular smooth muscles. The drug is well absorbed through the skin and mucous membranes. People with angina pectoris (chest pain) take nitroglycerin by putting a tablet under the tongue. In animals, nitroglycerin cream and nitroglycerin in patch form are applied to the skin to improve cardiac output and reduce pulmonary edema and ascites (abdominal fluid accumulation).

Nitroglycerin cream is applied every 8 to 12 hours to the hairless inner aspect of the pinna, thorax, or groin; the last area is used less frequently because the animal can easily lick it. The nitroglycerin patch provides drug for 24 hours and can be cut into smaller pieces to adjust the dose for smaller patients.

The site of nitroglycerin application should be changed with each dose. Clients should be instructed to always wear gloves when applying this drug because it can be absorbed through their skin as well as the animal's. Children and others should be instructed not to pet the animal where the cream or patch has been applied. As clarification of one point of curiosity, although this compound is the same chemical that is used in explosives, danger of explosion does not exist because the drug has been diluted with several other compounds (mainly dextrose, lactose, and propylene glycol).

Angiotensin-Converting Enzyme Inhibitors

Enalapril (veterinary product, Enacard) and captopril are vasodilators that exert their effects on arterial and venous vessels by blocking the angiotensin-converting enzyme and preventing formation of angiotensin II (a potent vasoconstrictor) and aldosterone. For this reason such drugs as captopril are sometimes referred to as *angiotensin-converting enzyme (ACE) inhibitors*. Many veterinary cardiologists believe that stimulation of the renin-angiotensin system has profound effects (beyond the vasoconstrictive effect) on cardiac disease. Therefore many cardiovascular therapeutic regimens now routinely include ACE inhibitors.

In normal animals the renin-angiotensin system has not been activated and angiotensin II vasoconstriction is not present. Therefore enalapril and captopril do not have much vasodilatory effect on the vasculature in normal animals because there is no ACE to inhibit. Hyperkalemia (high concentrations of K^+ in the blood) may occur if ACE inhibitors are used simultaneously with potassium-sparing diuretics or K^+ supplements. The hyperkalemia results from the ACE inhibitors blocking aldosterone production. Aldosterone normally causes Na^+ and water reabsorption at the expense of K^+ excretion; therefore if aldosterone production is blocked by ACE inhibitors, normal K^+ excretion is decreased. Because aldosterone normally enhances Na^+ reabsorption from the urine and ACE inhibitors would block Na^+ reabsorption, ACE inhibitors should be used with caution in animals that are hyponatremic (that is, animals that have low Na^+ concentrations in the blood).

Enalapril and captopril are "balanced" vasodilators that relax the smooth muscles of arterioles and veins, so they are useful in treating animals with cardiac disease that involves the right and left ventricles such as severe cardiac valvular disease and cardiomyopathy. As with other vasodilators the initial doses of captopril should be small and progressively increased to the most effective dose.

Prazosin

Prazosin is an α_1-receptor blocker that causes vasodilation on the arterial and venous sides of the cardiovascular system. Unlike hydralazine, prazosin does not usually cause reflex tachycardia or significantly reduce renal perfusion, thus preventing activation of the renin-angiotensin system to the degree of other vasodilator drugs. Prazosin may be indicated in animals with congestive heart failure, especially when failure is associated with poor mitral valve or aortic valve function, or in animals that are not responsive to other vasodilator medications.

Prazosin is difficult to obtain in dosage forms small enough for use in cats and small dogs and therefore is not used very often in these animals. Many veterinary cardiologists do not recommend use of prazosin because of greater success with other vasodilators, the difficulty in administering prazosin to smaller animals, and reports that people receiving prazosin do not live any longer than untreated patients.

DIURETICS

Diuretics increase urine formation and promote water loss **(diuresis).** In animals with congestive heart failure, Na^+ retention from aldosterone se-

Pharm Fact

Diuretics prevent resorption or enhance excretion of Na^+ and K^+ from the renal tubules, thereby promoting water loss.

cretion and concomitant retention of water in the blood and body tissue lead to pulmonary edema, ascites, and an increased cardiac workload. Removal of water from the body with diuretics reduces these deleterious conditions.

All diuretics act by the same basic mechanism. Diuretics prevent reabsorption of Na^+ or K^+ in the renal tubules or enhance their secretion into the tubules, thus creating an osmotic force that draws water into or retains water in the renal tubules and removes water from the body as urine. In animals with hypovolemia (low blood volume) or hypotension, diuretics should be used cautiously because they further decrease the fluid component of blood and reduce blood pressure.

Loop Diuretics

Loop diuretics such as furosemide (Lasix) are the most commonly used diuretics in veterinary medicine. The term *loop diuretic* refers to the way these drugs produce diuresis by inhibiting Na^+ reabsorption from the loop of Henle (Fig. 5-8). Retention of Na^+ in the forming urine osmotically retains water in the urine and prevents its reabsorption. In the distal convoluted tubule, K^+ is exchanged for Na^+ so that Na^+ is still reabsorbed and conserved by the body to some degree. The number of solutes (ions) in the urine remains the same and exerts the same degree of osmotic pressure to draw in or retain water. Because loop diuretics cause K^+ to be excreted in the urine, prolonged use of loop diuretics may result in hypokalemia.

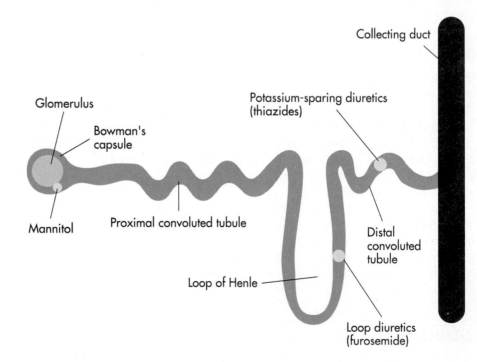

Fig. 5-8 Sites of diuretic drug activity in the nephron.

As previously mentioned, hypokalemia can increase the risk of digoxin toxicity.

Loop diuretics can be of some use in animals in the early stages of renal failure because they increase PgE_2, a naturally occurring vasodilator that increases renal blood flow. In the later stages of renal failure, loop diuretics are less effective because they are largely unable to reach their sites of action. Loop diuretics normally reach their sites of action by being secreted from the proximal convoluted tubule into the renal tubule lumen, where they pass with the urine to the loop of Henle. In the advanced stages of renal failure the proximal convoluted tubule cannot actively transport furosemide from the blood into the renal tubule.

Furosemide and other loop diuretics have been implicated in ototoxicity (toxicity associated with hearing or the inner ear). It is thought that ion imbalances, especially with use of large doses of furosemide in cats, change the electrolyte balance in the inner ear, resulting in loss of hearing. Hearing apparently returns after diuretic use is discontinued.

Thiazide Diuretics

Thiazide diuretics such as chlorothiazide are often not used in veterinary medicine because of the safety and effectiveness of furosemide. After administration, thiazides are secreted by the proximal convoluted tubule and pass to the initial segment of the distal convoluted tubule, where they decrease resorption of Na^+ and Cl^- (see Fig. 5-8). Because the Na^+ remaining in the tubule is exchanged for K^+ more distally in the nephron, thiazide diuretics can cause loss of K^+ with resultant hypokalemia.

Thiazides are less potent than loop diuretics because of the site of action in the distal convoluted tubule. Much of the excess Na^+ in the urine is normally resorbed in the loop of Henle (prior to the distal tubule), and the urine contains significantly less Na^+ when it reaches the distal tubule. Blocking reabsorption of Na^+ at that point only slightly increases the osmotic force within the urine compared to normal. With chronic use of thiazides, the body seems to adjust to the thiazide-induced Na^+ loss, resulting in a further reduction of the diuretic effect.

Potassium-Sparing Diuretics

Spironolactone is a diuretic that is a competitive antagonist of aldosterone, the hormone normally causing Na^+ reabsorption from the distal renal tubules and collection ducts (see Fig. 5-8). When aldosterone is inhibited, more Na^+ remains in the lumen of the renal tubules, osmotically retaining water and preventing its reabsorption. Because Na^+ is excreted and K^+ is conserved in the body, drugs like spironolactone are called *potassium-sparing diuretics*. These drugs depend on the presence of aldosterone and its Na^+ retention effect to promote diuresis. As described previously, aldosterone plays an important role in congestive heart failure by increasing blood volume and blood pressure. Therefore spironolactone can be useful for animals with excessive fluid retention associated with congestive heart failure.

Osmotic Diuretics

Mannitol is a carbohydrate (sugar) used as an osmotic diuretic. Unlike the other diuretics that work by inhibiting renal tubular resorption of Na^+ or K^+, mannitol retains water in the renal tubules by its physical presence within the lumen of the renal tubule. This sugar is freely filtered into the Bowman's capsule and poorly reabsorbed from the renal tubule, thus providing a solute that osmotically retains water in the renal tubular lumen. Mannitol is not used in treatment of cardiovascular disease but is used to reduce cerebral edema associated with head trauma and as a diuretic for flushing absorbed toxins from the body.

Carbonic Anhydrase Inhibitors

Carbonic anhydrase inhibitors such as acetazolamide are not often used as diuretics in veterinary medicine but may be used to decrease production of aqueous humor in the eye, which reduces intraocular pressure in animals with glaucoma. Because of its relatively weak diuretic effect and the ready availability of more effective diuretics, acetazolamide is not used to treat cardiac problems in veterinary patients. Veterinary ophthalmology texts contain information on use of this diuretic in treatment of glaucoma.

OTHER DRUGS USED IN TREATING CARDIOVASCULAR DISEASE

Aspirin

Aspirin (acetylsalicylic acid) inhibits formation of prostaglandins and thromboxanes. In so doing, it reduces aggregation (clumping) of platelets among other actions. This reduces the chances of clot formation and subsequent occlusion of blood vessels. Use of aspirin has been advocated for treatment of dogs with heartworm infection to reduce clot formation and retard proliferation of pulmonary arterial endothelium (see Chapter 11). In cats, aspirin can reduce thrombus formation associated with hypertrophic or congestive cardiomyopathy. However, aspirin must be used cautiously in cats because they do not metabolize the drug as readily as other species; therefore aspirin is usually given every other day. Daily use of aspirin in people is advocated to decrease the risk of stroke or myocardial infarction by reducing the chance for clot formation in the coronary arteries or vessels in the brain.

Bronchodilators

Aminophylline and theophylline dilate constricted bronchiole airways (see Chapter 6). These drugs may be used to increase perfusion of the lungs and decrease the workload on the right ventricle, which pumps the blood through the lungs. When increased oxygen reaches the alveoli, the vasculature associated with those alveoli dilates, allowing blood to flow more easily through that portion of the lung. This decreases the resistance against which the right ventricle must pump and thereby improves cardiac output.

Sedatives and Tranquilizers

Sedatives and tranquilizers are sometimes used to calm an anxious animal experiencing aerophagia ("air hunger") because of pulmonary edema associated with advanced congestive heart failure. The combination of tachycardia from increased sympathetic tone caused by fear and anxiety and insufficient oxygenation of the stimulated heart can result in death from arrhythmia. Sometimes merely calming the animal reduces the heart rate and allows the weakened heart to pump sufficient blood to meet the physiologic needs, thereby reducing the risk of fatal arrhythmias.

Cardiovascular Drug Categories and Names*

Antiarrhythmics

Sodium influx inhibitors
  Lidocaine
  Quinidine
  Procainamide
  Tocainide
β-Blockers
  Propranolol (Inderal)
  Atenolol
  Other "-olol" drugs (Timolol, Nadolol)
Calcium channel blockers
  Diltiazem
  Verapamil
  Nifedipine

Positive inotropes

Catecholamines
  Dobutamine
Digoxin

Vasodilators

ACE inhibitors
  Enalapril (Enacard)
  Captopril

Hydralazine
Nitroglycerin
Prazosin

Diuretics

Loop diuretics
  Furosemide (Lasix)
Thiazide diuretics
  Chlorothiazide
Potassium-sparing diuretics
  Spironolactone
Osmotic diuretics
  Mannitol

Other drugs

Aspirin
Aminophylline, theophylline
Sedatives, tranquilizers

*Brand names are in parentheses.

Recommended Reading

Bjorling DE, Keene BW: *The dyspneic cat,* Proceedings of the Waltham Feline Medicine Symposium, 1996.

Collatos C: Treating atrial fibrillation in horses, *Compend Cont Educ* (17)2: 243, Feb 1995.

Ettinger SJ: *Congestive heart failure treatment modalities: recent studies utilizing enalapril maleate,* Proceedings of the 18th Annual Waltham/Ohio State University Symposium for Treatment of Small Animal Diseases, Columbus, Ohio, Oct 1994.

Fox PR: *Feline thromboembolism,* Proceedings of the North American Veterinary Conference, Orlando, Fla, Jan 1996.

Henik RA: *Mixing and matching cardiopulmonary drugs,* Proceedings of the North American Veterinary Conference, Orlando, Fla, Jan 1996.

Keene BW: *Common problems in arrhythmia management,* Proceedings of the North American Veterinary Conference, Orlando, Fla, Jan 1996.

Keene BW: *Drug therapy of cardiac disease,* Proceedings of the North American Veterinary Conference, Orlando, Fla, Jan 1996.

Keene BW, Bonagura JD: Therapy of heart failure. In Bonagura JD, editor: *Kirk's current veterinary therapy XII,* Philadelphia, 1995, WB Saunders.

Kittleson MD: *The pathophysiology and treatment of mitral regurgitation in the dog,* Proceedings of the 18th Annual Waltham/Ohio State University Symposium for Treatment of Small Animal Diseases, Columbus, Ohio, Oct 1994.

Paddleford RR, Harvey RC: Anesthesia in cardiovascular dysfunction. In Thurman JC, Tranquilli WJ, Benson GJ, editors: *Lumb and Jones' veterinary anesthesia,* ed 3, Baltimore, 1996, Williams & Wilkins.

Reimer JM: Cardiac arrhythmias. In Robinson NE, editor: *Current veterinary therapy in equine medicine* 3, Philadelphia, 1992, WB Saunders.

Roth AL: Use of angiotensin-converting enzyme inhibitors in dogs with congestive heart failure, *Compend Cont Educ* (15)9:1240, Sept 1993.

Schlesinger DP, Rubin SI: Potential adverse effects of angiotensin-converting enzyme inhibitors in the treatment of congestive heart failure, *Compend Cont Educ* (16)3:275, Mar 1994.

Stepien RL: *Therapy of common cardiac arrhythmias,* Proceedings of the 18th Annual Waltham/Ohio State University Symposium for Treatment of Small Animal Diseases, Columbus, Ohio, Oct 1994.

Ware W: *Congestive heart failure: pathophysiology and therapeutic implications,* Proceedings of the 18th Annual Waltham/Ohio State University Symposium for Treatment of Small Animal Diseases, Columbus, Ohio, Oct 1994.

Review Questions

1. Describe the path of a red blood cell from its entrance to the heart via the vena cava through its exit via the aorta. Include the valves through which the cell passes.

2. Is the left or right ventricle larger? What is the reason for this difference in size?

3. On which side of the heart is the mitral valve?

4. What structure sets the pace for the heart's contraction rate? What effects do the sympathetic and parasympathetic nervous systems have on this structure?

5. Describe the path of a wave of depolarization from the SA node to the ventricles.

6. What wave form on the ECG represents depolarization of the atria? Of the ventricles? Of the AV node?

7. Describe ionic movement into and out of cardiac muscle cells during depolarization and repolarization.

8. The doctor comments that cats rarely develop atrial fibrillation because they have a small heart and the cardiac muscle cells are still in the refractory period when the impulse completes its circuit around the heart, thus preventing the wave of depolarization from setting off another wave of depolarization. What is meant by the term *refractory period?*

9. Explain the reason that the SA node inherently beats at a quicker rate than the AV node, which inherently beats faster than the cells in the bundle branches.

10. Describe the effect of each type of drug: β_1 agonist, β_2 antagonist, α_1 agonist, and parasympathetic agonist.
11. What effect would each of the drugs in the previous question have on an animal's blood pressure?
12. Classify the following arrhythmias according to heart rate (tachycardia or bradycardia) and the location of the problem (supraventricular or ventricular):
    a. Arrhythmia in a dog with ventricular contraction rate of 200/min caused by atrial fibrillation
    b. Arrhythmia in a dog with a ventricular contraction rate of 40/min caused by inability of the SA node to depolarize normally
    c. Arrhythmia in a dog with a series of PVCs that increases the heart rate to 150 beats/min for about 30 seconds
13. What is normally the drug of choice for emergency treatment of ventricular arrhythmias? By what route is it given? Can it be used in cats?
14. Ventricular arrhythmia in a dog has been controlled by emergency treatment with lidocaine; however, the doctor is concerned about recurrence of the problem after the dog is discharged. What oral drug should be dispensed to prevent recurrence of ventricular arrhythmias after the dog is discharged?
15. What is the difference between lidocaine (Xylocaine) used as an injectable local anesthetic and lidocaine used to treat arrhythmias?
16. A dog's medical chart indicates that the animal has been receiving digoxin to help increase contractility of the heart. The new associate veterinarian, a recent graduate, considers adding quinidine to the regimen to control the occasional PVCs seen on the ECG strip. What effect is quinidine likely to have in this dog?
17. The doctor asks you to dispense some sustained-release procainamide tablets for a client's dog. You calculate the required dose and determine that the dog needs 1½ of the sustained-release tablets per dose. The doctor tells you to label the vial and instruct the client to give only 1 tablet per dose rather than the 1½ tablets per dose that you calculated. Why did the doctor elect to reduce the dose rather than instruct the client to give 1½ tablets per dose?
18. β-Blockers are good antiarrhythmics when the cause is associated with high sympathetic tone as in animals with a weakened heart. Why, however, do β-blockers pose a risk in these animals?
19. The doctor comments that most antiarrhythmics are negative inotropes. What is the significance of this comment?
20. Explain the reason propranolol, an antiarrhythmic drug, may cause dyspnea (difficult breathing) in animals with respiratory disease.
21. Animals often develop resistance to β-blocking antiarrhythmics. How does such resistance to β-blockers develop?
22. Atropine is sometimes used to reverse bradycardia caused by a β-blocker. Why is atropine more effective in increasing the heart rate after a β-blocker overdose than epinephrine, which normally increases the heart rate?
23. In animals treated for long periods with drugs such as atenolol, why must drug administration be gradually tapered off rather than immediately halted?

24. Calcium channel blockers are used only occasionally as an antiarrhythmic in animals, but diltiazem is often used in cats. For what condition is diltiazem used in cats?

25. Catecholamines such as epinephrine stimulate the heart and seem to be ideal positive inotropes. Why are catecholamines not used more often to increase contractility of a weakened heart?

26. What is the drug of choice for increasing heart contractility in dogs and cats?

27. The doctor mentions that digoxin must be used carefully because there is "little room for error." What is the significance of this comment?

28. Why would digoxin, a positive inotrope, be used in a dog with atrial fibrillation if the problem in atrial fibrillation is the supraventricular tachycardia, not a weakened heart?

29. What early signs of digoxin toxicosis should pet owners be instructed to watch for?

30. How is digoxin toxicosis manifested on an ECG tracing?

31. Digoxin overdose can cause bradycardia and AV block. What drug is likely to be effective in reducing these effects of digoxin toxicity?

32. Furosemide (Lasix) and digoxin are often used together in patients with cardiovascular disease. What interaction should you watch for when using these two drugs simultaneously?

33. Why are animals with renal failure more predisposed to digoxin toxicosis than animals with normal renal function?

34. An animal is being treated with 0.2-mg tablets of digoxin and you want to switch the dosage form to digoxin elixir. What would be the equivalent elixir dose? What would be the equivalent tablet dose if you wanted to switch from 0.5 mg of elixir to a tablet form?

35. What effect does a slightly high dose of vasodilator have on capillary refill time?

36. Explain how the renin-angiotensin system causes vasoconstriction and water retention.

37. Which type of vessel is affected by hydralazine, nitroglycerin, and enalapril? How does each drug cause vasodilation? What is a clinical indication for each drug?

38. Because hydralazine is an arterial vasodilator, in theory it should benefit dogs with narrowed pulmonary arteries as a result of heartworm disease. Is hydralazine useful in such cases?

39. What are the signs of vasodilator overdose that pet owners should be warned about?

40. The doctor asks you to apply a nitroglycerin patch to the skin of a small dog to combat pulmonary edema related to heart disease. The patch, however, will deliver twice the recommended dose of nitroglycerin. How can you administer the appropriate dose of nitroglycerin to this dog?

41. What precautions should owners take to protect themselves when treating their animal with topical nitroglycerin products?

42. Why does enalapril cause vasodilation in animals with heart failure but have little effect in normal animals?

43. Why should plasma electrolyte (sodium, potassium, chloride, and so on) levels be monitored in animals being treated with enalapril? What electrolyte imbalance is most likely to cause problems during enalapril therapy?

44. Which diuretic seems to be most effective in veterinary patients? What is this drug's mechanism of action? How does this drug affect the body's electrolyte balance?

45. What cardiac drug is more likely to produce toxicosis if used simultaneously with large doses of furosemide or normal doses of furosemide for long periods? Why?

46. Explain the way the diuretics chlorothiazide and spironolactone differ in their mechanism of action and their effect on electrolyte balance.

47. Explain the differences between mannitol's mechanism of action and that of other diuretics such as furosemide, chlorothiazide, and spironolactone.

48. You overhear the doctor telling the owner of a cat with cardiomyopathy to administer aspirin. However, you remember that aspirin must be used with caution in cats. Is the doctor wrong to recommend aspirin for this cat?

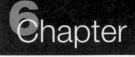

Drugs Affecting the Respiratory System

Key Terms

antihistamine
antimicrobials
antitussive drugs
β_1 receptor
β_2 receptor
bronchoconstriction
bronchodilation
centrally acting
   antitussive
cilia
cough center
cough suppressant
decongestant
diuretics
dyspnea
expectorant
hepatotoxic
histamine
hypoxic
inspissated
locally acting antitussive
mucociliary apparatus
mucolytic agent
nebulization
nonproductive cough
productive cough
prophylactic
synergistic
tachypnea
toxic synergism
volatile oils

Antitussives
   Butorphanol
   Hydrocodone
   Codeine
   Dextromethorphan
Mucolytics, Expectorants, and
   Decongestants
   Mucolytics
   Expectorants
   Decongestants
   Precautions in Using OTC Products

Bronchodilators
   β-Adrenergic Agonists
   Methylxanthines
Other Drugs Used to Treat Respiratory
   Problems
   Corticosteroids
   Antihistamines
   Antimicrobials
   Diuretics
   Oxygen

Learning Objectives

*After studying this chapter,
the veterinary technician should know the following:*

The ways antitussives work

The effects of mucolytics, expectorants, and decongestants

The types of bronchodilators and the ways they are used

The indications for use of corticosteroids, antihistamines, antimicrobials, diuretics,
   and oxygen in respiratory disease

The body has effective mechanisms for protecting the respiratory tract from injury or infection. These mechanisms include sneezing, coughing, increased mucus production in the nose and respiratory tree, and constriction of the bronchioles. In addition, the **mucociliary apparatus** facilitates removal of infective materials. The mucociliary apparatus consists of mucus and ciliated cells that line the respiratory tract. Unfortunately, under certain conditions these protective mechanisms may adversely affect the health of an animal. For example, a nonproductive cough that continues for months may lead to debilitation, pathologic changes in the airways, and ultimately, heart problems (a condition called *cor pulmonale*). Another example is extreme bronchoconstriction, which protects the alveoli from foreign substances but also prevents exchange of oxygen and carbon dioxide.

Normally these protective mechanisms benefit the animal and prevent respiratory damage or infection; inhibition of these mechanisms by drugs used to treat respiratory disease may counteract the animal's natural defenses. Therefore the veterinarian must weigh the potential benefit of the drug's effect against the potential for impairment of natural protective mechanisms when treating respiratory disease. (A box listing GI drugs can be found at the end of this chapter.)

Drugs Affecting the Respiratory System

Pharm Fact

The mucociliary apparatus traps dust and other respiratory debris and moves it out of the respiratory tract.

ANTITUSSIVES

Antitussive drugs block the cough reflex. The cough reflex is coordinated by a **"cough center",** which is a cluster of neurons located next to the respiratory centers in the medullary area of the brainstem. Cough or irritant receptor stimulation in the respiratory tree sends impulses to the brainstem, where the cough reflex causes contraction of the appropriate respiratory muscles to produce a sharp, forceful expiration (cough). Cough receptors are located throughout the respiratory tract from the pharynx to the smaller air passages in the lung.

The type of cough is determined by the location of the cough receptors that are stimulated. When stimulated by irritation or pressure from food or other materials, receptors in the larynx or pharynx send impulses to the brain via the vagus nerve, resulting in gagging, violent coughing, and constriction of the small terminal bronchioles. This is the type of choking cough observed when food is inhaled into the larynx or anything irritates the pharynx.

Receptors in the lower trachea and bronchi respond to mechanical and chemical irritation or release of histamine by producing a deep cough mediated by the cough center, **tachypnea** (rapid breathing), and reflex bronchoconstriction. This type of cough is associated with bronchitis, inhalation of irritating gases, allergic bronchoconstriction, or pressure of the bronchi from an enlarged heart. Because the characteristics of a cough vary with the location of the cough receptors, the type of cough can help determine the location of the problem in the respiratory tree.

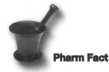

Pharm Fact

Cough suppressants may worsen the animal's condition in chronic respiratory disease.

The terms *productive cough* and *nonproductive cough* are often used to describe the clinical condition status of a cough. A **productive cough** refers to a cough that produces mucus and other inflammatory products. A **nonproductive cough** is dry and hacking with no mucus. A nonproductive cough may occur in the early stages of infection or inflammation, when the mucous glands lining the respiratory tree have not yet increased production of mucus. A nonproductive cough may also be associated with chronic conditions such as chronic bronchitis, in which the mucus produced becomes **inspissated** (dry and sticky) and accumulates in the bronchi, or the mucous glands become unable to produce mucus.

Antitussives suppress the coughing that normally removes mucus, cellular debris, exudates, and other products accumulating within the bronchi as a result of infection or inflammation. Therefore veterinarians should use antitussives cautiously and avoid large doses in animals with a very productive cough. In such situations, suppression of coughing with **cough suppressants** (antitussives) can result in accumulation of excessive mucus and debris. Cough suppressants should not be used routinely in animals with chronic bronchitis because coughing prevents obstruction of the small airways by sticky mucus.

Sometimes the terms *centrally acting* and *locally acting* are used to describe antitussive drug mechanisms. A **centrally acting antitussive** such as a narcotic reduces coughing by suppressing the cough center in the medulla. A **locally acting antitussive** such as a cough lozenge reduces coughing by soothing the mucosal irritation that is initiating the cough. Centrally acting antitussives are the only type used in veterinary medicine because veterinary patients are unwilling to hold lozenges in their mouth long enough to be effective.

Antitussives should be used in animals with a dry, nonproductive cough that produces little or no inspissated mucus. Often these coughs keep the pet and the owner from properly resting. Antitussives are commonly used to treat uncomplicated tracheobronchitis (kennel cough) in dogs. This retching cough is often punctuated by gagging of small amounts of mucus that the owner interprets as vomitus. This type of cough is extremely irritating to the upper airway mucosa. Such irritation stimulates more coughing, which further irritates the airway. This pattern can continue for weeks if the cough is left untreated. Cases of untreated tracheobronchitis can result in tracheal collapse, chronic bronchitis, secondary bacterial bronchitis or pneumonia, and even cardiac problems.

Butorphanol

Butorphanol, marketed as the veterinary product Torbutrol, is a centrally acting opioid cough suppressant that is not classified as a controlled substance in most states, unlike most other opioid cough suppressants. In antitussive doses, butorphanol causes little sedation as compared with stronger opioid drugs.

Hydrocodone

Hydrocodone (Hycodan) is a C-III narcotic available only by prescription from a veterinarian with a Drug Enforcement Administration (DEA) clearance for writing C-III prescriptions. Sedation is often noted in animals treated with hydrocodone. Long-term administration of this drug can result in constipation because opioids slow GI motility (see Chapter 4). All potent narcotics should be used with caution in animals with abdominal pain because their analgesic (pain-relieving) effect can mask pain, preventing observation of progression of clinical signs. Overdose of hydrocodone can cause severe respiratory and cardiovascular depression.

As with other controlled substances, hydrocodone has the potential for human abuse because of the psychologically and physiologically addictive qualities of opioids. Veterinary technicians should take notice of clients' repeated requests for strong opioid compounds to relieve their pet's cough. The technician should document these requests and inform the veterinarian.

Codeine

Codeine, a relatively weak opioid and narcotic, is a component of many cough suppressant preparations. Most products containing codeine are prescription preparations with a C-V controlled substance rating. The sedative effect of codeine is similar to that of hydrocodone. Although codeine has a low potential for abuse, continued use can become habit forming.

Dextromethorphan

Dextromethorphan is a common ingredient in OTC nonprescription cough, flu, and cold preparations. Although its actions are similar to those of the more potent narcotic antitussives, it is not a controlled substance. Dextromethorphan has a different chemical structure than the narcotics and does not cause addiction or have potential for abuse, hence its approval for OTC use.

Dextromethorphan is generally not as effective in controlling coughs in veterinary patients as butorphanol or other prescription antitussives; however, owners often initially use human cold products containing dextromethorphan to curtail coughing in their pets. Although dextromethorphan in OTC products is fairly harmless to animals, the other compounds in cold or flu preparations can cause significant harm. For example, acetaminophen can be very toxic in cats. Therefore the veterinary professional should not recommend use of OTC products to control coughing in pets.

MUCOLYTICS, EXPECTORANTS, AND DECONGESTANTS

In addition to coughing, the mucociliary apparatus helps remove materials from the respiratory tree (Fig. 6-1). Lining the respiratory tree are glands and mucous cells that secrete the blanket of bronchial mucus that traps in-

Lumen

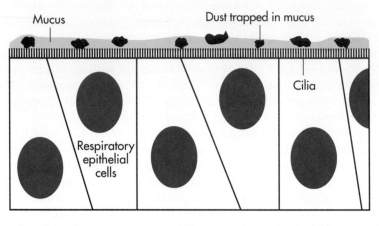

Fig. 6-1 The mucociliary apparatus traps dust particles and other debris in a blanket of mucus.

haled particulate matter. The epithelial cells lining the respiratory tree from the bronchioles to the laryngeal area have **cilia** (hairlike projections) on their exterior, or airway, surface. These hairlike appendages sweep mucus and particulate matter up to the oropharynx, where it is coughed up and swallowed or expectorated (spit out).

Mucolytics

Mucolytic agents are designed to break up, or lyse, mucus and reduce its viscosity so the cilia can move it out of the respiratory tract. With infection or inflammation, the inflammatory cells move into the affected area to combat the infectious agent or to help contain cellular damage. The DNA found in inflammatory cells or cellular debris reacts with mucus to increase its viscosity (make it more sticky). When this happens, the cilia cannot readily move the viscous mucus and the mucociliary apparatus becomes less effective. Acetylcysteine (Mucomyst) is a mucolytic agent that decreases the viscosity of mucus by breaking apart the DNA strands.

Acetylcysteine may be administered by **nebulization,** which is the inhalation of a fine mist containing the drug, or by mouth. If it is given by mouth, the unpleasant taste must be masked with flavoring agents or the drug must be administered by feeding tube). Although nebulization provides the potential to deliver drug to the surface of the bronchi and bronchioles, it is not very effective for veterinary patients because the animals resist deeply inhaling the mist. Because acetylcysteine is also irritating to the respiratory tree, it requires use of a bronchodilator before nebulization treatment to prevent reflex bronchoconstriction.

Acetylcysteine is also used as the intravenous antidote for acetaminophen (Tylenol) toxicity in cats. Acetylcysteine helps metabolize the **hepatotoxic** acetaminophen metabolite and reduces conversion of hemoglobin to nonfunctional methemoglobin.

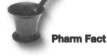

Pharm Fact

Expectorant and mucolytic drugs liquefy and expel respiratory secretions.

Owners sometimes treat a coughing pet by placing the animal in a steamy bathroom. Although this practice increases the fluidity of secretions in the upper respiratory tract, it does not increase the fluidity of the mucus in the lower airways because the comparatively large steam droplets are not inhaled deep enough to penetrate the lower airways. When oxygen is administered to animals with respiratory problems or other disease, the very dry nature of the gas can dehydrate the mucociliary apparatus and decrease its efficiency. Therefore moisture should be added to the oxygen, usually by bubbling oxygen through a container of water.

Expectorants

Expectorants also increase the fluidity of mucus in the respiratory tract and thereby improve the effectiveness of the mucociliary apparatus. As opposed to mucolytics, which reduce the viscosity of mucus by chemically altering it, expectorants increase the fluidity of mucus by generating liquid secretions by respiratory tract cells. Although expectorants are commonly included in human OTC cold preparations, they are of questionable benefit in veterinary patients. A more effective expectorant-like effect can be achieved by maintaining proper systemic hydration and increasing the humidity of inspired air. The benefits of expectorants must be weighed against the increased volume of fluid that would have to be removed from the respiratory tree by the mucociliary apparatus.

Guaifenesin (glycerol guaiacolate) and saline expectorants such as ammonium chloride, potassium iodide, and sodium citrate are given by mouth and increase watery secretions in the respiratory tree through stimulation of the parasympathetic nervous system. Guaifenesin is also given intravenously for muscle relaxation in equine anesthesia, but the expectorant action of guaifenesin is not related to the muscle relaxation mechanisms. In contrast to expectorants that act on gastric receptors, the **volatile oils** such as terpin hydrate, eucalyptus oil, and pine oil directly stimulate respiratory secretions when their vapors are inhaled.

Decongestants

Many OTC human cold preparations that contain expectorants also contain **decongestants** such as phenylephrine and phenylpropanolamine for relief of nasal congestion. Decongestants reduce congestion (vascular engorgement) by stimulating the sympathetic nervous system α_1 receptors on smooth muscle of blood vessels in the skin and mucous membranes. When stimulated, α_1 receptors cause vasoconstriction in the congested (swollen) mucous membranes of the nasal passages, reducing tissue edema and secretions by mucous glands.

Precautions in Using OTC Products

In addition to their decongesting effects, decongestants also stimulate the sympathetic nervous system's β_1 receptors, thereby increasing the heart rate. If an animal is **hypoxic** (that is, has low tissue oxygen tension) or has compromised respiratory function because of lung congestion and is treated with a decongestant, the animal's heart is forced to work harder without sufficient oxygen to supply the increased demand on the heart muscle. The result can be severe or even fatal arrhythmias. This is not usually a problem when OTC products are given to otherwise healthy animals, but it can cause complications in patients with impaired respiratory function.

In severely dehydrated animals the mucous membranes become dry and the overlying mucus becomes very sticky, impairing the action of the mucociliary apparatus. Therefore dehydrated animals often exhibit a nonproductive cough, which suggests that use of expectorants or mucolytic agents might improve mucociliary clearance. However, once the animal is properly rehydrated, the mucus regains its normal fluid consistency and the cough may become very productive. Thus the veterinary professional should correct for systemic dehydration before deciding whether or not an expectorant or mucolytic agent should be given.

A strong antitussive should not be used with an expectorant because the expectorant's action will increase the fluid in the respiratory tree that needs to be removed by coughing. Although cough suppressants such as dextromethorphan are commonly used with expectorants in OTC medications, the degree of cough suppression produced is not sufficient to impair removal of excess respiratory secretions.

Pet owners often treat illness in their animals with their own drugs. Because veterinary professionals are often asked questions regarding use of OTC cold preparations, they must understand the dangers involved with use of these products and be able to explain to pet owners the reasons these preparations should not be used in pets.

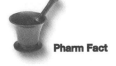

Pharm Fact

Veterinary professionals should inform animal owners of the dangers associated with giving their animal OTC cough and cold products.

BRONCHODILATORS

Bronchoconstriction is the contraction of smooth muscles surrounding the small terminal bronchioles deep within the respiratory tree. The stimulus for this contraction originates from several sources. Stimulation of the parasympathetic nervous system increases secretions in the respiratory tract and causes bronchoconstriction and subsequent **dyspnea** (difficult breathing). Drugs that stimulate release of the neurotransmitter acetylcholine or inhibit the activity of acetylcholinesterase, which breaks down acetylcholine, cause increased activity of the parasympathetic nervous system, resulting in bronchoconstriction and dyspnea. This is the common source of dyspnea associated with organophosphate insecticide toxicity.

A second mechanism of bronchoconstriction is release of **histamine** from mast cells. As shown is Fig. 6-2, stimulation of H_1-histamine receptors in smooth muscle cells causes smooth muscle contraction and subsequent reduced airway diameter. Other chemicals released by mast cells during inflammation may produce edema of the airways, excessive secretions, and migration of inflammatory cells onto the epithelial surface, where they may change mucus viscosity.

A third mechanism of bronchoconstriction involves blocking of the **β_2 re-**

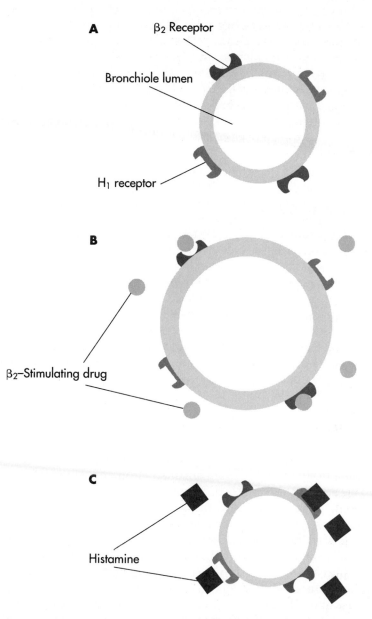

Fig. 6-2 Effects of β_2- and histamine receptor stimulation on bronchiolar smooth muscle. **A,** Smooth muscle layer surrounds the bronchiole. **B,** Smooth muscle relaxation and bronchiole dilation are caused by a predominance of β_2-stimulating drug. **C,** Smooth muscle contraction and bronchiole constriction are caused by a predominance of histamine.

ceptors found on smooth muscles and mast cells. β_2 Receptors are normally stimulated by the sympathetic nervous system neurotransmitters epinephrine and norepinephrine. These receptors cause the bronchiolar smooth muscles to relax, producing **bronchodilation** and vasodilation of coronary blood vessels and the vessels that supply blood to muscles (see Chapter 5). In addition to bronchodilation, stimulation of β_2 receptors also prevents mast cells from degranulating and releasing their mediators of inflammation (that is, histamine, prostaglandins, and leukotrienes). Thus if the β_2 receptors of the sympathetic nervous system are blocked by beta-blocker drugs such as antiarrhythmic drugs like propranolol, the bronchodilating effect is also blocked and the parasympathetic nervous system predominates, causing bronchoconstriction, excessive respiratory secretions, and edema within the airways.

β-Adrenergic Agonists

β-Adrenergic agonists (β agonists) are drugs that stimulate β receptors. Because β_2 receptors are involved in bronchodilation and stabilization of mast cells, drugs that stimulate β_2 receptors are bronchodilators. As discussed in Chapter 5, **β_1 receptors** are found in many parts of the body, most notably the heart. β-Adrenergic bronchodilators may not selectively stimulate only the β_2 receptors; they also stimulate the β_1 receptors. When stimulated by the sympathetic nervous system or nonselective β-adrenergic drugs, the β_1 receptors increase cardiac contractility, conduction speed of impulses through the heart, and the heart rate. If an animal is hypoxic because of bronchoconstriction, β_1 stimulation may result in cardiac arrhythmia or heart failure. Thus we prefer to use selective β_2 agonists to produce bronchodilation.

Terbutaline and albuterol are β-agonists that are selective for β_2 receptors and have *minimal* action on β_1 receptors. These drugs produce some stimulation of the heart, especially with the first few doses. Terbutaline has an additional value in treatment of bronchoconstriction and general bronchial congestion because it reduces mucus viscosity, thereby allowing the mucociliary apparatus to work more effectively. Both of these drugs are available in oral form and as inhalers; terbutaline is also available for SC injection.

Older β-agonists such as isoproterenol, ephedrine, and epinephrine (adrenaline), have significant β_1 effects; ephedrine and epinephrine also have α_1 effects such as vasoconstriction. Although isoproterenol is still occasionally used to treat bronchoconstriction, the more selective β_2 agonists terbutaline and albuterol are preferred. Ephedrine is sometimes used for treatment of urinary incontinence caused by a weak urethral sphincter in dogs and cats.

Methylxanthines

The methylxanthines include bronchodilators such as theophylline and aminophylline and the central nervous system (CNS) stimulants caffeine and theobromine (see Chapter 8). The difference between theophylline and

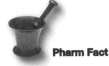

Pharm Fact

Terbutaline and albuterol are preferred over other β-adrenergic bronchodilators because of their selective β_2 stimulation.

aminophylline is that aminophylline consists of approxi-mately 80% theophylline and 20% ethylenediamine salt. The salt facilitates absorption of aminophylline and is better tolerated by the GI tract. Because 100 mg of aminophylline contains 80 mg of active theophylline, the dosages of aminophylline and pure theophylline differ based on the amount of active ingredient (theophylline) in the compound. The conversion formula is shown below. Various aminophylline products may contain different amounts of theophylline; therefore the 80% value (0.80 in the conversion formula that follows) may have to be changed to the percentage of theophylline in that aminophylline product:

$$\text{mg of theophylline} = \text{mg of aminophylline} \times 0.80$$

Conversion of 100 mg of theophylline to aminophylline is as follows:

$$100 \text{ mg of theophylline} = X \text{ mg of aminophylline} \times 0.80$$
$$100 \text{ mg of theophylline}/0.80 = X \text{ mg of aminophylline}$$
$$100 \text{ mg of theophylline} = 125 \text{ mg of aminophylline}$$
$$(80\% \text{ theophylline preparation})$$

Methylxanthines cause bronchodilation by affecting the smooth muscle cell's biochemical functions (Fig. 6-3). Normally, stimulation of the β_2 re-

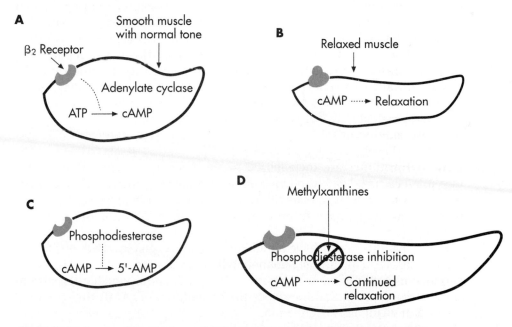

Fig. 6-3 Mechanism by which methylxanthines cause bronchodilation. **A,** β_2-Receptor stimulation results in the increased production of adenylate cyclase, which enhances increased production of cAMP. **B,** cAMP promotes relaxation of smooth muscle and hence bronchodilation. **C,** cAMP breaks down to 5'-AMP by phosphodiesterase, and the muscle returns to the normal state of tension. **D,** Methylxanthines inhibit phosphodiesterase, so cAMP is not broken down to 5'-AMP and muscle relaxation and bronchodilation continue.

ceptor results in production of cyclic AMP (cAMP), which promotes relaxation of the smooth muscle and hence bronchodilation. This cAMP is normally broken down within the cell by an enzyme called *phosphodiesterase,* which terminates smooth muscle relaxation. Methylxanthines inhibit phosphodiesterase and thus allow cAMP to accumulate and smooth muscle relaxation to continue.

Secondary benefits of methylxanthines in people include increased force of contraction of the respiratory muscles, slightly increased force of contraction of the myocardium, and dilation of coronary arteries. In most veterinary patients the effect on respiratory muscles is considered clinically insignificant.

Theophylline is available in sustained-release oral forms that prolong absorption of the drug over several hours. These preparations often have "sustained-release," or "SR," marked on the package. Generally, sustained-release preparations achieve lower peak plasma concentrations, but drug concentrations remain in the therapeutic range for a longer time. As discussed in Chapter 3, various factors affect absorption of sustained-release preparations, including the dissolving rate in the intestinal tract and the GI transit time. These tablets are formulated for human GI transit times, but in animals the tablets may pass through the GI tract before all the tablet has dissolved. The dissolving rate may differ for tablets made by different manufacturers. Therefore after an animal has initially been stabilized with a particular oral methylxanthine product, the animal should be maintained with that same manufacturer's product to ensure a more consistent clinical response.

Some CNS stimulation and GI upset may occur with use of methylxanthines. GI upset is especially common when theophylline is administered by mouth. Usually these effects are transient and resolve after a few days of administration. These drugs have a fairly narrow therapeutic index, meaning the therapeutic dose is very close to dosages that produce toxicity. Signs of overdose may occur with overstimulation of the CNS, cardiovascular system, and GI tract.

Methylxanthines are metabolized in the liver by enzymes that are induced by the presence of phenobarbital, primidone, phenytoin, and other barbiturates. Thus if theophylline is used with barbiturates, the theophylline dose may have to be increased to compensate for the increased metabolism.

Methylxanthines can have an additive, or **synergistic,** effect on the extent or duration of bronchodilation when used with a β_2-agonist bronchodilator. β_2 Stimulation increases cAMP production, which causes bronchodilation. Methylxanthines block the breakdown of cAMP, thus prolonging or enhancing bronchodilation.

Beta blockers (β antagonists such as propranolol) may antagonize the beneficial respiratory effect of theophylline if they block the β_2 receptor. β_1 Stimulants or some of the less specific β_2 agonists that also stimulate β_1 receptors could create a greater risk of cardiac arrhythmias because of methylxanthine's β_1 stimulatory effect. **Toxic synergism** refers to two drugs acting together to enhance a toxic effect.

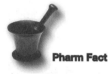

Pharm Fact

Sustained-release forms of theophylline may pass through an animal's GI tract before being fully absorbed.

Theophylline can interact with a wide variety of drugs; therefore the veterinary professional should refer to a pharmacology text before treating an animal simultaneously with theophylline and another drug. The veterinary professional should also investigate the addition of theophylline or aminophylline to IV fluids or other injectable medications before use because some combinations are incompatible.

OTHER DRUGS USED TO TREAT RESPIRATORY PROBLEMS

Corticosteroids

Corticosteroid use in treatment of respiratory disease remains controversial. The antiinflammatory effect of short-acting corticosteroids such as prednisone and methylprednisolone is beneficial when the swelling, inflammation, and congestion of the airways (that is, bronchoconstriction and obstruction) are life threatening. Corticosteroids have long been used for human treatment of asthma because they are thought to improve the activity of methylxanthine and β-agonist bronchodilators.

An appropriate use of corticosteroids is for acute respiratory problems in which inflammatory cells migrate to the bronchial surface and mast-cell inflammatory mediators cause swelling and edema of the bronchiolar tissues. The stabilizing effect of corticosteroids on mast cells and capillaries helps reduce swelling while reducing release of mediators that stimulate inflammatory cell migration. Insults to the lungs, such as with allergic responses, smoke inhalation, aspiration of chemicals, and eosinophilic bronchitis, could respond well to corticosteroids. Cats with feline asthma syndrome appear to respond well to corticosteroid treatment.

Considerable debate exists about whether corticosteroids should be used in treatment of chronic bronchitis or respiratory conditions involving a significant infectious component. Some veterinary internal medicine specialists who treat animals with chronic respiratory disease believe that corticosteroids are essential to maintain function of the respiratory tree; others are less adamant about the role of corticosteroids. Large doses of corticosteroids impair the immune system response to infection and delay healing (see Chapter 12). Therefore the veterinary professional should carefully weigh the benefits and risks before using corticosteroids.

Antihistamines

As discussed previously, histamine causes constriction of the bronchioles and is involved in the inflammatory responses of the respiratory tract. Because allergic reactions cause mast-cell degranulation and release of inflammatory mediators including histamine, **antihistamines** have been popular for use in people with hay fever and other allergies. However, histamine is not as much a factor in animal allergic respiratory problems. For example, histamine plays a minor role in feline asthma syndrome, as compared with its dominant role in human asthma. Nonetheless, histamine release is involved in chronic obstructive pulmonary disease ("heaves") in horses and other bronchial problems related to dust and particulate matter.

Unlike corticosteroids, which can reverse much of the damage caused by inflammation or allergic insult, antihistamines work effectively only if they reach the H_1 receptors on bronchial or vascular smooth muscles in large quantities *before* the arrival of histamines (see Fig. 6-2). Once histamine has stimulated the H_1 cell receptors, antihistamine drugs do little to reverse the histamine effects. If the allergic insult is a one-time event that is no longer present, corticosteroids are more appropriate than antihistamines to reverse the cellular damage and clinical signs. Theoretically the best use of antihistamines is either **prophylactically** before the histamine is released or when exposure to the allergic substance inducing release of histamine is continuous. This explains the reason antihistamines are used for heaves in horses that are continuously exposed to dust or molds in the barn environment.

Antimicrobials

Ideally the presence of a bacterial infection and the susceptibility pattern of the involved bacteria should be established before **antimicrobials,** which are drugs that combat infection by microorganisms, are used for treatment in respiratory diseases. Bacterial specimens can be obtained by transtracheal wash, bronchoscopic wash, or other sampling techniques. If culture and sensitivity tests are not used, the sample can be stained to determine the general type of bacteria involved, such as gram negative, gram positive, bacilli, or cocci. Based on the shape and gram stain of the bacteria, an antimicrobial can be selected that may be effective against that bacterial strain.

Although part of successful treatment of infectious respiratory disease depends on use of the appropriate antimicrobial, the other critical element is duration of therapy. Many animal owners stop giving their animal an antimicrobial after just a few days when clinical signs disappear. If they fail to give the full dose of the drug or do not give the medication for the recommended period, resistant bacteria can survive the shortened exposure to the antimicrobial. These resistant bacteria then multiply and become the predominant infectious bacteria in the respiratory tree. Thus animals with respiratory infections should be treated with antimicrobials for at least 7 to 10 days, with some treatments such as in chronic bronchitis lasting 4 to 6 weeks. A general rule is that antimicrobial use should be continued for 1 week after resolution of clinical signs in animals with chronic or severe infections.

Bacteria may propagate on the luminal, or airway, surface of the bronchioles. For an antimicrobial to reach the luminal surface of the bronchioles in significant concentrations, it must be secreted in the respiratory secretions. Many otherwise effective antimicrobials may not be effec-

Pharm Fact

Early cessation of antimicrobial therapy can lead to resistant bacteria.

tive when administered systemically (that is, by mouth, intramuscularly, or subcutaneously) because they do not reach the lumen infection site in concentrations sufficient to be bactericidal. In some of these cases the animal may benefit from administration of an antimicrobial by nebulization.

With nebulization the antimicrobial is suspended in a fine mist that the animal inhales into the airways. This technique deposits the drug directly on the surface of the bronchiolar epithelium. A disadvantage of nebulization is the need to use a mask or nebulizing chamber, which may cause stress to the animal and necessitate sedation. Another potential problem is the risk of reflex bronchoconstriction in response to introduction of the mist into the respiratory tree. Thus a bronchodilator is often given before nebulization is started. As mentioned earlier in this chapter, because animals do not deeply inhale the nebulized mist, most of the drug reaches only the trachea and primary bronchi but does not penetrate the smaller bronchioles.

Diuretics

Diuretics are used to remove accumulated fluid from the lungs, such as in animals with pneumonia or congestive heart failure. As explained in Chapter 5, diuretics promote loss of body water through diminished reabsorption by the kidneys. The decreased water content of the blood increases the osmotic forces within the capillaries and consequently attracts water from body tissues into the bloodstream. Through this mechanism the fluid of ascites or pulmonary edema is slowly moved into the blood and then out the body through the kidneys. Use of diuretics can be thought of as "therapeutic dehydration." A disadvantage of using diuretics to treat animals with respiratory disease is that they tend to dry the respiratory secretions, rendering the mucociliary apparatus less effective. This side effect must be measured against the potential benefits.

Oxygen

Oxygen administration with an oxygen cage or a mask is indicated in animals that are transiently hypoxic. For an animal, the stress of having the oxygen mask applied or being placed in an oxygen cage can sometimes precipitate collapse. Some cats and dogs tolerate a small diameter tube that is hooked to an oxygen source, placed into the nasal passages, and glued or taped to the hair of the head to hold it in place. Some veterinary professionals create a portable oxygen cage by placing an Elizabethan collar on the animal, *partially* covering the large end of the funnel with plastic wrap, and running an oxygen line into the inside of the collar. To allow for escape of heat, the opening of the Elizabethan collar funnel head should never be totally covered with plastic wrap. Oxygen is very dry so it should be humidified to prevent severe drying of the mucous membranes and mucociliary apparatus.

Respiratory Drug Categories and Names*

Antitussives

Butorphanol (Torbutrol)
Hydrocodone (Hycodan)
Codeine
Dextromethorphan

Mucolytics

Acetylcysteine (Mucomyst)
Water (steam)

Expectorants

Guaifenesin (glycerol guaiacolate)
Saline expectorants (ammonium chloride,
  potassium iodide, sodium citrate)
Volatile oils (terpin hydrate, eucalyptus oil, pine oil)

Bronchodilators

β Adrenergics
  Terbutaline
  Albuterol
Methylxanthines
  Theophylline
  Aminophylline

Other Respiratory Drugs

Corticosteroids
Antihistamines
Antimicrobials
Diuretics
Oxygen

*Brand names are in parentheses.

Recommended Reading

Bjorling DE, Keene BW: *The dyspneic cat,* Proceedings of the Waltham Feline Medicine Symposium, Ohio State University, Columbus, Ohio, 1996.

Boothe DM, McKiernan BC: Respiratory therapeutics, *Vet Clin North Am Small An Pract* 22(5):1231, 1992.

Dixon PM: Therapeutic of the respiratory tract. In Robinson NE, editor: *Current veterinary therapy in equine medicine* 3, Philadelphia, 1992, WB Saunders.

Ford RB: Infectious tracheobronchitis. In Bonagura JD, editor: *Kirk's current veterinary therapy XII,* Philadelphia, 1995, WB Saunders.

Hawkins EC: *Antibiotic therapy for respiratory infections in clinical practice,* Proceedings of the North American Veterinary Conference, Orlando, Fla, Jan 1996.

Murtaugh RJ: Acute respiratory distress, *Vet Clin North Am Small An Pract* 24(6):1041, 1994.

Padrid P: Diagnosis and therapy of canine chronic bronchitis. In Bonagura JD, editor: *Kirk's current veterinary therapy XII,* Philadelphia, 1995, WB Saunders.

Review Questions

1. A dehydrated animal with a nonproductive cough caused by acute bronchitis is admitted to the clinic. The veterinarian wants to correct the dehydration and determine whether character of the cough changes before deciding on therapy for the cough. Why does the veterinarian want to rehydrate the animal before starting therapy for the cough?

2. Why does bronchial inflammation (bronchitis) cause coughing but inflammation and infection in the alveoli (pneumonia) do not always?

3. A veterinary pharmaceutical sales representative is offering a special price on locally acting antitussives for your animal patients. Is it advisable to make such a purchase?

4. Name some antitussives that are approved for veterinary use. Which are available OTC and which are by prescription only? Which have the most potent antitussive effect?
5. The doctor mentions that the same protective mechanism of inflammation that helps attack bacteria also causes a complication in respiratory disease. He plans to use acetylcysteine to counteract this complication. What complication is the doctor talking about?
6. Nebulizers are commonly used to treat people with respiratory disease. Why are nebulizers not commonly used to treat animals?
7. How does an expectorant differ from a mucolytic?
8. You notice that an OTC cough and cold product contains guaifenesin. You remember that guaifenesin is also used in anesthetic protocols for horses. In what way does the effect of guaifenesin in anesthesia differ from its effect in treatment of respiratory disease?
9. How do decongestants cause tachycardia? What effect would an owner likely see if her cat lapped up several milliliters of the owner's spilled liquid decongestant?
10. Why is using a potent antitussive with a potent expectorant unwise?
11. Atropine blocks receptors for acetylcholine and therefore tends to block parasympathetic stimulation. What effect does atropine have on the respiratory tract? Is atropine used therapeutically for respiratory problems? Why or why not?
12. Why are terbutaline and albuterol used more commonly for bronchodilation than epinephrine, since they have similar mechanisms of action?
13. Why should β-blocking antiarrhythmics be used cautiously in animals with respiratory disease?
14. Explain how β_2 agonists such as terbutaline can act synergistically (produce a greater effect) with methylxanthine bronchodilators such as theophylline.
15. A dog being treated for a respiratory disease with a methylxanthine develops GI upset. The doctor decides to switch the animal's treatment from 200 mg of theophylline to an equivalent dose of aminophylline. Why would the doctor make such a change? What is the equivalent dose of aminophylline?
16. Why are antihistamines used in horses that have allergic respiratory problems related to a dusty environment but not usually used in dogs experiencing laryngeal swelling from an allergic reaction to penicillin?
17. A client calls and asks whether it is okay to stop giving his cat the amoxicillin tablets the doctor dispensed 2 days previously. The cat appears to be doing much better, and the owner is having to struggle with the cat to give the medication twice daily. What is your recommendation to the client?
18. Diuretics help remove excessive fluid from the lungs (such as in pulmonary edema). What is a disadvantage of using diuretics for this purpose?
19. Oxygen administration can be very beneficial to hypoxic animals. Why does oxygen therapy often reduce an animal's ability to remove inflammatory products, cellular debris, or excess mucus from the respiratory tract?

Drugs Affecting the Endocrine System

Key Terms

anabolic
analog
aplastic anemia
catabolic
contraception
corpus luteum (CL)
diabetes mellitus
endocrine system
endogenous
estrus synchronization
exogenous
foal heat
follicular phase
glucosuria
goiter
hyperglycemia
hyperthyroidism
hypoglycemic agent
hypothyroidism
luteal phase
milk (let-down)
mismating
negative feedback
    mechanism
seasonal anestrus
superovulation
synchronized estrous
    cycle
transitional estrus

The Negative Feedback System
Drugs Used to Treat Thyroid Disease
    Drugs used to treat hypothyroidism
    Drugs used to treat hyperthyroidism
Endocrine Pancreatic Drugs
Drugs Affecting Reproduction
    Hormonal control of the estrous
        cycle

Types of reproductive drugs
Drugs used to control estrous
    cycling
Drugs used to prevent, maintain, and
    terminate pregnancy
Other uses of reproductive drugs

Learning Objectives

*After studying this chapter,
the veterinary technician should know the following:*

The way hormone secretion is regulated

Drugs used to treat thyroid disease and their effects

Types and effects of insulin

Drugs that regulate the estrous cycle and their mechanism of action

Drugs that regulate pregnancy and their mechanism of action

The **endocrine system** is composed of the thyroid gland, ovaries, testicles, pancreas, adrenal glands, and other glands that produce hormones. The proper balance of hormonal activity is essential to maintain normal physiologic functions. This balance is easily upset by disease or drugs that increase or decrease the amount or effectiveness of different hormones. Hormonal therapy, which is the therapeutic use of hormone or hormonelike substances, plays an important role in certain diseases and health conditions. Therefore veterinary technicians should understand the ways basic hormone mechanisms work and the effects specific hormonal therapies have on the body. (A box listing endocrine drugs can be found at the end of this chapter.)

THE NEGATIVE FEEDBACK SYSTEM

All endocrine systems are regulated by a feedback mechanism in much the same way as ambient temperature and a thermostat regulate the activity of a furnace. The furnace produces heat until the thermostat detects that the interior environment is warm enough and turns off the furnace. When the temperature drops below a certain point again, the thermostat turns on the furnace, which in turn produces heat. The increased temperature shuts down the furnace by a **negative feedback mechanism.** A negative feedback mechanism is a particular factor that stops or decreases some activity.

As shown in Fig. 7-1, *endocrine gland A* produces a hormone when concentrations of that hormone fall below a certain level, similar to the way the furnace produces heat when the temperature drops below a certain point. As concentrations of hormone increase to desired levels, the negative feedback mechanism shuts off, or inhibits, additional hormone production. When the body metabolizes the available hormone and concentrations drop below the critical concentration again, the inhibiting feedback effect is removed and the gland begins to secrete hormone again.

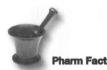

Pharm Fact

The negative feedback mechanism that regulates endocrine hormone secretion is similar to a thermostat regulating heat output from a furnace.

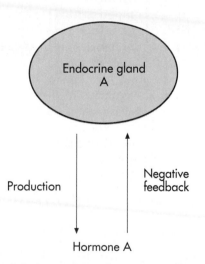

Fig. 7-1 Negative feedback loop regulating hormone production.

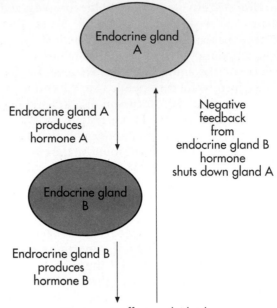

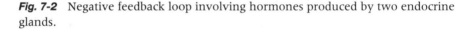

Fig. 7-2 Negative feedback loop involving hormones produced by two endocrine glands.

Often more than one endocrine gland is involved in the feedback loop. As shown in Fig. 7-2, *endocrine gland A* stimulates *endocrine gland B,* which in turn produces the hormone that provides the negative feedback to shut down gland A. This situation is common when the pituitary gland is involved in a particular endocrine function. Although the arrangement illustrated in Fig. 7-2 involves an intermediate step, it functions in the same way as the previously described arrangement.

If an **exogenous** drug (a compound that "originates from outside the body") is chemically similar to an **endogenous,** or naturally occurring, hormone, it can produce similar physiologic effects and exerts the same negative feedback effect as the hormone. Endocrine systems are finely balanced; therefore large doses of exogenous hormone or hormonelike drugs can easily upset the balance and produce unintended effects.

This chapter discusses thyroid, pancreatic, and reproductive hormones because these endocrine systems are the targets for most endocrine-related drugs used in veterinary medicine. Corticosteroids also affect the endocrine system and are discussed in Chapter 12.

DRUGS USED TO TREAT THYROID DISEASE

Drugs Used to Treat Hypothyroidism

Thyroid gland function is illustrated in Fig. 7-3. Under the influence of thyroid-stimulating hormone (TSH) produced in the pituitary gland, follicular cells of the thyroid gland produce two thyroid hormones: triiodothyro-

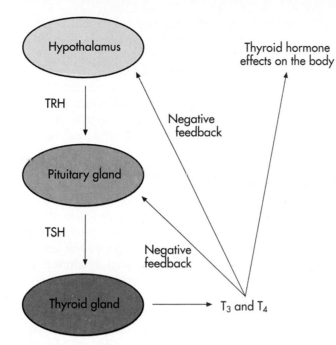

Fig. 7-3 Regulation of thyroid hormone production.

nine (T_3) and tetraiodothyronine, or thyroxine (T_4). T_3 is responsible for the cellular changes associated with normal thyroid function. T_4 is converted by tissues to T_3 in amounts required by that tissue. Increasing levels of T_4 produce the negative feedback that curtails secretion of thyroid-releasing hormone (TRH) from the hypothalamus and TSH from the pituitary gland.

Thyroid drugs (including antithyroid drugs) and thyroid supplements are used to treat thyroid hormone imbalances in dogs, cats, and occasionally horses and ruminants. Dogs are prone to develop **hypothyroidism,** which is an insufficiency of thyroid hormone, and cats are prone to develop **hyperthyroidism,** which is an excessive amount of thyroid hormone. Horses and cattle can be affected by hypothyroidism but to a lesser extent than dogs.

The terms *primary* and *secondary* refer to the site of dysfunction in some endocrine diseases. For example, primary hypothyroidism is a decrease in thyroid hormone production that is associated with disease or destruction of the thyroid gland. Canine thyroid tumors usually produce primary hypothyroidism because the thyroid tumor cells often do not produce thyroid hormones while they proliferate and destroy normal thyroid tissue. In contrast, secondary hypothyroidism is a drop in thyroid hormone production associated with decreased secretion of TSH by the pituitary gland, which consequently decreases thyroid function. Secondary hypothyroidism may be caused by malformation of the pituitary gland, destruction of the pituitary gland by a tumor, or suppression of pituitary function by a variety of illnesses. Thus in secondary hypothyroidism the pituitary gland is diseased and the thyroid gland is normal.

Goiter is a hypothyroid condition in which the thyroid gland enlarges because of a lack of iodine in the diet. Without iodine the thyroid cannot manufacture T_3 or T_4 and these thyroid hormone concentrations fall. The hypothalamus and pituitary gland detect the low circulating levels of thyroid hormone and increase output of TRH and TSH in an attempt to raise T_3 and T_4 levels. In response to this stimulation from TSH, the thyroid cells proliferate and the gland increases in size to produce a goiter. In spite of the increased number of thyroid cells, without the required iodine the thyroid gland cannot manufacture thyroid hormones, and the hypothyroid condition remains uncorrected. Goiter is easily treated by feeding iodinated foods and is now rare because of the wide availability of commercially prepared, well-balanced animal feeds.

Because T_3 and T_4 are the main regulators of energy production and metabolism in the body, a lack of T_3 or T_4 causes signs associated with a decreased basal metabolic rate. Signs of hypothyroidism include lethargy, weight gain despite normal consumption of food, need for heat, bradycardia, lack of estrous cycling, decreased growth in young animals, hair loss (alopecia), and dry and scaly skin, which is a result of altered dermal metabolism. Contracted tendons and poor development of respiratory epithelium have been reported in foals of mares with hypothyroidism. These offspring often have poor central nervous system (CNS) development, resulting in lethargic, uncoordinated ("dull") young animals. These signs are evident when hypothyroidism has progressed to a fairly advanced stage. Signs may be subtle or absent in the earlier stages.

Thyroid drugs in the form of hormone supplements are used to correct hypothyroidism. Drugs used to treat hypothyroidism include thyroid extract, synthetic levothyroxine (T_4), and synthetic liothyronine (T_3). Thyroid extracts are no longer commonly used, but some products are still available through veterinary drug suppliers. Thyroid extracts are made from bovine or porcine thyroid glands acquired from slaughterhouses. The potency of these extracts is often based on the iodine content of the extract, not the actual amounts of T_3 or T_4; therefore the amount of thyroid hormone in an extract product may vary considerably among batches.

The synthetic T_4 product levothyroxine (Synthroid, Soloxine) is the drug of choice for treatment of hypothyroidism. One of the key advantages of T_4 therapy is that it provides each tissue with its required amount of thyroid hormone for the individual organs. For example, the CNS has a high requirement for thyroid hormone; thus it normally uses all the T_3 presented to it and also converts any available T_4 to T_3 as needed. In contrast, other organs with lower metabolic demands such as the liver and kidney convert less T_4 to T_3. Supplementing a hypothyroid animal with levothyroxine provides each organ and tissue with the appropriate amount of thyroid hormone because each organ or tissue converts just enough T_4 to T_3. With T_3 supplementation the local tissue regulation of thyroid hormone conversion is bypassed. Another advantage of synthetic levothyroxine is its ability to trigger the natural negative feedback mechanism, thus emulating the normal regulatory mechanism for thyroid hormone production.

Some endocrinologists recommend initially using a well-known brand name of T_4 such as Soloxine to regulate the animal because these products produce a more predictable effect than some generic brands of T_4. Regardless of the brand of T_4 used, the dose should be regulated according to blood

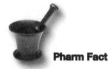

Pharm Fact

The potency of thyroid extracts can vary considerably among batches.

T_4 concentrations, and the product used should not be arbitrarily changed. Changing from one brand to another may alter the blood concentrations of thyroid hormone and possibly cause recurrence of hypothyroid signs. The drug is usually given once daily, although some animals improve more when given levothyroxine twice daily initially.

The effects of T_4 overdose are generally not as severe in veterinary patients as they are in people, thereby providing the veterinarian with a wider therapeutic (safety) index. People being treated with thyroid supplements may experience periodic thyroid "storms," or thyrotoxicosis, in which even a small overdose can cause signs consistent with hyperthyroidism, such as tachycardia, agitation, nervousness, and polyuria. Most dogs are fairly resistant to thyrotoxicosis. However, thyroid drugs should still be used with caution in animals with cardiac disease because of the potential for increased cardiac stimulation.

The effects of thyroid hormone include increases in glucose absorption from the gastrointestinal (GI) tract, conversion of protein to glucose (gluconeogenesis), and mobilization of glycogen stores to glucose (glycogenolysis). Therefore insulin requirements of diabetic animals that also are being treated for hypothyroidism must be adjusted after initiation of thyroid supplementation.

Synthetic liothyronine (T_3), which is available as the human product Cytomel and the veterinary product Cytobin, is generally not the first choice for treatment of hypothyroidism in dogs because T_3 supplementation bypasses local conversion of T_4 to T_3 according to individual tissue needs. Theoretically the T_3 dose would be based on the T_3 needs of the CNS, which has the highest demand for thyroid hormone. If an animal is given that dose, however, other organs with lesser requirements may be overdosed. In addition, T_3 products are more expensive than T_4 products and must be administered 3 times daily rather than once daily.

Occasionally liothyronine is used if levothyroxine therapy fails to produce adequate blood concentrations of thyroid hormone. Lack of T_4 efficacy may be related to the way it more readily combines with intestinal contents than T_3, thus reducing the amount of T_4 absorbed into the body. Normally T_3 has a bioavailability of 0.95, so 95% of T_3 is absorbed from the GI tract, versus only 40% to 80% absorption of T_4. However, consultation with a veterinary endocrinologist or internal medicine specialist is recommended before switching from T_4 to T_3.

Products are available that contain both liothyronine and levothyroxine. The ratio of T_3 to T_4 in these products is designed to meet the needs of people with hypothyroidism. Dogs require a slightly different ratio. Also, T_3 is metabolized more quickly than T_4, which is reflected in the three times daily dosage of T_3 versus once daily for T_4. Thus the T_3 component is metabolized before the T_4 component. For these reasons, use of combination thyroid drugs is not recommended.

Drugs Used to Treat Hyperthyroidism

Hyperthyroidism is an increase in levels of thyroid hormone. It is most common in cats and is associated with a hormone-secreting thyroid tumor. In contrast to hypothyroidism, hyperthyroidism is manifested by increased physical activity, diarrhea from increased GI motility, weight loss despite a voracious appetite, tachycardia (with heart rates exceeding 240 beats/minute), polyuria (increased urination), and polydipsia (increased water intake). Owners of hyperthyroid cats often do not bring their animals for treatment early in the course of disease because the animal appears healthy and fit (lean), is alert, and eats well.

Hyperthyroidism in cats is generally best treated by thyroidectomy, which is the removal of the thyroid gland. However, some clients may decline such surgery or the cat may not be a good surgical or anesthetic risk because of the effects of hyperthyroidism on the cardiovascular system. As an alternative to surgery these animals may be treated with antithyroid drugs, which decrease thyroid hormone production or destroy the thyroid tissue.

Methimazole (Tapazole) and propylthiouracil have been used to control hyperthyroidism in cats by blocking the thyroid tumor's ability to produce T_3 and T_4. These drugs block incorporation of iodine into the thyroid hormone molecule and thus prevent manufacture of a functional thyroid hormone molecule. Of the two drugs, methimazole causes fewer complications and is preferred over propylthiouracil for decreasing functional thyroid hormone production.

Because methimazole only prevents hormone formation but does not destroy existing T_3 and T_4 molecules, signs of hyperthyroidism do not abate until body stores of thyroid hormones have been metabolized. Cessation of methimazole treatment results in recurrence of hyperthyroid signs because the mechanism for producing thyroid hormones is not permanently disabled by the drug. Cats with hyperthyroidism must receive this drug for the rest of their lives to control the hyperthyroid signs.

Side effects occur in about 20% of cats treated with methimazole. The most common side effects are vomiting and anorexia; however, these signs may resolve after a few weeks of methimazole treatment. Although rare side effects such as liver problems, bleeding, and changes in white blood cell counts are seen in less than 3% of treated cats, when they do occur they are serious enough to require withdrawal of methimazole and reevaluation of the animal.

If the owner is reluctant or unable to give oral medication or the risk of side effects is unacceptable to the owner, use of radioactive iodine (I-131) is an alternative. The radioactive iodine is injected intravenously. The iodine, a normal component of thyroid hormone, is taken up and concentrated by the active thyroid tumor cells, which are then destroyed by the radioactivity. Generally, normal thyroid tissue is not destroyed by standard doses of radioactive iodine because the high levels of T_3 and T_4 produced by the tumor cells produce negative feedback to the pituitary gland and hypothalamus, shutting down TRH and TSH production and subsequently removing stimulation of normal thyroid tissue. Normal thyroid tissue atrophies, so it does not take up much radioactive iodine and is spared from the radiation effects.

Advantages of radioactive iodine include death of the tumor cells as opposed to just control of hormone production with methimazole treatment, less stress imposed on the patient than with surgery or daily administration of oral drugs, no anesthetic risk, and destruction of metastatic thyroid tumors with a single injection. However, iodine-131 can only be administered at institutions with facilities licensed to perform radioactive treatments and dispose of radioactive material. The pet owner should weigh the significant financial cost of I-131 treatment and its prolonged hospital stay of 1 to 3 weeks against the benefits and disadvantages of alternative treatments.

Another drug sometimes used to control signs of hyperthyroidism is propranolol, which is a β-blocker drug that helps reduce the tachycardia associated with hyperthyroidism in cats. In hyperthyroidism the elevated levels of thyroid hormones produced by the thyroid tumor increase the number of β_1 receptors on cardiac cells, making the heart more sensitive to sympathetic stimulation. Thus normal sympathetic stimulation produces tachycardia with heart rates exceeding 240 beats per minute. β_1-Blockers such as propranolol decrease the effect of sympathetic stimulation by preventing the normal sympathetic neurotransmitter molecules of epinephrine and norepinephrine from combining with the β_1 receptors. The heart then beats more slowly, pumps blood more efficiently, has less demand for oxygen, and is less likely to develop arrhythmias.

ENDOCRINE PANCREATIC DRUGS

The pancreas plays a role in both endocrine (hormone) and exocrine (digestive enzyme) functions in the body. Insulin, glucagon, and somatostatin are the hormones normally produced by the pancreas. Insulin is the only pancreatic hormone that is used for therapeutic purposes with any regularity.

The major effect of insulin is the movement of glucose from the blood into tissue cells. Insulin causes the liver to store glucose as glycogen and facilitates deposition of fat in adipose tissue. The net effect of insulin is to decrease blood glucose concentrations by enhancing distribution of glucose to body tissues. Lack of insulin results in **diabetes mellitus,** a disease characterized by high blood glucose levels, or **hyperglycemia,** and passage of glucose in the urine, or **glucosuria.**

The most common cause of diabetes mellitus in veterinary patients is destruction of the pancreatic beta cells, which produce insulin. This type of diabetes, Type I diabetes mellitus, can cause rapid or gradual onset of clinical signs associated with progression of the beta-cell destruction. Type II diabetes mellitus results from a decreased number of insulin receptors on tissue cells, rendering these cells insensitive to the effects of insulin.

Insulin-dependent (Type I) diabetics require subcutaneous injection of insulin. (In these patients blood glucose can only be controlled by insulin administration.) Insulin is a protein and thus would be destroyed by gastric acid if given orally. Even if it passed through the stomach intact, the insulin molecule is too large to be absorbed through the bowel mucosa. Therefore most diabetic animals must have one or two insulin injections every day for the rest of their lives. Pet owners must administer these injections at home. The veterinary technician often plays a critical role in educating the client about proper administration and storage of insulin and methods for monitoring the animal's blood glucose concentrations.

Various types of insulin are available. They are classified according to the species from which the insulin is derived, such as beef, pork, or human by genetic engineering, and the duration of activity. The more common classification is the duration of activity and includes the short-acting Regular (crystalline) and Semilente insulins, intermediate-acting NPH and Lente insulins, and the long-acting Ultralente insulin. Protamine zinc insulin (PZI) was formerly the most commonly used long-acting insulin for cats. However, the manufacturer of PZI stopped producing it in 1991. The duration of activity of the different insulins relates to their differences in absorption based on the crystal size of the insulin. Generally, the larger the crystal size, the more slowly the insulin is absorbed and the longer the duration of activity.

Insulin derived from beef, pork, or a combination of beef and pork were the main types available to both the human and veterinary markets for many years. Development of genetically engineered human insulin (recombinant human insulin) at a reasonable price has resulted in discontinued production of most beef and combination insulins. Only recombinant human insulin (Humulin) and purified pork insulin are likely to be available in the future.

The most commonly used insulins for maintaining the health of diabetic dogs are NPH and Lente insulin, which are of intermediate duration. The beef and pork combinations of NPH and Lente insulin are preferred over the recombinant human forms because they may have a longer duration of activity in dogs, sometimes allowing once-daily injections, which is more convenient and improves client compliance in treating the animal. Diabetic cats require the longer-acting Ultralente insulin, which is only available in human insulin form and is administered once or twice daily. Regular insulin is not commonly used to maintain diabetic cats or dogs because its short duration of activity requires multiple doses during a 24-hour period. However, because Regular insulin is the only type that can be given intravenously, it is used initially to stabilize the glucose concentrations of animals with severe, uncontrolled diabetes or diabetic ketoacidosis.

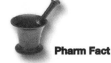

Pharm Fact

Insulin doses must be carefully calculated, properly administered at a well-perfused site, and coordinated with feeding times.

Insulin doses must be carefully calculated, properly administered at a well-perfused site to allow adequate absorption, and timed to be coordinated with a strict feeding regimen. The onset and duration of insulin action and ability to regulate blood glucose levels would vary considerably if the insulin were injected intramuscularly one time and subcutaneously the next time or into an area of fat. (See Chapter 3 for more information regarding the role of tissue perfusion and its effect on absorption.) Because a delicate balance exists between the amount of insulin administered and the relatively narrow range of normal glucose concentrations, consistent administration of insulin is essential to the health of the insulin-dependent diabetic patient.

Use of other drugs in diabetic patients can alter the insulin requirement and may necessitate changing the insulin dosage. For example, corticosteroids such as prednisone and dexamethasone mobilize glycogen stores, elevate blood glucose levels, and interfere with insulin receptors, all of which can produce significant hyperglycemia in a diabetic animal. Other drugs that elevate blood glucose levels include thiazide diuretics, phenothiazine tranquilizers (such as acepromazine), progesterone, and catecholamines such as epinephrine.

Clients often ask about use of human oral **hypoglycemic agents** for their pets as an alternative to daily injections of insulin. These sulfonylurea compounds such as glipizide are often used to treat adult-onset or non–insulin-dependent diabetes in people. They stimulate additional insulin production by pancreatic beta cells (the main effect), increase binding of insulin to peripheral tissue insulin receptors, or enhance the cellular response to insulin. These hypoglycemic agents are used in humans who have the non–insulin-dependent form of diabetes.

Although human patients with non–insulin-dependent diabetes may respond to hypoglycemic agents, most veterinary patients (especially dogs) have very few functional beta cells by the time diabetes mellitus is diagnosed, so compounds that stimulate beta cells cannot significantly increase insulin production. Some small percentage of cats may present with a non–insulin-dependent form of diabetes during the early stages of the disease. Because these cats may have some functional beta cells, some endocrinologists recommend a trial of glipizide as an alternative to euthanasia for these cats if the owner is unable or unwilling to administer insulin injections.

Veterinary technicians must understand the dynamics of diabetes mellitus and insulin regulation because they play an important role in educating owners of diabetic animals, helping owners regulate their pets' blood glucose levels, and answering questions related to diabetes mellitus.

DRUGS AFFECTING REPRODUCTION

Hormone drugs, either natural or synthetic, are used in food animals and horses to synchronize estrous cycles, terminate pregnancies, and induce ovulation. In dogs and cats, these drugs are used primarily to prevent pregnancy or alter the state of the uterus. Because the degree of response to reproductive hormone therapy varies among species, the dosage regimen in one species should not be assumed to produce the same effect in another species. The following discussion describes the most common ways drugs are used to treat reproductive problems. The reader is encouraged to review the literature to learn more about the ways these drugs are used in the treatment of specific reproductive problems in a particular species.

Hormonal Control of the Estrous Cycle

In female animals, hormone therapies often block or enhance the effect of endogenous reproductive hormones. Because reproductive hormones increase and decrease at various times in the estrous cycle, the veterinarian must determine (before treatment) the animal's stage in the estrous cycle to ensure the presence of the required hormone or physiologic process on which the therapy acts. Hence reproductive hormone drugs can be effective or ineffective, indicated or contraindicated at different stages of the estrous cycle (that is, proestrus, estrus, diestrus, and anestrus).

The estrous cycle is sometimes described as having two phases: the **follicular phase,** in which hormones produced by the ovarian follicle exert predominant control, and the **luteal phase,** in which hormones of the corpus luteum on the ovary predominate. The follicular phase includes the proestrus and estrus stages, whereas the luteal phase usually includes diestrus (metestrus).

Early in the follicular phase, the pituitary gland, under the influence of gonadotropin-releasing hormone (GnRH) from the hypothalamus, releases follicle-stimulating hormone (FSH), which in turn stimulates the ovary to produce follicles containing egg cells, or oocytes (Fig. 7-4). Under the influence of FSH the follicular tissue also begins to produce estrogens. The behavioral and physical changes associated with estrus ("heat") are largely related to changes in estrogen levels.

Estrogen production usually peaks near the time of estrus, although considerable variation exists among species on this point. A second hormone, inhibin, or folliculostatin, is also produced by the developing follicular tissue and serves as a negative feedback mechanism to decrease release of GnRH and FSH. By decreasing the release of FSH, inhibin allows only the most developed follicle to continue maturation until it can release an ovum. Thus inhibin helps prevent development of multiple follicles and decreases the potential for multiple births in animals that normally have only one or two offspring per birth.

The follicular phase terminates with the release of luteinizing hormone (LH) from the pituitary gland. Luteinizing hormone lyses (aids rupture of) the mature follicle(s), releases the ova, and transforms the ruptured follicle into a **corpus luteum (CL).**

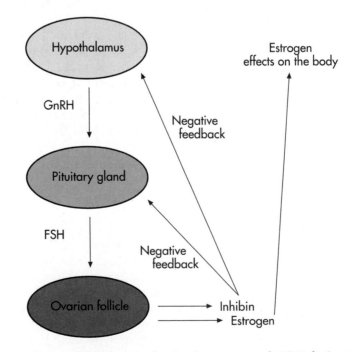

Fig. 7-4 Regulation of female reproductive hormone production during the follicular phase of the estrous cycle.

In the luteal phase of the estrous cycle (Fig. 7-5), the principal hormone produced by the CL is progesterone, which is considered the hormone of pregnancy. Progesterone causes the lining of the uterus to thicken and secrete a nutrient-rich fluid in preparation for implantation of the ovum or ova. In addition, progesterone keeps the uterine smooth muscles (myometrium) in a quiescent, noncontractile state and provides negative feedback to the hypothalamus and pituitary to inhibit further release of GnRH, FSH, and LH. If the released ova are not fertilized and do not implant in the receptive uterus within a certain time, the CL degenerates, causing a drop in progesterone production and subsequently reduced progesterone concentrations. This decrease in progesterone removes the inhibition on hypothalamic GnRH production and release of pituitary FSH and LH, resulting in initiation of a new estrous cycle.

A pregnant animal must have adequate levels of progesterone produced by the CL and the placenta to maintain the pregnancy. At the end of pregnancy the fetus initiates parturition (the birth process) by producing adrenocorticotropic hormone (ACTH), which results in elevated levels of cortisol (a natural corticosteroid) in both the fetal and maternal circulations. In response to the cortisol the uterus begins to produce estrogens and prostaglandins, both of which make the myometrium more prone to contraction and produce physical changes in the cervix and birth canal that favor passage of the newborn.

The prostaglandins produced by the uterus cause lysis (degeneration) of the CL, which terminates its production of progesterone. Together, estrogen

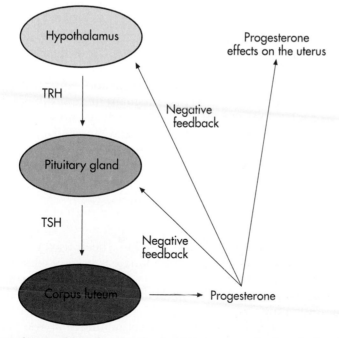

Fig. 7-5 Regulation of female reproductive hormone production during the luteal phase of the estrous cycle.

and prostaglandins increase the number of oxytocin receptors on the myometrial cells, making these smooth muscle cells more sensitive to the powerful contracting effect of oxytocin. Stimulation of the cervix or vagina such as from entry of the fetus into the birth canal or stimulation of the nipples from a nursing animal causes the pituitary gland to release oxytocin, which produces the forceful uterine contractions associated with labor and postpartum contractions and release of **milk (let-down)** from the mammary gland.

Types of Reproductive Drugs

Gonadotropin-releasing Hormone and Synthetic Analogs

Manufactured GnRH drugs stimulate release of LH and FSH similar to the way endogenous GnRH does. GnRH drugs include synthetic GnRH (Cystorelin), which has the same chemical structure as endogenous GnRH, and GnRH **analogs,** which are structurally different from endogenous GnRH but have similar effects. Because endogenous GnRH is released in pulses from the hypothalamus, injections of synthetic GnRH are usually not as effective as endogenous GnRH. The GnRH analogs may be more effective than synthetic GnRH, but they tend to be very expensive and are not readily available to the private practitioner.

Gonadotropins

FSH and LH are gonadotropins produced by the pituitary gland. Gonadotropin drugs consist of a powder made from the pituitary glands of food animals; they generally have more FSH effect than LH effect. In addition to pituitary gonadotropins, some species produce chorionic gonadotropins from the placenta. These can be used as drugs and include human chorionic gonadotropin (HCG), a hormone produced by pregnant women that has LH-like effects with little or no FSH effects, and equine chorionic gonadotropin (eCG), formerly known as "pregnant mare serum gonadotropin (PMSG)," which has FSH and LH effects. These drugs are sometimes used in food animals to induce **superovulation** (release of ova from multiple follicles) and occasionally in dogs and cats to induce estrus. Chorionic gonadotropins are also sometimes used to stimulate testicular descent in cryptorchid males with undescended testicles.

Estrogen

Estrogen drugs such as estradiol cypionate have been used to induce estrus in anestrual mares. In cows, estradiol cypionate is used in conjunction with other drugs to stimulate uterine contraction to expel purulent contents. The most common use of this drug in small animals is for prevention of pregnancy after mismating.

Diethylstilbestrol (DES) is an estrogen compound that was used extensively in food animals as a growth-promoting, or **anabolic,** steroid. After DES was found to have significant carcinogenic (cancer-producing) potential in people, the drug was banned from use in food animals. DES is no longer available in the injectable form; however, it is still available in an oral form. The drug is used to treat mismating in female dogs, reduce urinary incontinence, and treat perianal adenomas in male dogs.

Progestins

Progestins are reproductive hormones that are similar to progesterone. Use of progestin drugs during the follicular phase can slow or halt progression of the estrous cycle by inhibiting release of GnRH, FSH, and LH, further slowing development of the follicles. When used in this manner, progestins can prevent an animal from coming into full estrus. Use of progestins during the luteal phase can prolong diestrus beyond the time when the CL has regressed by providing the progesterone normally produced by the CL in this phase. Progestin drugs used in veterinary medicine are often recognizable by the stem *gest* in the nonproprietary (generic) name, such as altrenogest (Regu-Mate) and norgestomet.

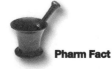

Pharm Fact

Veterinary professionals must use progestins carefully and advise animal owners of the potential adverse effects of progestin treatment.

The veterinary professional should be aware of certain precautions when using progestins. Progesterone causes the endometrium (uterine lining) to produce secretions ("uterine milk") that favor implantation of ova after fertilization. These progesterone-induced changes also provide an environment conducive for bacterial growth in the uterus. Thus use of progestins at higher than normal levels or for extended periods predisposes the uterus to infection such as metritis or pyometra. Even if the uterus does not become infected, prolonged treatment with progestins can result in cystic endometriosis with subsequent decreased fertility. Progestins may also cause mammary hyperplasia, which may increase the risk of mammary tumors. Orally administered liquid forms of progestins can be readily absorbed through the skin of the person administering the drug, producing systemic effects of progesterone. Because of these serious potential adverse effects, progesterone compounds should be used with great caution in intact females. In addition, the animal owner must be informed of the risks and signs associated with uterine infection.

Prostaglandins

Synthetic prostaglandin drugs are often used to lyse an active CL in an animal in the diestrus period of the luteal phase. Lysis of the CL causes progesterone levels to drop and a new estrous cycle to begin. During the estrus or proestrus period of the follicular phase, no CL is present, so prostaglandins administered during this phase do not have the desired effect. This emphasizes the importance of knowing the estrous cycle phase of an animal before administration of drugs to alter the reproductive cycle.

Prostaglandins are marketed under a variety of trade names. Most can be recognized by the stem *prost* in the chemical or generic name. Common prostaglandin drugs include dinoprost tromethamine (Lutalyse), cloprostenol (Estrumate), fluprostenol (Equimate), and fenprostalene (Bovilene).

Endogenous prostaglandins affect many body systems, and exogenous prostaglandins similarly cause a wide variety of effects. The most common side effects include unintended abortion in pregnant animals because of CL lysis, bronchoconstriction in animals with respiratory disease (such as horses with heaves), vomiting (in dogs and cats), colic and sweating (in horses), and in larger doses, CNS effects such as anxiety, hyperpnea, and pupillary dilation.

Technicians who handle prostaglandins should be aware that these drugs are easily absorbed through the skin and can easily produce CL lysis and bronchoconstriction in people as well as animals. Therefore the technician should take precautions such as wearing latex surgical gloves when handling these drugs. Women of childbearing age and asthmatics should completely avoid handling these drugs at any time.

Drugs Used to Control Estrous Cycling

Prostaglandins

Livestock breeders use **estrus synchronization** in female animals so that artificial insemination can be planned in advance and a number of animals can be inseminated at the same time. By synchronizing heat and insemination dates, all offspring are born at approximately the same time, which facilitates management at parturition and better neonatal care.

Injecting cows with prostaglandins during diestrus results in CL lysis, which subsequently causes progesterone concentrations to fall and the animal to return to estrus within 2 to 5 days of prostaglandin administration. Prostaglandins are used similarly in mares but with more variable results because, among other reasons, the equine CL is less sensitive to the lysing effects of prostaglandins for up to 5 days after ovulation and CL formation. Prostaglandins are not used in this manner in small animals because it is not common practice to synchronize groups of animals for breeding, and the CL of cats and dogs tends to be very resistant to the effects of exogenous prostaglandin for most of the luteal phase.

Progestins

Another way to synchronize estrus in a herd of livestock in varying stages of diestrus is to administer progestins several times to prolong the luteal phase beyond its normal termination, then abruptly terminate treatment to mimic CL lysis and bring the animals back into heat. In mares, injectable progesterone in oil or oral progestin altrenogest (Regu-Mate) are administered for 2 weeks to mimic diestrus, suppress LH stimulation, and allow subsequent regression of the CL. When the exogenous progestin is withdrawn after 2 weeks, no CL is present to maintain progesterone levels and the cycle returns to proestrus and estrus. Estrogen is sometimes added to the progestin regimen in mares to suppress follicular development and provide a more predictable return to estrus. In some mares the CL persists beyond the 2 weeks of treatment with progestin, resulting in failure to return to estrus.

Therefore prostaglandins may be used at the time of the progestin withdrawal to lyse any CL that has not already regressed.

Gonadotropins

Use of gonadotropins in an attempt to stimulate follicle growth or ovulation in animals has not been consistently successful. eCG has been used to stimulate follicle growth because of its FSH and LH effects. In contrast, HCG, because of its predominantly LH effect, has been used to lyse normal, developed follicles or those that persist such as occur in cows with prolonged estrus (nymphomania).

Drugs Used in Foal Heat

Mares that come into heat soon after foaling generally have a significantly lower conception rate than mares that come into heat at a later time. Many breeding managers delay this **foal heat** to increase the chances of conception at a later breeding. Because progesterone inhibits release of FSH and LH, administration of exogenous progestin drugs halts progression of the estrous cycle, delaying the onset of foal heat. This delay facilitates recovery of the uterus from the recent pregnancy so that it can support the embryo of the next pregnancy. A second technique to increase conception rates in mares that have recently foaled is to shorten the diestrous phase of the first cycle by using prostaglandins to lyse the CL and initiate a new cycle.

Drugs Used to Treat Anestrus

As the days grow shorter in autumn and the photoperiod decreases, mares stop cycling and their reproductive hormones are produced in minimum amounts, causing the mare to enter a period of **seasonal anestrus,** which is characterized by absence of heat. Because equine breed registries encourage birth of foals as soon as possible after January 1, breeders often ask veterinarians to help mares conceive during the spring, when the animals are in transition from seasonal anestrus to full reproductive capacity. During this period of **transitional estrus,** several follicles grow and regress, causing periods of estrus that are frequently long and during which the exact time of ovulation is unknown. To stimulate more predictable ovulation, progesterone or a progestin drug is administered for 10 to 14 days to mimic diestrus and then halted to mimic CL lysis. This technique is only used after rectal palpation reveals multiple, large follicles on the ovaries.

The progesterone drug blocks release of LH from the pituitary gland but does not significantly decrease production of LH, causing LH to accumulate in the pituitary gland. When progesterone administration is halted, the stored LH is released in sufficient quantities to lyse the large follicles, thereby releasing the ova. Concomitant use of estrogens seems to enhance this effect on LH. HCG may also be used because of its predominantly LH activity. Such hormonal therapy is often coupled with exposing the mares to artificial lighting in the stalls to lengthen the photoperiod. This causes the mare to go through the estrous cycle as it would during the summer.

Drugs Used to Prevent, Maintain, and Terminate Pregnancy

Contraceptives for Use in Preventing Pregnancy

Pregnancy can be prevented by suppressing the estrous cycle or preventing implantation of the fertilized ova in the uterine wall. Prevention of pregnancy is known as **contraception.**

Megestrol acetate (Ovaban) is an orally administered progestin used for contraception in female dogs and cats. The drug is similar to progesterone and is thought to suppress release of GnRH and subsequent release of FSH and LH, causing cessation of cycling. Because megestrol is a progestin, it causes endometrial changes such as thickened, increased secretions that are consistent with progesterone stimulation. Use of megestrol increases the risk of cystic hyperplasia of the endometrium, endometritis, or pyometra, although the risk of pyometra appears to be fairly low. Prolonged use of megestrol can result in mammary hyperplasia (that is, proliferation of mammary tissue). For these reasons, megestrol acetate is contraindicated in animals with any disease of the reproductive organs, mammary tumors, or mammary growth. Megestrol is contraindicated in pregnant females because the drug can have a masculinizing effect on female fetuses and can delay parturition.

Like progesterone and other progestins, megestrol has an antagonistic effect on insulin and reduces its ability to move glucose into cells. This effect of progestins helps explain the hyperglycemia and gestational diabetes seen in pregnant women and females in other species. Because of their insulin antagonism, progesterones, megestrol, and other progestins should not be used in diabetic animals. Long-term therapy with megestrol may predispose female dogs and cats to diabetes mellitus.

The adrenal gland in cats is apparently sensitive to the suppressive effects of megestrol acetate. Plasma cortisol levels in cats treated with megestrol can drop well below normal, producing a syndrome resembling hypoadrenocorticism. Most cats treated with megestrol do not show severe signs with this effect; however, administration of prednisone or other corticosteroids should be considered if such cats are to have surgery, be hospitalized, or be subjected to other stress.

Mibolerone (Cheque Drops) is another contraceptive used in female dogs. This is an androgen hormone similar to testosterone and interrupts estrous cycling by inhibiting LH release. Follicles develop to a point but do not lyse and consequently do not release their ova. The manufacturer lists several precautions for use of mibolerone, and veterinary professionals are strongly advised to review these before using this drug.

Because mibolerone is a testosterone analog and therefore has a similar structure to testosterone, it produces effects similar to those of high levels of endogenous testosterone. These include increased production of anal sac secretions, masculinization of developing female fetuses, and increased vulvar discharge. Mibolerone is contraindicated in dogs with perianal adenoma or perianal adenocarcinoma because these types of tumors are stimulated by androgen (male) hormones such as testosterone. Some dogs develop icterus (jaundice) while receiving this drug; therefore mibolerone should not be used in dogs with a history of liver disease. Female dogs treated for longer

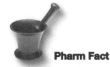

Pharm Fact

Prolonged use of megestrol can produce mammary tissue proliferation.

than 8 months should have tests to monitor liver function. Although mibolerone is relatively effective in female cats, it is generally contraindicated in this species because of reports of liver toxicosis and thyrotoxicosis.

Estrogens are used in large doses to prevent implantation of fertilized ova. Estradiol cypionate (ECP) is an injectable estrogen used in dogs after mismating occurs. Estrogens prevent pregnancy by increasing the number and thickness of folds within the oviducts, thereby preventing passage of the ova to the uterus.

The timing of estradiol cypionate injection is important. The egg must have been released from the follicle but not yet arrived in the uterus. If the animal has not yet ovulated, estradiol injection may delay ovulation and prolong estrus. In this case the animal could mate again a few days later and become pregnant. If the animal is in diestrus, the fertilized egg may already be in the uterus and would be unaffected by the estradiol injection.

Although estradiol injection is often successful when used properly, such estrogen therapy can have potentially life-threatening side effects. One potentially severe side effect is the increased risk of open-cervix pyometra. This uterine infection usually occurs 3 to 6 weeks after use of estrogen. As mentioned, progesterone creates an environment within the uterus that favors bacterial growth. Estrogens increase the number of progesterone receptors on uterine cells. After a large dose of estrogen the uterus becomes more sensitive to the natural effects of progesterone and subsequently becomes more susceptible to infection. Owners of animals treated with estrogen should watch for and report polyuria (increased urination), polydipsia (increased water intake), lethargy, anorexia, or any abnormal vulvar discharge because these constitute the early signs of open-cervix pyometra.

A second and more deadly side effect of estrogens, even when used at normal dosages, is bone marrow suppression with subsequent suppression of blood cell production. The resulting **aplastic anemia,** which usually appears 2 to 8 weeks after estrogen administration, is manifested as low platelet counts (thrombocytopenia), pinpoint hemorrhages in the skin or mucous membranes, evidence of bruising, leukopenia (low white blood cell count), and severe anemia. Aplastic anemia may slowly resolve after discontinuation of estrogen therapy; however, the anemia often progresses, resulting in death of the animal.

For all these reasons, the manufacturer of ECP has not approved the use of the drug in dogs for any purpose. Therefore any use of ECP in this manner is considered extra-label use. In addition, because safer alternatives to estradiol therapy exist, such as ovariohysterectomy (spaying) or allowing the pregnancy to progress to parturition, many theriogenologists (specialists in animal reproduction) do not recommend use of estradiol in dogs and some consider it a form of malpractice.

Progesterone and Progestin

Because progesterone is the normal hormone that maintains pregnancy, progestins and progesterone have been advocated for use in maintaining pregnancy in mares prone to abortion. These drugs may help if the problem is related to low progesterone levels because of a poorly functioning CL. Altrenogest has been used with varying success in mares to prevent premature parturition. Because altrenogest is slightly different from progesterone, it does not produce negative feedback on endogenous progesterone production and thus can be given as an oral progesterone supplement. Unfortunately because abortion and premature parturition have multiple causes, the success of progestin therapy in maintaining pregnancy varies considerably.

Prostaglandins

Several drugs are used to induce abortion or initiate parturition. These drugs are used in animals carrying a dead fetus, mares carrying twins, or heifers that have been bred too young to safely deliver a live calf. Prostaglandins are the most commonly used drugs for termination of pregnancy. Prostaglandin administration causes CL lysis, resulting in a decrease in progesterone levels and subsequent fetal death.

The effectiveness of $PgF_{2\alpha}$ and its analogs varies among species because of the resistance of some CLs to prostaglandin and the placenta's role in providing some progesterone necessary to maintain pregnancy. In cows the CL continues to produce progesterone for the entire pregnancy; however, the placenta can produce sufficient progesterone to maintain pregnancy after the fourth or fifth month. Therefore prostaglandins are only effective in cows if given before the fourth month of pregnancy.

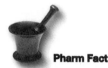

Pharm Fact

Prostaglandins can cause transient respiratory distress, salivation, vomiting, diarrhea, tachycardia, and polyuria.

In dogs the CL is relatively resistant to the lytic effects of prostaglandins during the first 2 to 4 weeks of pregnancy. Canine CL sensitivity to prostaglandin increases after this time. Although $PgF_{2\alpha}$ is quite effective in terminating pregnancy, it often causes side effects such as panting, salivation, respiratory distress, GI stimulation (that is, vomiting and diarrhea), tachycardia, and increased urination. If side effects occur, they last only about 20 minutes. If needed, the GI stimulation and respiratory distress can be alleviated by giving the animal atropine.

The $PgF_{2\alpha}$ analogs fluprostenol (Equimate) and dinoprost tromethamine (Lutalyse) are both approved for termination of pregnancy in mares. As in dogs, side effects include increased respiratory and heart rates, sweating, transient fever, and some abdominal discomfort. These signs usually disappear about 1 hour after administration.

Corticosteroids

Corticosteroids may induce abortion in mares or cows by mimicking the elevated levels of cortisol that occur at the beginning of normal parturition. In dogs, corticosteroids such as dexamethasone have been reported to cause intrauterine death and fetal resorption if given after 30 days of gestation (pregnancy) and abortion if given during the last 3 weeks of gestation. When used as abortifacients (drugs that induce abortion), corticosteroids are unpredictable in their efficacy. Corticosteroid use in cows is associated with a fairly high incidence of retained placenta. Because prostaglandins are usually much more effective, corticosteroids are not used very often for inducing parturition or abortion. However, the inadvertent administration of a significant dose of a corticosteroid in a pregnant animal for a problem unrelated to pregnancy, such as joint inflammation and immune-mediated diseases, can induce unintended abortion.

Ergot alkaloids

Ergot alkaloids such as bromocriptine are potent vasoconstrictors and inducers of parturition through stimulation of dopamine secretion. Dopamine suppresses secretion of prolactin, a hormone necessary for maintaining pregnancy in some species. By stimulating dopamine secretion, bromocriptine indirectly suppresses prolactin secretion and terminates the pregnancy. In dogs, prolactin is normally secreted in significant quantities after about 30 days of gestation and is needed to maintain pregnancy from midgestation afterward. Any suppression of prolactin production after midgestation could result in abortion.

Ergot alkaloids are not very predictable in inducing parturition and generally produce more severe vomiting and depression than prostaglandins. Ergot alkaloids may be found in rye, tall fescue grass, and other grains infected with endophyte fungi. If ingested in the grain of horses and cattle, these ergot alkaloids can produce abortion.

Various other drugs are being investigated for termination of pregnancy in dogs, including the controversial experimental drug, RU486.

Other Uses of Reproductive Drugs

Oxytocin is an endogenous hormone released from the pituitary gland and causes contraction of the uterus. Normally the uterus becomes sensitized to oxytocin by release of prostaglandins and estrogens just prior to parturition. Exogenous oxytocin is most commonly used to increase uterine contractions in animals with dystocia (difficult labor) related to a weakened or fatigued uterus. Calcium gluconate is sometimes given in conjunction with oxytocin to facilitate uterine contraction in these dystocia cases. Veterinarians may also give an oxytocin injection to a female to increase expulsion of placental materials after birth and to decrease uterine hemorrhage. Controversy exists as to whether this is of any significant benefit. Administration of oxytocin causes both contraction of mammary smooth muscles and milk letdown and therefore may also result in dripping of milk from the teats after administration for uterine contraction.

In mares with endometritis, $PgF_{2\alpha}$ is sometimes used to shorten the estrous cycle through lysis of the CL, causing a return to proestrus. It is thought that this "short cycling" improves the health of the uterus because of the estrogen effects. Prostaglandins are used to evacuate the uterine contents of cows with metritis or pyometra. Although $PgF_{2\alpha}$ has been advocated as a nonsurgical treatment of pyometra in dogs, results are not consistent due to the resistance of the canine CL to the effects of prostaglandin. This resistance, combined with the side effects, makes $PgF_{2\alpha}$ a second choice to surgical correction of pyometra, except to salvage the breeding capacity of a breeding female.

Many reproductive hormones such as testosterone and progesterone have **anabolic** effects. (That is, they enhance production of muscle and body tissue.) Corticosteroids have **catabolic** effects. (That is, they favor breakdown of muscle and tissue.) Anabolic steroids such as forms of testosterone and progesterone have been used in the food animal industry to increase the weight and conditioning of feedlot cattle. Use of anabolic steroids to increase muscularity in food animals is controversial. Anabolic steroids are also used

Pharm Fact

Progestins are sometimes used to treat behavior problems in cats.

to improve the appetite and condition of dogs or cats subjected to surgery or stress. In humans, some anabolic steroids are used to improve muscle tone and conditioning of geriatric patients. Again, some controversy exists as to the effectiveness of these compounds in producing significant benefits.

Progestins, especially megestrol acetate, have been used to modify behavior in cats. Megestrol has been used in treatment of urine spraying by male cats, changes in litterbox behavior, neurodermatitis (excessive self-grooming), and feline hyperesthesia syndrome (hypersensitivity to touch). The veterinary professional must weigh the possible long-term effects on the uterus and mammary tissue against any benefit with prolonged use of these hormones.

Small doses of estrogens have been used to treat urinary incontinence in spayed dogs on the premise that estrogen increases smooth muscle tone and partly compensates for loss of estrogen after the ovaries have been removed. Estrogens are also used as adjunctive chemotherapy for perianal adenomas or perianal adenocarcinomas in male dogs. As mentioned previously, growth of these tumors is stimulated by testosterone. Castration and estrogen therapy greatly enhance the remission rate. Estrogens have also been used to decrease prostatic inflammation in noncastrated male dogs and to stimulate passage of a retained placenta in cattle.

Reproductive hormones have a wide variety of effects on the body. Because many of the uses described are extra label and have not been approved by the Food and Drug Administration, clients must be warned of po-

Endocrine Drug Categories and Names

Thyroid hormones

Thyroid-stimulating hormone
Triiodothyronine
Tetraiodothyronine (thyroxine)
Levothyroxine (Synthroid, Soloxine)
Liothyronine (Cytobin)

Antithyroid drugs

Methimazole (Tapazole)
Radioactive iodine
Propranolol

Endocrine Pancreatic Drugs

Regular insulin
Semilente insulin
Lente insulin
Ultralente insulin
Recombinant human insulin

Drugs used to regulate the estrous cycle

Prostaglandin $F_{2\alpha}$

Altrenogest
Equine chorionic gonadotropin (eCG)
Human chorionic gonadotropin (HCG)
Gonadotropin-releasing hormone (GnRH)
Gonadotropins (FSH, LH)
Estrogens

Drugs used to prevent, maintain, or terminate pregnancy

Megestrol acetate (Ovaban)
Mibolerone (Cheque Drops)
Estradiol cypionate (ECP)
Prostaglandin $F_{2\alpha}$
Corticosteroids
Ergot alkaloids (bromocriptine)

Other reproductive drugs

Oxytocin
Anabolic steroids

tential side effects and adverse reactions. In addition, the veterinary professional handling these hormone drugs must prevent these compounds from entering the human food chain and prevent accidental exposure to these compounds during administration.

Recommended Reading

Thyroid Drugs

Feldman EC, Nelson RW: *Canine and feline endocrinology and reproduction,* ed 2, Philadelphia, 1996, WB Saunders.

Graves TK: Complications of treatment and concurrent illness associated with hyperthyroidism in cats. In Bonagura JD, editor: *Kirk's current veterinary therapy XII,* Philadelphia, 1995, WB Saunders.

Merchant SR, Wofsheimer KJ: *Common questions concerning canine hypothyroidism,* Proceedings of the North American Veterinary Conference, Orlando, Fla, 1996.

Peterson ME: Radioactive iodine (Radioiodine) treatment for hyperthyroidism in cats. In Bonagura JD, editor: *Kirk's current veterinary therapy XII,* Philadelphia, 1995, WB Saunders.

Endocrine Pancreatic Drugs

Broussard JD, Wallace MS: Insulin treatment of diabetes mellitus in the dog and cat. In Bonagura JD, editor: *Kirk's current veterinary therapy XII,* Philadelphia, 1995, WB Saunders.

Feldman EC, Nelson RW: *Canine and feline endocrinology and reproduction,* ed 2, Philadelphia, 1996, WB Saunders.

Peterson ME, Sampson GR: CVT update: insulin and insulin syringes. In Bonagura JD, editor: *Kirk's current veterinary therapy XII,* Philadelphia, 1995, WB Saunders.

Nelson RW, Feldman ED: Treatment of feline diabetes mellitus with the oral sulfonylurea glipizide. In Bonagura JD, editor: *Kirk's current veterinary therapy XII,* Philadelphia, 1995, WB Saunders.

Reproductive Drugs

Blanchard TL, Varner DD: Manipulating estrus in the mare, part 1, *Vet Med* 90(2): Feb 1995.

Blanchard TL, Varner DD: Manipulating estrus in the mare, part 2, *Vet Med* 90(3): Mar 1995.

Braakman A, Okkens AC, van Haaften B: Medical methods to terminate pregnancy in the dog, *Compend Cont Educ* 15(11):1505, 1993.

Cain JL: The use and misuse of reproductive hormones in canine reproduction. In Bonagura JD, editor: *Kirk's current veterinary therapy XII,* Philadelphia, 1995, WB Saunders.

Concannon PW: Use of progesterone-suppressing drugs for termination of unwanted pregnancy in dogs. In Bonagura JD, editor: *Kirk's current veterinary therapy XII,* Philadelphia, 1995, WB Saunders.

Davidson AP: Medical treatment of pyometra with prostaglandin F2 alpha in the dog and cat. In Bonagura JD, editor: *Kirk's current veterinary therapy XII,* Philadelphia, 1995, WB Saunders.

Feldman EC, Nelson RW: *Canine and feline endocrinology and reproduction,* ed 2, Philadelphia, 1996, WB Saunders.

Godke RA, Ryan DP: Synchronization of estrus. In Howard JL, editor: *Current veterinary therapy 3—food animal practice,* Philadelphia, 1993, WB Saunders.

Ley BL: Prefoaling management of the mare and induction of parturition. In Robinson NE, editor: *Current therapy in equine medicine,* Philadelphia, 1992, WB Saunders.

Plumb DC: *Veterinary drug handbook,* ed 2, Ames, 1995, Iowa State University Press.

Root MV, Johnston SD: Pregnancy termination in the bitch using prostaglandin F2 alpha. In Bonagura JD, editor: *Kirk's current veterinary therapy XII,* Philadelphia, 1995, WB Saunders.

Whitmore HL: Bovine ovarian cysts. In Howard JL, editor: *Current veterinary therapy 3—food animal practice,* Philadelphia, 1993, WB Saunders.

Youngquist RS: Therapeutic management of reproduction. In Howard JL, editor: *Current veterinary therapy 3—food animal practice,* Philadelphia, 1993, WB Saunders.

Review Questions

1. What is the difference between an exogenous hormone and an endogenous hormone in terms of definition, effect on the body, and effect on negative feedback mechanisms?

2. If an animal has primary hypothyroidism, would you expect the serum T_3/T_4 level to be increased or decreased? What about serum TSH and TRH levels?

3. What is the biologically active form of thyroid hormone? Is this form the supplement of choice for hypothyroid dogs?

4. Some combination T_3 and T_4 products are available for use in human medicine. Why are these not used to treat hypothyroid animals, since they would apparently provide both the active hormone and the precursor hormone?

5. Why are most hyperthyroid cats not brought to the veterinarian until the disease has greatly progressed?

6. Which drugs are used to treat hyperthyroidism in cats? Why are they not used more often?

7. Why is propranolol, a heart medication, sometimes used to treat hyperthyroid cats?

8. An insulinoma is a pancreatic tumor that produces excessive amounts of insulin. Would the clinical signs of insulinoma resemble those of diabetes mellitus? What signs do insulinomas cause?

9. What are the differences among regular, Lente, and Ultralente insulins? Which type of insulin is most appropriate to initially infuse intravenously to quickly reduce the blood glucose level in a dog with uncontrolled diabetic ketoacidosis? Which type is most likely to be dispensed to the client after a diabetic dog is well regulated? Which type is most likely to be dispensed to a client for home treatment of a diabetic cat?

10. Why should insulin not be injected into adipose tissue (fat)?

11. Why are oral hypoglycemics not used in animals to control diabetes mellitus?

12. The package insert for a drug used to correct reproductive problems states that the drug is only effective during the luteal phase. What does this mean? What hormones normally predominate during the luteal phase? When does estrus occur relative to the luteal phase?

13. What is the difference between gonadotropin-releasing hormone and a gonadotropin?

14. What is the difference between progesterone and progestin drugs? What are examples of progestins?

15. What are some potentially dangerous side effects of progesterone and progestin drugs?

16. What drugs are used to lyse the CL, and why is this done?

17. Why should veterinary professionals handle prostaglandins very carefully? Which group of people is especially at risk of prostaglandin side effects?

18. Explain how progestins may be used in a mare in transitional anestrus to induce estrus during the spring months.

19. The chances for conception after breeding a mare during foal heat increase with the interval between foaling and the onset of foal heat. What drug might be used to suppress the onset of foal heat by suppressing the follicular phase of the estrous cycle?

20. What drug is sometimes given to mares, especially those with a history of abortion, to facilitate a full-term pregnancy? Is this drug very effective?

21. How does the contraceptive megestrol acetate work? Do any significant side effects occur?

22. The veterinarian is reluctant to give an older female dog megestrol for treatment of a behavior problem (megestrol sometimes being used for that purpose) because the animal has diabetes mellitus. Why should megestrol not be given to diabetic animals?

23. How is mibolerone different from megestrol in its composition and mechanism of action?

24. What type of drug is used as a "mismating" injection? By what physiologic mechanism does this drug prevent pregnancy? Why are these injections of limited efficacy?

25. Why does the doctor spend considerable time explaining the side effects of estrogen therapy to prevent pregnancy?

26. The veterinarian tells a client that drugs like estradiol cypionate can cause pyometra. You had previously been told progesterones cause pyometra. How can you explain this apparent contradiction?

27. What drug is most commonly used to terminate pregnancy in livestock and horses? How does it work? Does this drug work in preventing pregnancy in dogs and cats?

28. A heifer has exhausted itself trying to deliver a near-term dead calf. You remember that prostaglandins are used to initiate labor in dogs and cats. Would prostaglandins be appropriate to use in this heifer?

29. A horse owner calls to say her pregnant mare is slightly lame in a front leg. The injury does not appear to be serious, but she asks whether it is safe to give some dexamethasone intramuscularly to reduce the swelling and inflammation. What is an appropriate response?

30. A Chihuahua female gave birth to one pup yesterday, strained all yesterday afternoon and last evening, and then stopped. Today the veterinarian palpated another puppy in the uterus and decided to induce labor by administering a drug. What drug might be helpful in this situation? Would prostaglandins be effective?

31. Progestins are sometimes used in behavior modification. For what type of behavior problems are progestins most likely to be effective?

32. An old, castrated male dog has numerous small tumors in the perianal area. The doctor elects to treat the tumors medically rather than surgically removing them. What type of drug is most likely to be effective in reducing the size of these tumors?

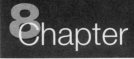

Drugs Affecting the Nervous System

Key Terms

acidosis
α_2 receptor
analgesic
anesthesia
anticonvulsant
apnea
bradypnea
convulsion
diffusion hypoxia
disinhibition
drug-induced
  hepatopathy
epilepsy
focal seizure
general anesthesia
generalized seizure
grain
grand mal seizure
hypothermia
ictus
idiopathic epilepsy
idiosyncratic reaction
κ-opioid receptor
local anesthesia
malignant hyperthermia
mixed-function oxidase
  enzyme system
μ-opioid receptor
partial agonist
petit mal seizure
postictal phase
preictal phase (aura)
sedative
seizure
σ-opioid receptor
tranquilizer

Anesthetics
  Barbiturates
  Propofol
  Dissociative anesthetics
  Inhalant anesthetics
Tranquilizers and Sedatives
  Acepromazine
  Droperidol
  Diazepam, zolazepam, midazolam,
    and clonazepam
  Xylazine detomidine, and medetomi-
    dine
Analgesics
  Narcotic or opioid analgesics
  Neuroleptanalgesics

Anticonvulsants
  Phenobarbital
  Primidone
  Phenytoin
  Diazepam
  Clonazepam
  Potassium bromide
  Valproic acid
Central Nervous System Stimulants
  Methylxanthines
  Doxapram
  Yohimbine, tolazoline, and
    atipamezole

Learning Objectives

*After studying this chapter,
the veterinary technician should know the following:*

Different types of anesthetics and their effects

Different types of tranquilizers and sedatives and indications for their use

Different types of analgesics and their effects

Numerous drugs used in veterinary medicine alter the function of the nervous system. The categories of these drugs include anesthetics, tranquilizers, sedatives, analgesics, anticonvulsants, and stimulants. For a more complete description of the uses of anesthetic agents, readers should consult textbooks of anesthesiology. This chapter discusses drugs of these five categories, their mechanisms of action, and problems encountered when using these drugs. (A box listing nervous system drugs can be found at the end of this chapter.)

ANESTHETICS

Anesthesia means "without sensation." An anesthetized animal or person cannot feel such stimulation as pain, cold, heat, pressure, or touch. **General anesthesia** is the reversible loss of sensation associated with unconsciousness, and **local anesthesia** is the reversible loss of sensation in a regional area of the body without loss of consciousness.

Anesthetics should not be confused with analgesics, which are compounds designed to decrease the perception of pain but not necessarily cause total loss of sensation. For example, aspirin is an analgesic because it decreases the pain associated with inflammation; however, it is not an anesthetic because it does not produce anesthesia.

Sedatives and tranquilizers are often used in their injectable forms with other drugs as part of anesthetic protocols because they can produce profound sedation or deep hypnosis, which contributes to anesthesia. The statement "the closest you are likely to come to death and survive is when you have been anesthetized" emphasizes the importance of understanding the ways anesthetics affect the body so that potential problems can be prevented and anesthetic emergencies and deaths can be avoided.

Barbiturates

Barbiturates are frequently used in veterinary medicine to produce short-term anesthesia, induce general anesthesia, control seizures, and euthanize animals. Barbiturates are frequently used accordingly to their duration of action:

Type	Duration of Action	Example
Ultra short acting	10 minutes	Thiamylal sodium
		Thiopental sodium
		Methohexital sodium
Short acting	1 hour	Pentobarbital
Long acting	6 to 7 hours	Phenobarbital

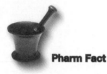

Barbiturates are also divided into thiobarbiturates, which contain a sulfur molecule on the barbituric acid molecule, and oxybarbiturates, which contain an oxygen molecule. Thiamylal and thiopental are thiobarbiturates; methohexital, pentobarbital, and phenobarbital are oxybarbiturates. Thiobarbiturates are more lipid soluble than oxybarbiturates and therefore have a more rapid onset but shorter duration of action than oxybarbiturates.

Generally, barbiturates depress the central nervous system (CNS); however, animals given a bolus injection of ultra–short-acting barbiturates (entire dose injected at one time) experience a momentary excitatory phase before passing into unconsciousness. Doses of ultra–short-acting barbiturates insufficient to induce anesthesia may result in hyperactivity (for example, paddling and vocalizing).

The CNS depressant effects of barbiturates account for their major side effect—respiratory and cardiac depression. Animals injected with thiobarbiturates may experience transient apnea (cessation of breathing). Because of the rapid redistribution of these drugs to other tissues, spontaneous breathing usually resumes within seconds to minutes. Barbiturates are also used as euthanasia solutions because they produce unconsciousness before they cause respiratory and cardiac arrest. Barbiturates should generally be used with caution in cats because of the reduced ability of this animal to metabolize these drugs.

Repeated use of barbiturates, such as for long-term control of seizures, induces accelerated hepatic metabolism of barbiturates and a subsequent decrease in plasma concentrations, a phenomenon called *drug tolerance* (see Chapter 3). Induction of hepatic enzymes produces tolerance to phenobarbital but also can reduce the effectiveness of corticosteroids, chloramphenicol, propranolol, doxycycline, and quinidine.

Barbiturates are highly protein bound, and the circulating plasma proteins act as reservoirs of active drugs. In animals with hypoproteinemia (low plasma protein levels), dosages of barbiturates should be decreased to prevent excessive sedation or respiratory depression. This binding of barbiturates by plasma proteins can be decreased by **acidosis,** in which the blood becomes more acidic than the normal pH of 7.4. In animals experiencing acidosis associated with shock, diabetes mellitus, hypoxia from lung disease (such as pneumonia), or some toxins (such as antifreeze poisoning), any barbiturate given for anesthesia is less bound by plasma proteins, making more drug available to affect the CNS. Thus in any condition in which acidosis is likely to be present, the normal barbiturate dosage should be reduced to prevent overdosing.

Thiopental (Pentothal) and thiamylal (Surital), both ultra–short-acting thiobarbiturates, are widely used in veterinary practice for induction of anesthesia. Although thiamylal was very popular as an induction agent, in 1993, Parke-Davis discontinued Surital, and Bio-Ceutics and Fermenta Animal Health recalled their thiamylal products because of problems with the precursor of thiamylal. As of this printing, thiamylal is not available to veterinarians; however, thiopental is still available.

Thiobarbiturates can be given only intravenously because they are extremely irritating to tissues. If accidentally injected perivascularly (in the area around the vein), thiobarbiturates can produce severe inflammation, swelling, and necrosis (tissue death). After accidental perivascular injection the area should immediately be infiltrated with 1 or 2 ml of procaine or lidocaine (local anesthetics) to prevent tissue sloughing. Injection of additional saline into the site, injections of corticosteroids or nonsteroidal antiinflammatory drugs, and application of cold packs and later hot packs also have been advocated to reduce tissue inflammation and necrosis.

Because these drugs are quickly distributed and easily penetrate the blood-brain barrier, onset of anesthesia is rapid. As mentioned, animals given a bolus injection of thiobarbiturates recover quickly (within minutes) as the drug distributes to less perfused tissue (for example, adipose tissue and inactive muscle) and concentrations in the brain decrease as the drug is redistributed to these other tissues. The drug has not left the body in these few minutes but rather has been redistributed to and begun to fill up these other body compartments. Therefore if a second dose of thiobarbiturate is given to reanesthetize the animal, these secondary body compartments are saturated and cannot absorb as much redistributed drug. After injection of the second dose, anesthetic drug concentrations in the brain are higher and remain higher for a longer time than after the first injection. If the second dose is not significantly smaller than the first, brain concentrations may be elevated to the point where respiratory arrest occurs.

These dynamics are similar in obese patients. When thiobarbiturates are initially injected, the drug readily enters well-perfused tissues such as the brain. In a sense, the brain and other well-perfused tissues receive nearly the entire dose because the drug does not enter fatty tissues very rapidly. If the dose of thiobarbiturates calculated for an obese animal is based on its total body weight, much of that total dose is delivered initially to the brain, resulting in excessive CNS depression, respiratory depression, and possibly cardiac depression. For this reason, obese animals should be given several small doses based on their estimated lean weight (actual weight less estimated weight of excess fat) so that the drug has time to enter poorly perfused adipose tissue and the brain is not overly affected. Because the barbiturates enter poorly perfused tissues slowly, they also leave poorly perfused tissues slowly, providing a continuing source of anesthetic that may prolong barbiturate anesthesia in obese animals for hours after drug administration.

A common side effect of ultra–short-acting barbiturates is cardiac arrhythmias (abnormal heart rhythms). Cardiac arrhythmias can be precipitated by concurrent administration of any two of the following: xylazine, halothane, methoxyflurane, and epinephrine. Excitement before anesthetic induction also predisposes an animal to cardiac arrhythmias from release of norepinephrine. On an electrocardiogram (ECG) monitor, one of the most common abnormalities is bigeminy, in which a normal QRS complex alternates with an abnormal complex (Fig. 8-1). Generally, bigeminy is not life threatening and spontaneously disappears or is lessened with administration of oxygen or lidocaine. As long as the animal is otherwise healthy and adequately oxygenated during anesthesia, this arrhythmia poses no significant risk.

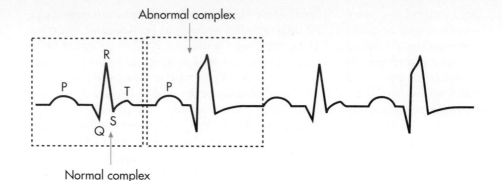

Abnormal complex

Normal complex

Fig. 8-1 Bigeminy is characterized by normal QRS complexes alternating with premature ventricular contractions.

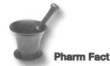

Pharm Fact

Sight hounds metabolize thiobarbiturates more slowly than do other breeds.

Greyhounds and other sight hounds metabolize thiobarbiturates much more slowly than they metabolize methohexital (Brevital), an ultra–short-acting oxybarbiturate. For this reason, some veterinarians prefer to use methohexital rather than thiobarbiturates in these dogs. Surgical anesthesia is usually maintained for 5 to 15 minutes after the initial injection of methohexital. Recovery is rapid and often accompanied by paddling, excitement, and muscle tremors. Methohexital is probably better used as an induction agent for gas anesthesia rather than as the sole anesthetic agent.

If the technician is cautious and aware of the animal's body condition and species and breed predisposition to adverse reactions to barbiturates, anesthetic accidents with these compounds can be minimized.

Propofol

Propofol is an injectable anesthetic agent unrelated to barbiturates. It is marketed as an emulsion of drug, egg lecithin, and soybean oil. Because of the nature of this emulsion, bacteria readily grow and produce endotoxins if the propofol emulsion is contaminated. For this reason, propofol is supplied in sterile glass ampules designed for a single use. Keeping an open ampule overnight for use the next day runs the risk of introducing iatrogenic (doctor-caused) sepsis.

Propofol is usually injected as an IV bolus and provides rapid induction of anesthesia and a short period of unconsciousness. Recovery time after a single bolus injection is about 20 minutes for dogs and 30 minutes for cats. The IV dosage is 3 to 8 mg/kg depending on whether the animal has been premedicated with a tranquilizer, sedative, or opioid. Propofol provides sedation and only minimal analgesic activity at dosages that do not induce full anesthesia. Even in an unconscious state, animals often respond to painful stimuli unless other analgesics such as xylazine and oxymorphone also are administered.

People given propofol sometimes complain of pain on injection; this may also occur in veterinary patients. This discomfort can be minimized by first using an analgesic such as xylazine or injecting the propofol into the larger veins. Fortunately, propofol, unlike thiobarbiturates, does not cause tissue inflammation or necrosis if injected perivascularly.

Propofol has the potential to enhance arrhythmias caused by epinephrine release associated with fear or stress, but it does not seem to generate arrhythmias alone. Because propofol is a phenol type of chemical, it is not conjugated and metabolized as readily by cats and can produce a Heinz-body anemia if given repeatedly.

Propofol is relatively expensive. If used as an anesthetic agent, it costs 15 to 20 times the cost of an equivalent period of anesthesia using halothane and approximately 5 times the cost of using isoflurane. However, because thiamylal is no longer available to veterinarians, propofol may gain favor for induction of anesthesia or short surgical or diagnostic procedures in small animals.

Dissociative Anesthetics

Ketamine and tiletamine (a component of Telazol) are short-acting injectable anesthetics that produce a rather unique form of anesthesia in which the animal feels dissociated (apart) from its body. A veterinary technician in a university veterinary teaching hospital accidentally received a dose of ketamine while attempting to inject a cat. She described feeling as though she were walking down the hall ahead of herself, in effect, dissociated from her body.

This dissociative effect is thought to be associated with overstimulation of the CNS, resulting in a cataleptic state. Catalepsis is characterized by a heightened emotional response, maintenance of many reflexes (laryngeal, pharyngeal, and corneal), a general lack of muscular relaxation (often increased muscle tone or rigidity), and an increased heart rate. The lack of muscular relaxation makes ketamine unsuitable as a sole anesthetic agent for major surgery. Both drugs are commonly used with a tranquilizer or sedative to reduce some of the CNS stimulation effects.

Ketamine and tiletamine produce good somatic (peripheral tissue) analgesia and are suitable for superficial surgery; however, they are much less effective in blocking visceral pain and should not be used alone as anesthesia for internal procedures.

In cats given ketamine, the eyes remain open and unblinking, which can dry the cornea. Therefore when using ketamine in cats, the veterinary professional should apply an ophthalmic lubricant or ointment to prevent corneal damage.

Some cats recovering from ketamine anesthesia develop seizures. Such seizures can be controlled with diazepam (Valium) administered intravenously. Most cats recovering from ketamine anesthesia and dogs recovering from tiletamine anesthesia appear delirious. The term "tennis match cats" is sometimes used to describe cats recovering from ketamine anesthesia. Their heads move in a rhythmic bobbing motion from one side to the other during this period. These recovering animals are best placed in areas with little visual or auditory stimulation; loud noises or bright lights may precipitate violent reactions or even seizures.

Pharm Fact

An ophthalmic lubricant should be applied to prevent corneal drying in cats anesthetized with ketamine.

Ketamine is well absorbed through the mucous membranes of the mouth and nasal cavity. The drug is sometimes squirted through the cage bars into the mouth of a hissing, fractious cat to subdue the animal enough to properly anesthetize it.

Another dissociative drug with hallucinogenic activity is phencyclidine, which has become well known as a widely abused drug known as *PCP* or *angel dust.* Because of its similarity to phencyclidine, ketamine has gained popularity in the past few years among drug users. Liquid ketamine, known on the streets as "special K," is evaporated to a white powder and then inhaled by the abuser. Ketamine is not classified as a controlled substance, so C-II, C-III, or C-IV is not inscribed on the label. Therefore the drug is often not locked up with the other substances subject to abuse. However, with ketamine's increasing popularity among drug users, veterinary hospitals have become targets for burglary by those eager to obtain the drug.

Tiletamine is commercially packaged with zolazepam, a benzodiazepine tranquilizer, in a product marketed as Telazol. Zolazepam reduces some of the CNS excitation and side effects produced by tiletamine. The product is used for restraint or anesthesia for minor procedures lasting less than an hour in cats and less than 30 minutes in dogs. As with ketamine, animals given tiletamine have open eyes (with the potential for corneal drying), poor muscle relaxation, and analgesia insufficient to prevent visceral pain. The zolazepam in Telazol reduces CNS excitation and provides some degree of muscle relaxation. Tiletamine anesthesia lasts longer and produces better analgesia than ketamine; however, even when tiletamine is combined with zolazepam in Telazol, the drug should be used for restraint or minor surgical procedures only.

Inhalant Anesthetics

Nitrous Oxide

Also referred to as "laughing gas," nitrous oxide is very safe when used properly and has much weaker analgesic qualities than other inhalant anesthetics. The major role of nitrous oxide is to decrease the amount of the more potent inhalant anesthetics needed to achieve a surgical plane of anesthesia.

Nitrous oxide alone enhances spontaneous breathing and may produce transient anxiety or excitement in people and animals. The gas diffuses through the body very rapidly and enters gas-filled body compartments such as the stomach, rumen, and loops of bowel. When a gas diffuses into a compartment, it increases the overall pressure within that compartment. Under normal conditions, this causes no ill effects. However, if the animal has a distended rumen, twisted necrotic bowel, dilated stomach (gastric dilation), or gas-filled thoracic cavity (pneumothorax), the increased pressure from nitrous oxide diffusion can rupture devitalized tissue or compress adjoining structures. Therefore nitrous oxide is contraindicated for use under these conditions.

At the end of surgery when the flow of inhalant anesthetic gas is ended, 100% oxygen should be administered at a high flow rate as the animal recovers with the endotracheal tube in place. When the flow of nitrous oxide ceases at the end of a surgical procedure, nitrous oxide rapidly diffuses out of tissues, into the blood, and then into the alveoli, diluting the oxygen concentration within the alveoli. If the flow of 100% oxygen has been turned off and the animal is receiving oxygen only from room air, which contains 15% to 17% oxygen, the oxygen concentration in the lungs can be diluted enough by the nitrous oxide to produce hypoxia. This phenomenon, called **diffusion hypoxia,** or the *second-gas effect,* is the reason for maintaining a high rate of oxygen flow for at least 5 to 10 minutes after the end of nitrous oxide administration.

Methoxyflurane

The inhalant anesthetic methoxyflurane (Metofane, Penthrane) is characterized by good muscle relaxation, a relatively slow rate of anesthetic induction compared with the rates of halothane and isoflurane, and a prolonged recovery period. Unlike halothane and isoflurane, methoxyflurane does not require a precision vaporizer for administration.

Up to 50% of methoxyflurane in the body is metabolized by the liver to various metabolites, including fluoride ions. These fluoride ions are excreted by the kidney and are nephrotoxic (toxic to the kidneys). Exposure to methoxyflurane has been implicated in acute renal failure in people and animals. For this reason, methoxyflurane should not be used with any other nephrotoxic drugs such as gentamicin, amikacin, or tetracycline. In addition, methoxyflurane should not be used or should be used only with great caution in older animals, dehydrated animals, and animals with renal disease because of their decreased ability to eliminate fluoride ions and decreased functional kidney reserve if renal toxicity occurs.

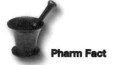

Pharm Fact

Methoxyflurane should not be used with other nephrotoxic drugs.

Because of the risk of nephrotoxicity from repeated methoxyflurane exposure, a methoxyflurane anesthetic machine should have an efficient and leak-free scavenger system to capture and remove the gas from the surgery suite and the building. Some veterinary anesthesiologists believe that for their own health, technicians should not work in a practice where methoxyflurane anesthetic gas is not properly scavenged from the surgery room.

Methoxyflurane is highly soluble in adipose tissue and diffuses easily into body fat deposits. Because fat is poorly perfused, the anesthetic can remain in these tissues for a long time. Thus obese animals tend to take longer to recover from methoxyflurane anesthesia than animals with less fat.

In addition to being soluble in fat, methoxyflurane is also soluble in rubber, such as that found in the Y tubes or the nonrebreathing apparatus attached to the anesthetic machine. Even after the methoxyflurane vaporizer has been turned off, methoxyflurane that has dissolved in the rubber leaches out of the rubber and into the tube's lumen, providing additional anesthetic gas to the animal. A quick sniff of these rubber hoses an hour after a surgical procedure verifies that the methoxyflurane impregnating the rubber tubes is still evaporating to the environment. Thus the anesthetic recovery period is prolonged if the animal continues to breathe through the rubber anesthetic machine hoses after the need for anesthesia has ended.

Halothane

Like methoxyflurane, halothane (Fluothane) is a nonflammable, nonirritating inhalant anesthetic that can be used in all species. Anesthesia is induced much more rapidly with halothane than with methoxyflurane. Because of its chemical and physical properties, halothane should be administered with a precision vaporizer. A much lower percentage of halothane is metabolized by the liver than methoxyflurane. However, the fluoride and bromide metabolites of halothane have been implicated in producing hepatotoxicity in human patients repeatedly anesthetized for extended periods with halothane. Although the potential for this exists in veterinary patients, similar syndromes have rarely been reported in the veterinary literature.

A more common disadvantage of halothane is that it sensitizes the heart to epinephrine and predisposes to arrhythmias caused by excitement or stress associated with fear or struggling during anesthetic induction. The effects of stress and fear can be reduced by administration of tranquilizers or sedatives before induction of anesthesia.

An abnormal thermoregulatory response has been reported in people, horses, pigs, and occasionally dogs and cats anesthetized with halothane. This condition, called **malignant hyperthermia,** occurs in a small number of animals and is characterized by sudden onset of an extremely elevated body temperature that can result in brain damage or death. Rapid recognition of the condition and aggressive treatment to lower the core body temperature can save some animals experiencing malignant hyperthermia. The more common effect of halothane on body temperature is **hypothermia,** or subnormal body temperature, which is caused by halothane's inhibition of the thermoregulatory centers in the brain, reducing the normal reflexes that maintain body temperature such as shivering and vasoconstriction.

Although animals anesthetized with methoxyflurane can almost regulate anesthetic depth themselves because methoxyflurane depresses respiration, halothane often produces tachypnea (an increased rate of breathing) by a mechanism that is not well understood. Tachypnea causes more halothane to be taken into the body, producing a deeper plane of anesthesia. Therefore halothane anesthesia generally requires closer monitoring than that required with methoxyflurane anesthesia.

Isoflurane

The inhalant anesthetic isoflurane (Forane, AErrane) has gained popularity in veterinary practices because of its rapid, smooth induction of anesthesia and short recovery period. Other inhalant agents with similar properties of isoflurane include enflurane (Ethrane), desflurane (Suprane), and sevoflurane (Ultane). Isoflurane is not metabolized to any significant amount and therefore does not produce toxic metabolites as methoxyflurane and halothane do.

Unlike halothane, isoflurane produces much less sensitization of the myocardium to epinephrine or similar sympathomimetic compounds. Some anesthesiologists have stated that halothane-related arrhythmias may resolve if the anesthesia is switched to isoflurane. Nonetheless, reducing excessive stress, which produces sympathetic nervous system stimulation, and avoiding the use of catecholamine drugs such as epinephrine, norepinephrine, and dopamine before or during isoflurane use is prudent.

Isoflurane and related anesthetics require use of a precise, temperature-compensated vaporizer and vigilant patient monitoring during anesthesia. The rapid recovery from isoflurane anesthesia in cats has sometimes resulted in delirium and a somewhat stormy recovery. Use of a tranquilizer or sedative before anesthetic induction with isoflurane can smooth the recovery period.

TRANQUILIZERS AND SEDATIVES

Acepromazine

Acepromazine maleate is a phenothiazine **tranquilizer** that reduces anxiety and produces a mentally relaxed state. It is often used to calm animals for physical examination or transport. Unlike xylazine, detomidine, or medetomidine, which relieve pain, phenothiazine tranquilizers have no analgesic effect. In addition to its tranquilizing effect, acepromazine is commonly used to decrease vomiting associated with motion sickness or stimulation of the chemoreceptor trigger zone by drugs such as cancer chemotherapeutic agents and narcotic analgesics. Acepromazine and other phenothiazines have little effect in preventing vomiting caused by irritation or direct stimulation of the gastrointestinal (GI) tract.

Although phenothiazine tranquilizers are generally very safe, in some situations they should be used with caution or should not be used at all. Acepromazine reduces the threshold of seizure activity in animals with epilepsy, making seizures more likely and making it contraindicated for use in animals with a history of seizures. Acepromazine also should not be used to tranquilize animals before myelography, a procedure commonly used to assess the spinal cord in which contrast material is injected into the cerebrospinal fluid for a radiographic contrast study. The contrast material predisposes the animal to seizures, and concurrent use of acepromazine increases that risk.

In addition to their other activities, phenothiazines also block the α_1 receptors found on smooth muscle cells of peripheral blood vessels (see Chapter 5). Stimulation of these receptors normally causes vasoconstriction (constriction of blood vessels). Hence blocking these receptors results in relaxation of smooth muscle and vasodilation. This blocking activity, combined with acepromazine's direct relaxation of vascular smooth muscles and depression of some normal blood pressure regulatory mechanisms, causes a marked drop in blood pressure. For this reason, phenothiazines should be used with caution or not used in animals with hypotension (decreased blood pressure) associated with shock, blood loss, or dehydration.

A common effect of phenothiazine tranquilizers is protrusion of the nictitating membrane (third eyelid). This can be alarming to clients using the drug for the first time to control their dog's motion sickness. It also makes ophthalmologic examination more difficult.

Another side effect of phenothiazine tranquilizers includes transient or permanent penile prolapse in stallions, reducing or preventing the animal's use in breeding. Additional side effects that should be considered include an antihistaminic effect that can interfere with intradermal (allergy) testing

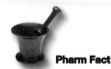

Pharm Fact

Phenothiazine tranquilizers should be used cautiously in animals with hypotension.

procedures and the occasional frenzied or aggressive behavior seen in cats and dogs receiving the drug.

Droperidol

Droperidol tranquilizer is very similar to the phenothiazine tranquilizers but belongs to another class of drugs called the *butyrophenones*. Like acepromazine, it has an α-adrenergic blocking effect and should be used with caution in animals that are hypotensive. It has much more potent **sedative** and antiemetic effects than most phenothiazine tranquilizers. Droperidol has been combined with fentanyl, a strong narcotic analgesic with emetic activity, and marketed as a neuroleptanalgesic product called Innovar-Vet.

Diazepam, Zolazepam, Midazolam, and Clonazepam

Diazepam (Valium), zolazepam (contained in Telazol), midazolam (Versed), and clonazepam (Klonopin) are benzodiazepine tranquilizers often used with other agents as part of a preanesthetic protocol for their calming and muscle-relaxing effects. Zolazepam is combined with tiletamine, the dissociative anesthetic described previously, in the short-acting, sedative-analgesic product Telazol. Diazepam is often combined with ketamine to provide similar actions. Midazolam is a good alternative to diazepam for use with dissociative anesthetics. Clonazepam is not used as preanesthetic but is used in anticonvulsant therapy for seizure control.

Unlike the phenothiazine tranquilizers, benzodiazepines have little effect on the brain's chemoreceptor trigger zone and therefore are not useful in preventing motion sickness. Unlike phenothiazines, benzodiazepines decrease the risk of seizure activity. For this reason, diazepam and clonazepam are used in conjunction with phenobarbital to control seizure activity. Diazepam is the intravenous drug of choice for control of status epilepticus, the actual state of seizing.

Because of their stimulatory effects on the appetite center in the brain, diazepam and midazolam have been used to increase the appetite in anorectic cats. Overall, the benzodiazepines are very safe compounds and have few side effects of clinical significance. (The anticonvulsant aspects of these drugs are discussed in greater detail later in this chapter.)

Xylazine, Detomidine, and Medetomidine

Xylazine (Rompun, Anased), detomidine (Dormosedan), and medetomidine (Domitor) are sedatives classified as α_2 agonists because they exert their effect by stimulating **α_2 receptors** located on neurons that normally release norepinephrine. These compounds produce a calming effect and somewhat decrease an animal's ability to respond to stimuli. All three drugs also have some analgesic activity.

When these drugs attach to and stimulate α_2 receptors located on the terminal bouton of norepinephrine-secreting neurons (Fig. 8-2), they decrease norepinephrine release. Norepinephrine is part of the sympathetic nervous system and plays a role in maintaining general alertness; therefore inhibition of norepinephrine release by xylazine, detomidine, or medetomidine results in sedation.

Xylazine alone is used in most species for sedation or analgesia or may be combined with other drugs in a preanesthetic regimen. Xylazine is marketed in a large animal concentration (100 mg/ml) and a small animal concentration (20 mg/ml). Because the bottles containing the different concentrations appear similar, an animal could be overdosed or underdosed if the wrong concentration is used.

A disadvantage of xylazine is that sedative doses produce vomiting, or emesis, in about 90% of cats and 50% of dogs. Some veterinarians use xylazine as a routine part of a preanesthetic regimen to induce emesis in animals that may have eaten before surgery. If vomiting is induced while the animal is still conscious rather than after it has been anesthetized, it is not as likely to aspirate vomitus into the lungs. Because of its emetic effect, xylazine is contraindicated in animals with gastric torsion, bloat, ingestion of caustic substances, or other circumstances in which vomiting is dangerous. In such cases, vomiting may be prevented to some degree by use of phenothiazine tranquilizers such as acepromazine.

Occasionally, intravenous (IV) or intramuscular (IM) administration of xylazine in large-breed dogs can produce acute abdominal distention. The distention is caused by either aerophagia (swallowing air) or decreased gastric tone with subsequent accumulation of gas. Deep-chested, large-breed dogs given xylazine should be observed closely; dogs with this body configuration are predisposed to gastric dilation and volvulus, which is a twisting of the stomach on its attachments.

In horses, xylazine and detomidine are used for relieving pain associated with GI and other abdominal conditions such as colic. The analgesic effect of detomidine lasts longer than that of xylazine; the analgesic effect of either drug is of shorter duration than the sedative effect. These drugs can be used to control visceral pain associated with intestinal disease, but their analgesic

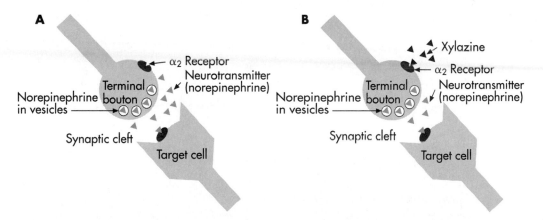

Fig. 8-2 Mechanism of action for α_2-agonist drugs. **A,** Normally, epinephrine is released and travels across the synaptic cleft to receptors on the target cell. When the receptors are filled, the extra norepinephrine released provides negative feedback to prevent further release by attaching to the α_2 receptor on the terminal bouton. **B,** When xylazine is present, it attaches to the α_2 receptors on the terminal bouton. This simulates the negative feedback provided by the extra norepinephrine and decreases its release.

effect on somatic (or nonvisceral) tissue is limited, and pain perception on the limbs or skin may even be increased, a condition called *hyperalgesia.*

Accidental injection of xylazine in the carotid artery of horses or an IV overdose can produce violent seizures and sudden death resulting from overstimulation of α_1 receptors in the CNS. Detomidine is less likely to produce this effect because it selectively stimulates α_2 receptors, which does not cause seizures, and has much less effect on the α_1 receptors in the CNS associated with these violent reactions. Medetomidine is only approved for use in dogs at the time of this publication, but like detomidine, it is more selective for the α_2 receptor.

Cattle are very sensitive to the effects of α_2 agonists like xylazine. Only 10% of the equivalent equine dose produces a similar degree of sedation in cattle. As with the gastric distention that occurs in dogs, cattle are predisposed to rumen stasis (decreased rumen motility), with subsequent development of gas, a condition known as *tympany.* In cattle and other ruminants, xylazine can cause contraction of uterine smooth muscle. If given to pregnant ruminants, xylazine can induce premature onset of parturition. This effect has not been noted in horses or small animals.

Swine appear to be quite resistant to the effects of xylazine and require much higher dosages to produce any sedative effect. For this reason, α_2 agonists are not used in swine.

Detomidine, medetomidine, and xylazine cause fairly predictable changes in cardiovascular function. After injection of an IV bolus, blood pressure initially increases in response to stimulation of α_1 receptors on vascular smooth muscle and subsequent precapillary vasoconstriction (see Chapter 5). As the normal reflexes to the increased blood pressure slow the heart and as the sympathetic nervous system is blocked, the heart rate slows, producing bradycardia, and blood pressure drops to normal or subnormal levels.

With increasing doses of medetomidine, detomidine, or xylazine, the risk of first- or second-degree atrioventricular block increases (see Chapter 5). In heart block, impulses traveling from the depolarized atrium to the ventricles are slowed or blocked entirely. As shown in Fig. 8-3, first-degree heart block

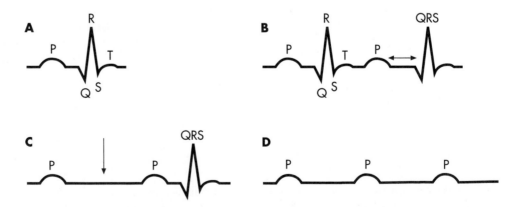

Fig. 8-3 ECG manifestations of the different types of atrioventricular (heart) block. **A,** Normal complex. **B,** First-degree AV block (increased distance between P and QRS). **C,** Second-degree AV block (loss of QRS complex). **D,** Third-degree AV block (P waves without QRS). Ventricular escape complex not shown.

is manifested on the ECG as an increased interval between the P wave and QRS complex and second-degree heart block is indicated by an occasional P wave without the QRS complex. Atropine may be used to reverse or decrease the bradycardia or atrioventricular block but should not be used in horses with colic because of the possibility of atropine-induced ileus, a cessation of intestinal motility.

With the administration of xylazine, medetomidine, or detomidine, increasing the dose does not proportionally increase the depth of sedation or analgesia but only increases the duration of activity. Therefore if an animal has received an effective dose of either drug but is still responding to pain or is displaying agitation, administration of another analgesic drug should be considered rather than increasing the dose of xylazine, medetomidine, or detomidine. Stress or fear in the animal before administration of α_2-agonist drugs is a common reason for failure to achieve desired levels of sedation. Catecholamines such as norepinephrine and epinephrine released from the sympathetic nervous system stimulation compete for sites on the α_2 receptor and can prevent the xylazine, medetomidine, or detomidine molecules from reaching these sites and producing the desired sedation.

The effects of medetomidine, xylazine, or detomidine sedation can be reversed with α_2 antagonists such as yohimbine, atipamezole, and tolazoline. Yohimbine and atipamezole are marketed as veterinary formulations (Yobine and Antisedan respectively), and tolazoline is available as a human formulation (Priscoline). Doxapram (Dopram) is sometimes recommended for reversal of respiratory depression associated with α_2 antagonist use; however, it should be used with caution or avoided altogether because it may result in unpredictable or aggressive behavior.

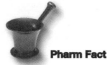

Pharm Fact

Increasing the dose of xylazine increases the duration of action but not necessarily the analgesic or sedative effect.

ANALGESICS

Analgesics are drugs that reduce the perception of pain without loss of other sensations. Some sedatives mentioned previously have analgesic effects, but the most potent analgesics generally include the opioids.

Narcotic or Opioid Analgesics

Narcotic or opioid analgesics derive their name from the narcosis, or stuporous state of disorientation, produced by opium-related compounds. Opioids, a name that means "opium-like", are often used as part of a preanesthetic or general anesthetic regimen to reduce the need for other anesthetic agents. Butorphanol, pentazocine, and buprenorphine are classified as **partial agonists** (see Chapter 3) and generally have weaker opioid effects than oxymorphone, meperidine, codeine, and morphine sulfate. Because they are partial agonists, drugs such as butorphanol are sometimes used to partially reverse oxymorphone narcosis.

Opioids act by attaching to opioid receptors in the CNS, GI tract, urinary tract, and smooth muscle. The effects of a given opioid can vary tremendously between species. The veterinary professional should *never* assume that because a particular opioid is safe for use in one species, it is safe for use in another. These differences in opioid effects among species are related to the multiple classes and subclasses of opioid receptors, of which only three are responsible for the bulk of observable effects. Veterinary technicians can better understand the way opioids work by studying a drug's package insert, closely observing animals medicated with narcotics, and learning the specific actions each drug has on the species treated.

Mu (μ) receptors are found throughout the brain and are primarily responsible for the analgesia and euphoria associated with narcosis. These μ receptors are also thought to be associated with respiratory depression, miosis (pupillary constriction), and hypothermia. Therefore an opioid drug with strong analgesic effects is also likely to cause significant respiratory depression, a common side effect of opioid analgesia. Codeine and butorphanol are commonly used as cough suppressants because of their μ activity.

When stimulated by an opioid drug, **kappa (κ)** receptors also produce analgesia as well as sedation and miosis without respiratory depression. The **sigma (σ)** receptors are responsible for the dysphoria (excitement and struggling), hallucinations, mydriasis (pupillary dilation), and cardiac and respiratory stimulation seen in cats, horses, cattle, and swine that are given opioids.

The proportions of the three classes of opioid receptors found in a species and an opioid drug's affinity for these different receptors determine whether that opioid is an effective analgesic or has such severe side effects that it should not be used. Ideally, an opioid should have strong κ-receptor activity and fairly good μ-receptor action because these receptors are associated with the desirable effects of analgesia, sedation, and euphoria. Opioids with a significant σ receptor effect are more likely to have adverse effects. An additional receptor, called a *delta (δ) receptor,* may play an important but as yet undefined role in the activity of other opioid receptors.

Because of their central parasympathetic effects, opioids often cause salivation, vomiting, and defecation. Opioids also increase segmental intestinal contractions and muscle tone of the alimentary sphincters, which is the reason these drugs are used as antidiarrheals (see Chapter 4). The central parasympathetic effect can also slow the heart rate and, when combined with the decreased activity of α receptors on the blood vessels, can result in hypotension, syncope (fainting), and prolonged capillary refill time (see Chapter 5). Some effects may not be evident if the opioid produces cardiac stimulation through σ-receptor stimulation. In general, opioids should not be used in animals with severe bradycardia. Parasympathetic-induced bradycardia is reversed through the administration of atropine to block vagal nerve stimulation.

Opioids produce analgesia through their action on opioid receptors, but most opioids do not induce anesthesia. Therefore animals given opioids can still respond to sound, cold, heat, taste, and visual stimuli. Some animals medicated with opioids may appear to become hypersensitive to sound, resulting in an exaggerated response to noise. Animals recovering from significant doses of opioids should be placed in a quiet room to avoid a stormy recovery.

An advantage of using opioids for analgesia or in anesthetic regimens is that their effects are reversible with narcotic antagonists. These drugs reverse some of the effects of opioid narcosis by competing for sites on the μ receptors. Naloxone is considered a "pure" narcotic antagonist because when it combines with μ and κ receptors, it has little or no intrinsic activity (meaning no effect on the cell) and thus reverses the sedation, analgesia, and respiratory depression of potent opioids (such as oxymorphone) without producing sedation of its own. Naloxone is not very effective in reversing the emetic effects of apomorphine, which is a dopamine receptor effect, and has little effect in blocking σ receptors.

Nalorphine is another reversal agent with very good antagonistic action on μ receptors, but it causes some sedation through stimulation of κ receptors. Because nalorphine reverses the stronger effects of oxymorphone but contributes some sedation of its own, it is considered a partial antagonist and also a *partial agonist.* Butorphanol, pentazocine, and buprenorphine are sometimes used to partially reverse some of the respiratory depression and sedation caused by stronger narcotic agents.

Oxymorphone (Numorphan) is one of the more potent opioids commonly used for preanesthesia and anesthesia. It has a much greater analgesic effect than morphine sulfate and does not stimulate vomiting or defecation. This drug should be used with caution in neonates, geriatric animals, and animals with severe liver disease because elimination of oxymorphone may be delayed in these cases. When combined with acepromazine, oxymorphone is safe for induction of anesthesia in dogs and cats, although larger doses in cats can produce a frenzied state. This dysphoria is commonly referred to as "morphine mania."

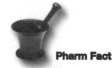

Pharm Fact

Narcotic drugs can produce frenzied behavior in cats, a condition termed "morphine mania."

Butorphanol (Torbutrol, Torbugesic) is a synthetic opioid with partial agonist and partial antagonist activity that is used for cough control in small animals and for reduction of colic pain in horses. Larger doses of butorphanol occasionally cause excitement in "high-strung" horses if not administered with a sedative such as xylazine or detomidine. This is usually true for most larger opioid doses in horses. Because it is a partial agonist and antagonist, butorphanol can be used to reverse some narcotic effects of such drugs as oxymorphone while providing some analgesia and sedation of its own.

Fentanyl is a potent opioid with an analgesic effect 250 times greater than that of morphine. Whereas most narcotics are respiratory depressants, the respiratory effects of fentanyl vary from apnea, which is cessation of breathing, to panting. Fentanyl often produces bradycardia through stimulation of the vagus nerve. Such vagally mediated bradycardia can be combatted with atropine or glycopyrrolate administration, which blocks parasympathetic stimulation. Fentanyl does not cause vomiting; however, it relaxes anal sphincter tone. Dogs anesthetized with Innovar-Vet (fentanyl and droperidol) frequently defecate or have flatus (gas).

Meperidine (Demerol) is a fairly weak analgesic and sedative and is fairly safe when injected subcutaneously to restrain cats. An advantage of meperidine is that like atropine, it reduces salivary and respiratory secretions and does not cause vomiting or defecation.

Pentazocine (Talwin) is a weak analgesic with partial agonist and antagonist activity. It is indicated for use in horses with colic and for dogs recovering from painful surgery. Its use in cats is controversial. Some researchers believe that the drug should not be used in cats because of the dysphoria associated with pentazocine. Others state that the drug is safe to use in cats if given in small doses.

Buprenorphine (Buprenex) is a partial agonist and antagonist with moderately strong analgesic properties. It is most commonly combined with sedatives or tranquilizers such as acepromazine, xylazine, and detomidine for neuroleptanalgesia. It is also used alone in dogs and cats as an analgesic, both for its potency, which is 30 times the analgesic potency of morphine, and its 8- to 12-hour period of analgesia through μ-receptor stimulation.

Etorphine (M-99) is used to sedate and capture wildlife or zoo animals. It is an extremely potent narcotic, with 1000 times the analgesic potency of morphine, and for that reason must be handled with great caution to avoid accidental injection of animal handlers. Failure to administer a narcotic antagonist after accidental self-injection can result in death from CNS depression and respiratory arrest.

Neuroleptanalgesics

Neuroleptanalgesia refers to a state of CNS depression and analgesia induced by a combination of a sedative such as xylazine or tranquilizer such as acepromazine and an analgesic such as oxymorphone. Phenothiazine tranquilizers or butyrophenone tranquilizers such as droperidol calm the animal and also decrease or block the emetic side effect of a narcotic analgesic. Innovar-Vet is a neuroleptanalgesic product containing droperidol and fentanyl, the latter of which is a narcotic analgesic. Side effects are most commonly associated with the narcotic component of the neuroleptanalgesic.

ANTICONVULSANTS

Seizures are periods of altered brain function characterized by loss of consciousness, increased muscle tone or movement, altered sensations, and other neurologic changes. **Convulsions** are seizures characterized by spastic muscle movement. In the following discussion, use of the term *seizure* also includes convulsions.

Seizures can be caused by various pathologic states such as hypoxia (low tissue oxygen tension), hypoglycemia (low blood sugar level), hypocalcemia (low blood calcium level), and toxicity such as that caused by lead, strychnine, and organophosphates. Infectious diseases such as canine distemper, or conditions such as hydrocephalus, neoplasia, and parasitic migration involving the CNS also may precipitate seizures.

Recurrent seizures are referred to as **epilepsy,** whereas recurrent seizures of unknown cause are referred to as **idiopathic epilepsy.** *Status epilepticus* refers to the state of being in the seizure activity and often is used to describe the condition of animals with prolonged seizure activity.

Seizures typically have three phases. The **preictal phase (aura)** occurs before a seizure begins and may be characterized by pacing, panting, anxiety, apprehension, and other behavioral changes. This phase may last for minutes or hours before a seizure. The seizure, or **ictus,** itself lasts only 1 to 2 minutes and may be **focal,** (involving only a limited area such as one limb), or **generalized** (involving the entire body).

Generalized seizures in animals are usually described as **grand mal** and involve spastic muscle contractions such as paddling, leg extension, and opisthotonos. **Petit mal seizures** are uncommon in animals and are characterized by brief loss of consciousness. The **postictal phase** occurs after the seizure activity has subsided. During this phase, which can last from seconds to hours, the animal may appear tired, confused, anxious, or even blind depending on the nature and location of the seizure activity within the CNS and the type of seizure experienced.

Drugs used to control seizures are called **anticonvulsants.** Most seizures, although frightening to the animal's owner, are usually not life threatening. However, the underlying cause may eventually be life threatening. Therefore a dog that has minor seizures twice a year with 6 months of normal behavior between episodes may not be a candidate for daily anticonvulsant therapy. On the other hand, if the client is upset by the seizures and is willing to medicate the animal daily to prevent them, no reason exists to oppose this decision. Seizure activity in a horse or livestock usually warrants euthanasia because of the potential for injury to animal handlers and others near the animal during a seizure.

Phenobarbital

Phenobarbital is the drug of choice for long-term control of seizures in dogs and cats. This barbiturate is inexpensive and, because of its long half-life, may be given orally once or twice a day. Phenobarbital acts by decreasing the likelihood of spontaneous depolarization in brain cells. If such depolarization occurs, phenobarbital helps prevent its spread throughout the brain, resulting in a milder seizure.

Phenobarbital is biotransformed by a specific family of enzymes found primarily in the liver. This group of enzymes, sometimes referred to as the **mixed-function oxidase enzyme system,** is also responsible for metabolism of a number of commonly used drugs. As discussed previously, this enzyme system can be induced, resulting in the rate of drug metabolism increasing with repeated doses of phenobarbital. The net effect of induction is that phenobarbital and any other drugs metabolized by the mixed-function oxidase system are broken down more rapidly and circulating concentrations are lower. This is the reason animals and people develop tolerance to repeated doses of barbiturates and require an increasingly larger dose to achieve the same effect. Similarly, in epileptic animals treated with phenobarbital, the dose of any other drugs using the same metabolic pathway must be increased to compensate for their increased metabolism.

In contrast to induced metabolism, use of the antibiotic chloramphenicol may inhibit phenobarbital metabolism, resulting in elevated barbiturate concentrations and consequent increased sedation and ataxia. If chloramphenicol is temporarily used in dogs being treated with phenobarbital for seizure control, the dose of the barbiturate may need to be decreased until chloramphenicol use is discontinued.

As with most other barbiturates, phenobarbital is highly protein bound. When plasma protein levels are decreased such as from liver disease, more

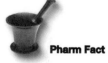

Pharm Fact

Concurrent use of certain other drugs may increase or decrease the required dose of phenobarbital.

phenobarbital becomes available in the free form and more phenobarbital molecules are free to diffuse into the brain, producing its clinical effect (see Chapter 3). Thus animals with hypoproteinemia may require lower dosages of phenobarbital. Use of salicylates such as aspirin or sulfonamide antimicrobials also increases the amount of free phenobarbital by displacing the barbiturate from sites on plasma proteins.

Cats have less ability than dogs to metabolize phenobarbital. Consequently, phenobarbital dosages in cats are about half those used in dogs. Plasma concentrations of phenobarbital vary widely depending on the drug's degree of absorbtion and the speed of its metabolism and elimination. As much as a sixfold difference in plasma drug concentrations may be presents in dogs of similar weights, ages, and breeds.

When a veterinarian begins treating an animal with phenobarbital, past experience is often used in estimating the dosage to prevent seizure activity. Because plasma phenobarbital concentrations vary considerably, they should be checked periodically by a veterinary diagnostic laboratory. Without such monitoring, some veterinarians continue to increase a phenobarbital dose if seizures are not well controlled without knowing whether the dosage previously used was inadequate or whether the poor control is associated with underlying disease that is resistant to barbiturate. The only way to determine this is to measure the plasma concentration of the barbiturate.

Serum activity of liver-derived enzymes such as alkaline phosphatase and alanine aminotransferase may be mildly increased after an animal has received phenobarbital. Serum activity of alkaline phosphatase may be increased fourfold above normal ranges. As long as the activity of other liver enzymes is not markedly increased, this finding is acceptable. Serum activity of liver-derived enzymes returns to normal a few weeks after phenobarbital therapy is discontinued.

Occasionally a dog receiving phenobarbital becomes excitable or hyperactive instead of lethargic or sedated. This may occur at a subtherapeutic dose, and an increase in the dose of phenobarbital does not seem to decrease this effect. This **idiosyncratic reaction** to phenobarbital is individual and erratic and is not dose dependent. That is, as the dose increases, signs do not increase in severity. Therefore these animals must be treated with a different anticonvulsant.

The dose of phenobarbital is often measured in **grains,** with 1 grain equaling approximately 60 mg. Tablets are usually available in ¼-, ½-, 1-, and 2-grain sizes, which roughly correspond to 15, 30, 60, and 120 mg, respectively.

Primidone

Primidone has been used for a number of years in veterinary medicine to control seizure activity. Although primidone itself has some anticonvulsant activity, most of its efficacy is attributable to phenobarbital produced by metabolism of primidone. The other primidone metabolite, phenylethylmalonamide, has weak anticonvulsant activity in dogs. Because

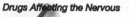

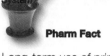

Pharm Fact

Long-term use of primidone with phenytoin may cause hepatopathy.

the efficacy of primidone largely depends on its metabolism to phenobarbital, many clinicians simply give phenobarbital rather than primidone.

The side effects and drug interactions of primidone are similar to those seen with phenobarbital. Long-term use of large doses of primidone, especially if used in conjunction with the anticonvulsant phenytoin (Dilantin), has been implicated in **drug-induced hepatopathy.** This syndrome is characterized by diffuse inflammation and destruction of the liver. Unfortunately, once the signs become apparent, the prognosis for recovery is poor.

If a veterinarian is considering switching anticonvulsants from primidone to phenobarbital, a reasonable dosage conversion rate is 60 mg of phenobarbital for each 250 mg of primidone. Plasma concentrations of phenobarbital should be measured in treated dogs 1 to 2 weeks after conversion to phenobarbital to determine the plasma concentration relative to the normal therapeutic range.

Phenytoin

Phenytoin (Dilantin) is a human anticonvulsant that was once popular for use in treating epilepsy in animals. The major disadvantage of phenytoin is that maintaining therapeutic plasma concentrations of drug is difficult in dogs. The drug is poorly and erratically absorbed from the GI tract and, once absorbed, is rapidly eliminated by the liver. Phenytoin must be given at least 3 times daily to maintain therapeutic levels in plasma.

Another disadvantage of phenytoin is that at doses necessary to achieve and maintain therapeutic plasma concentrations, the enzyme system that eliminates phenytoin becomes saturated. For most drugs, as concentrations increase, the rate at which the drug leaves the blood also increases (see Chapter 3). Therefore very high plasma concentrations of drugs tend to drop rapidly. For phenytoin, this occurs until drug concentrations rise high enough to saturate the enzyme system. At that point, the elimination system, which is working at its maximum rate, is overwhelmed, resulting in accumulation of the drug in the body.

As with primidone, phenytoin has also been implicated in drug-induced hepatopathy, usually when the drug is used in conjunction with primidone. Because of its poor absorption, short half-life, saturation kinetics, and risk of liver damage, phenytoin is not generally recommended for use in controlling idiopathic epilepsy.

Diazepam

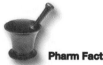

Pharm Fact

Diazepam is effective in controlling seizures if injected intravenously, but it has a short duration of action.

Diazepam (Valium) is the drug of choice for emergency treatment of convulsing animals. Benzodiazepine tranquilizers such as diazepam and clonazepam control seizures by enhancing the inhibitory effect of the CNS neurotransmitter γ-aminobutyric acid (GABA). GABA helps counter the effect of stimulatory neurotransmitters in the brain such as acetylcholine, norepinephrine, and others. By enhancing the GABA effect, benzodiazepines "quiet" the activity of the CNS.

Diazepam is very effective when given intravenously but poorly effective when given by mouth. Only about 2% to 5% of the diazepam given orally to dogs enters the systemic circulation because of the first-pass effect (see Chapter 3). The first-pass effect occurs when drugs absorbed from the intestinal tract pass via the hepatic portal system to the liver and are eliminated before they reach the systemic circulation. This rapid elimination also explains diazepam's fairly short duration of activity when it is given intravenously.

In animals with underlying conditions that continue to produce seizures such as strychnine poisoning, IV administration of diazepam every 10 to 20 minutes to control the seizures is often necessary. These animals may be more practically treated with IV pentobarbital or phenobarbital because these drugs control the seizures for a longer time than diazepam. Seizures of this nature are sometimes treated with IV fluid drips containing diazepam; the drip bottle or bag should be inverted several times to distribute the diazepam in the solution, since it does not mix well with most fluids.

Diazepam is absorbed irregularly if injected subcutaneously or intramuscularly. Because cats are less efficient at eliminating diazepam than dogs, this drug tends to be more effective in the former when given orally. Diazepam is sometimes used as an appetite stimulant in cats.

Clonazepam

Clonazepam (Klonopin) is a benzodiazepine tranquilizer related to diazepam. It is occasionally used with phenobarbital in animals in which plasma concentrations of barbiturate are in the therapeutic range but the seizures are not adequately controlled. Clonazepam is less rapidly eliminated than diazepam and is better absorbed when administered orally.

A disadvantage of clonazepam is that it is expensive, and the recommended dosage of 0.1 to 0.5 mg/kg 3 times daily often requires administration of a large number of tablets each day. For example, an 88-lb German Shepherd requires between 4 to 20 mg of clonazepam 3 times a day. Clonazepam is available only in ½-, 1-, and 2-mg tablets, requiring administration of 6 to 30 tablets a day in this large dog. For smaller dogs, clonazepam may be a reasonable alternative to phenobarbital and has few side effects. Unfortunately, most animals develop a tolerance to clonazepam within the first year of treatment.

Potassium Bromide

Potassium bromide may be used daily in conjunction with phenobarbital to control seizures. Like phenobarbital, potassium bromide has a very long half-life; thus several days of drug administration are needed to achieve therapeutic levels and steady-state plasma concentrations (see Chapter 3).

Potassium bromide has a narrow therapeutic index, meaning that the dose producing therapeutic effects is very close to the dose causing toxicity. The most common side effects are GI irritation in the form of anorexia, vomiting, and diarrhea; sedation; stupor; and skin rash, which is more commonly associated with chronic toxicity.

Potassium bromide is not available from pharmaceutical distributors but must be obtained as a chemical from supply companies or special pharmacies. The powder is mixed with dextrose or corn syrup and administered once daily by mouth.

Several laboratories in the United States can measure plasma concentrations of potassium bromide. Animals treated with potassium bromide may show a false elevation of serum chloride levels because of the insensitivity of some blood chemistry analyzers to differentiate between chloride and bromide ions.

Valproic Acid

Valproic acid (sodium valproate) may be used as an adjunct to phenobarbital in dogs that do not respond to other anticonvulsants used alone. The drug has a short half-life of 1.7 to 3.1 hours.

CENTRAL NERVOUS SYSTEM STIMULANTS

CNS stimulants are primarily used to stimulate respiration in anesthetized animals or to reverse CNS depression caused by anesthetic or sedative agents. Therapeutic or toxic CNS stimulants act by any of several mechanisms:

- Promote release of excitatory neurotransmitters such as acetylcholine and norepinephrine
- Delay separation of excitatory neurotransmitters from their receptors
- Inhibit release of inhibitory neurotransmitters such as GABA and adenosine
- Facilitate the breakdown or removal of inhibitory neurotransmitters after their release
- Inhibit processes that prevent release of excitatory neurotransmitters such as by blocking α_2 receptors

The processes described in the last three items are often referred to as **disinhibition** because they inhibit an inhibitory process, resulting in CNS stimulation. Common toxicants that operate by one of these mechanisms include strychnine, which blocks GABA activity; theobromine, the component in chocolate that increases norepinephrine release and inhibits adenosine activity; caffeine, which has a mechanism of action similar to that of theobromine and is commonly found in "diet pills"; and amphetamines or cocaine, drugs that are commonly abused.

Methylxanthines

Caffeine and theobromine belong to a broad group of drugs known as *methylxanthines,* which include the respiratory drugs theophylline and aminophylline (see Chapter 6). Because "chocolate toxicity" in dogs has been a popular topic in magazines and newspapers, veterinary technicians should be aware of facts surrounding this syndrome. The active ingredient in chocolate is theobromine. A dosage as low as 90 mg/kg (41 mg/lb) can

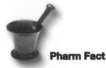

produce toxicity in dogs, although some sources say that the dosage at which half of the animals given that dosage will die (LD_{50}) for theobromine is 250 to 500 mg/kg (114 to 228 mg/lb).

A typical chocolate bar contains 2 or 3 ounces of milk chocolate, and 4 ounces of milk chocolate contain about 240 mg of theobromine. A 10-lb dog would have to ingest two or three candy bars to produce serious toxicity. Fortunately, ingestion of that much chocolate by such a small dog would likely produce vomiting, thus decreasing the amount of theobromine absorbed.

A greater danger comes from ingestion of unsweetened baking chocolate, which usually contains 390 mg of theobromine per ounce. Thus a single ounce of baking chocolate could be enough to produce severe toxicity and even kill a susceptible 10-lb dog. An additional source of theobromine intoxication in horses is cocoa bean hulls, which are sometimes used as stall bedding.

Treatment of chocolate toxicity is induction of emesis and supportive care. Animals that ingest amounts of milk chocolate sufficient to cause toxicity usually vomit spontaneously and develop diarrhea. Removal of a large mass of chocolate by gastric lavage using a stomach tube is difficult because the soft chocolate tends to form into a ball within the stomach.

Doxapram

Doxapram (Dopram) is a CNS stimulant that works primarily at the medulla of the brainstem to increase respiration in animals with **apnea,** which is cessation of breathing, or **bradypnea,** which is slow breathing. Because many anesthetic, sedative, and analgesic drugs depress the medullary respiratory centers as part of their overall CNS depression effect, doxapram is most often used in animals that have received large amounts of these respiratory depressant drugs. For example, doxapram is commonly needed when opioids have been used as part of the anesthetic regimen for cesarean section or dystocia. The neonates, which receive the opioid drug via the placenta, usually have depressed respiratory function. After removal from the dam, the neonates can be given doxapram via the umbilical vein or sublingually (under the tongue).

Doxapram also stimulates other parts of the brain in addition to the medullary area, but this stimulation is significantly weaker. Still, when combined with the effects of such drugs as xylazine, this stimulation of the cerebral cortex or emotion and behavior areas of the brain may produce aggressive behavior, muscle tremors, catatonic rigidity, and signs that have been attributed to "hallucinogenic behavior." These effects are fortunately transient and subside within a few minutes after administration of doxapram.

Doxapram should be used with caution in animals that are predisposed to seizures. Overstimulation of the CNS by doxapram may precipitate seizures in susceptible animals.

Yohimbine, Tolazoline, and Atipamezole

Yohimbine, tolazoline, and atipamezole which are α_2 antagonists bind to α_2 receptors on the terminal bouton of norepinephrine-releasing neurons and prevent the negative feedback that normally decreases release of more excitatory neurotransmitter. This is another example of disinhibition; yohimbine, tolazoline, and atipamezole inhibit an inhibitory process at the α_2-receptor site.

Because α_2 receptors are found in the cardiovascular system, GI tract, and genitourinary system, yohimbine, tolazoline, and atipamezole may cause increased heart rate, increased blood pressure, and an antidiuretic effect resulting from sympathetic tone causing vasoconstriction of renal arteries, thereby decreasing urine formation. Respiration is increased through stimulation of respiratory centers in the CNS. Although the effects of yohimbine, tolazoline, and atipamezole on animals predisposed to seizures are not well documented, cautious use of these drugs in these animals is prudent.

Nervous System Drug Categories and Names

Anesthetics

Barbiturates
  Thiopental (Pentothal)
  Thiamylal (Surital)
  Methohexital (Brevital)
Propofol
Dissociative anesthetics
  Ketamine
  Tiletamine
Inhalant anesthetics
  Nitrous oxide
  Methoxyflurane (Metofane, Penthrane)
  Halothane (Fluothane)
  Isoflurane (Forane, AErrane)

Tranquilizers and Sedatives

Phenothiazine tranquilizers
  Acepromazine maleate
Droperidol
Benzodiazepine tranquilizers
  Diazepam (Valium)
  Zolazepam
  Midazolam (Versed)
  Clonazepam (Klonopin)
α_2 Agonists
  Xylazine (Rompun, Anased)
  Detomidine (Dormosedan)
  Medetomidine (Domitor)
α_2 Antagonists
  Yohimbine (Yobine)
  Tolazoline (Priscoline)
  Atipamezole (Antisedan)

Analgesics

Narcotic analgesics
  Nalorphine
  Oxymorphone (Numorphan)
  Butorphanol (Torbutrol, Torbugesic)
  Fentanyl
  Meperidine (Demerol)
  Pentazocine (Talwin)
  Buprenorphine (Buprenex)
  Etorphine (M-99)
Neuroleptanalgesics

Anticonvulsants

Phenobarbital
Primidone
Phenytoin (Dilantin)
Diazepam (Valium)
Clonazepam (Klonopin)
Potassium bromide
Valproic acid

CNS stimulants

Methylxanthines
  Caffeine
  Theobromine
  Aminophylline
  Theophylline
Doxapram (Dopram)
Yohimbine
Tolazoline
Atipamezole

Recommended Reading

Benson GJ, Tranquilli WJ: Advantages and guidelines for using opioid agonist-antagonist analgesics. In *Veterinary clinics of North America: small animal practice—opinions in small animal anesthesia,* Philadelphia, 1992, WB Saunders.

Hubbell JA, Bednarski RM, Muir WW: Practical methods of anesthesia. In *Saunders manual of small animal practice,* Philadelphia, 1994, WB Saunders.

Ilkiw JE: Other potentially useful new injectable anesthetics agents. In *Veterinary clinics of North America: small animal practice—opinions in small animal anesthesia,* Philadelphia, 1992, WB Saunders.

LeBlanc PH: Chemical restraint for surgery in the standing horse, *Vet Clin North Am Equine Pract* 7(3):521, 1991.

Plumb DC: Propofol monograph. In *Veterinary drug handbook,* ed 2, Ames, Iowa, 1995, Iowa State University Press.

Robinson EP, Sanderson SL, Machon RG: Propofol: a new sedative-hypnotic anesthetic agent. In Bonagura JD, editor: *Kirk's current veterinary therapy XII,* Philadelphia, 1995, WB Saunders.

Smith JA, Gaynor JS, Bednarski RM: Adverse effects of administration of propofol with various preanesthetic regimens in dogs, *JAMA* 202:1111, 1993.

Thurmon JC, Tranquilli WJ, Benson GJ: *Lumb and Jones' veterinary anesthesia,* ed 3, Baltimore, 1996, Williams & Wilkins.

Wagner AE, Muir WW, Hinchcliff KW: Cardiovascular effects of xylazine and detomidine in horses, *Am J Vet Res* 52(5):651, 1991.

Weaver BM, Raptopoulos D: Induction of anesthesia in dogs and cats with propofol, *Vet Record* 126:617, 1990.

Review Questions

1. A dog with a fractured pelvis is given a sedative and seems to be resting comfortably. Will this make it easier for you to position the animal for radiographs?

2. What is the difference between pentobarbital and phenobarbital?

3. Why is thiopental (Pentothal) given intravenously and not intramuscularly or subcutaneously?

4. If a thiobarbiturate is accidentally injected outside the vein, what is the appropriate procedure?

5. How is the dose of thiobarbiturate adjusted for obese animals as compared with that used in lean animals?

6. An animal is anesthetized with an injectable agent and the ECG is being monitored. The doctor comments about the bigeminy arrhythmia. What is the most appropriate action with regard to heart function in this anesthetized animal?

7. The doctor wants to use a different agent rather than thiopental to induce anesthesia in a Whippet. Why is this recommended, and what would be a suitable alternative?

8. Can painful procedures be safely performed using propofol as the only anesthetic agent? Does extravascular injection of propofol cause tissue sloughing?

9. The doctor comments that Telazol is basically Valium plus ketamine. What is the significance of that comment?

10. Why is applying an ophthalmic ointment to the eyes of a cat injected with ketamine or tiletamine important?

11. The veterinarian has told you to keep the ketamine locked up with the narcotic injectables. The label of the ketamine vial mentions no such special handling. Why should this drug be locked up?

12. Does ketamine or tiletamine with zolazepam provide adequate chemical restraint and analgesia for such procedures as ovariohysterectomy?

13. Which agent is known as "laughing gas"? How is it used in inhalant anesthesia protocols?

14. Name some contraindications for use of nitrous oxide. What procedures are recommended when terminating anesthesia in which nitrous oxide is used?

15. Of the commonly used gas anesthetics (halothane, methoxyflurane, and isoflurane), which induces anesthesia most rapidly and which provides the greatest degree of muscle relaxation?

16. Under what conditions is use of methoxyflurane contraindicated?

17. Why should cardiac function be monitored during halothane anesthesia?

18. What is malignant hyperthermia? What causes it and how can it be prevented?

19. What type of anesthetic agents are desflurane, sevoflurane, and enflurane, and what are their effects?

20. Which drug can be used to control motion sickness, as a tranquilizer, and as a preanesthetic agent? How can a single drug have all these uses?

21. Why is acepromazine less likely to be used in stallions than in mares?

22. The doctor has referred a dog to a veterinary ophthalmologist and the owner requests a tranquilizer for the car ride. Why does the doctor avoid dispensing the usual acepromazine and instead dispenses another tranquilizer?

23. What is the difference between an α_2 agonist and an α_2 antagonist? What effects do these drugs have?

24. Under what conditions is use of xylazine contraindicated in dogs? Which species is very sensitive to the effects of xylazine?

25. A dog has severe abdominal pain after ingesting a liquid alkali drain cleaner. There are burns on the oral mucosa and tongue. In this case, why is xylazine not a good choice for sedation and analgesia?

26. A Great Dane has been sedated with xylazine for radiography. The doctor tells you to watch for any signs of abdominal distention. Why is this observation recommended?

27. Equine practitioners know that they must be cautious when performing painful procedures such as suturing on horses sedated with α_2 agonists. Why is this caution warranted?

28. The doctor advises her new associate to be especially careful when injecting xylazine or detomidine into the jugular vein. Why is this warning necessary?

29. What effect does detomidine have on the heart rate and pulse strength in a horse?

30. A dog is given xylazine and the ECG shows an atrioventricular block. Is this something commonly seen with xylazine? With what drug is this usually treated?

31. A livestock producer telephones and says he is worried because he gave xylazine to two calves and they are extremely depressed. The doctor says he will drive out to the farm immediately to try to reverse the effects of xylazine. Which drug is the doctor most likely to use in reversing the effects of xylazine?

32. A dog with a badly fractured pelvis is admitted to the hospital and the doctor gives the dog oxymorphone (Numorphan) as an analgesic instead of the usual xylazine. Why did she select oxymorphone rather than xylazine? Would oxymorphone be an appropriate choice for a cat with a similar fracture?

33. Promotional information for a narcotic analgesic states that the drug has "κ-receptor agonist" activity, which provides fewer respiratory side effects and is superior to other narcotic analgesics with "σ-receptor activity." What is the significance of this information?

34. Why are animals recovering from sedation or anesthesia in which a narcotic was used often placed in a dark, quiet room?

35. Which drug is used as a cough suppressant and an analgesic?

36. In what situations are mixed agonist/antagonist narcotic agents used? Give an example of a mixed or partial agonist/antagonist.

37. What is a potential adverse effect of large doses of opioids in cats?

38. What is a neuroleptanalgesic?

39. What is the drug of choice for control of status epilepticus in dogs? What drug is used for long-term control of seizures in dogs? Why are two different drugs necessary?

40. An epileptic dog was initially treated with phenobarbital and is now doing fine. The doctor cautions the owners that the seizures could recur 3 to 6 weeks after therapy was started. Why would the seizures recur if they are now under control?

41. Why is phenobarbital preferred over primidone as an anticonvulsant?

42. A client brings in a container of phenobarbital dispensed by a local drug store according to the veterinarian's prescription. The label shows that the bottle contains 0.5-grain tablets, with two tablets to be given every 8 hours. The client is concerned because the doctor specified that her dog was to receive 60 mg of phenobarbital 3 times a day. Are the dosage instructions on the drug container correct?

43. The blood chemistry profile of a dog that has been receiving phenobarbital for several months shows high serum alkaline phosphatase activity. You remember that alkaline phosphatase is associated with liver function and that liver problems can occur with use of some anticonvulsant drugs. The other liver enzymes on the blood chemistry profile are normal. How should you interpret this finding?

44. An owner wants to know whether her epileptic dog will be treated with Dilantin, just like her cousin. What is an appropriate response?

45. What compound is sometimes used with phenobarbital to control seizures? What are the most likely adverse effects of this compound?

46. A drug reference describes a particular drug as a CNS disinhibitor. What effects will this drug have?

47. What is a common source of theobromine intoxication?

48. A client telephones and asks if his Siberian Husky will become ill from the chocolate bar it just ate. What is an appropriate response?

49. What drug is used to stimulate breathing in apneic animals?

Chapter 9

Antimicrobials

Key Terms

aerobic
anaerobic
antibacterial
antibiotic
antimicrobial
bacterial cell membrane
bacterial cell wall
bacterial nucleic acids
bactericidal
bacteriostatic
cephalosporinases
chelate
cross-resistance
crystalluria
Fanconi's syndrome
fungicidal
fungistatic
hepatotoxic
β-lactam ring
β-lactamase
minimum inhibitory
     concentration (MIC)
myelosuppression
nephrotoxicosis
ototoxic
penicillinase
protozoistatic
residue
resistance
ribosome
spectrum of activity
virucidal

Types of Antimicrobials
Goals of Antimicrobial Therapy
Resistance of Microorganisms to
     Antimicrobial Therapy
Concern Over Antimicrobial Residues
Mechanisms of Antimicrobial Action
     Effects against the cell wall
     Effects against the cell membrane
     Effects at the ribosomes
     Effects against cell metabolism
     Effects against nucleic acids
Classes of Antimicrobials
Penicillins
     Mechanism of action
     Pharmacokinetics of penicillins
     Bacterial resistance to penicillins
     Precautions for use of penicillins
     Considerations for use of specific
          penicillins
Cephalosporins
     Mechanism of action
     Pharmacokinetics of cephalosporins
     Precautions for use of
          cephalosporins
Bacitracins
Aminoglycosides
     Mechanism of action
     Pharmacokinetics of
          aminoglycosides

Precautions for use of
     aminoglycosides
Quinolones
     Mechanism of action
     Pharmacokinetics of quinolones
     Precautions for use of quinolones
Tetracyclines
     Mechanism of action
     Pharmacokinetics of tetracyclines
     Precautions for use of tetracyclines
Sulfonamides and Potentiated
     Sulfonamides
     Mechanism of action
     Pharmacokinetics of sulfonamides
     Precautions for use of sulfonamides
Other Antimicrobials Used in Veterinary
     Medicine
     Lincosamides
     Macrolides
     Metronidazole
     Nitrofurans
     Chloramphenicol
     Rifampin
Antifungals
     Amphotericin B and nystatin
     Ketoconazole and itraconazole
     Griseofulvin

Learning Objectives

*After studying this chapter,
the veterinary technician should know the following:*

The types and classes of antimicrobials

Strategies for antimicrobial use

The way and locations at which antimicrobials exert their effect

The way bacteria develop resistance to antimicrobials

Precautions for using various antimicrobials

ntimicrobials are drugs that kill or inhibit the growth of microorganisms, or microbes, such as bacteria, protozoa, viruses, and fungi. The term **antibiotic** is often used interchangeably with the term **antimicrobial.** Technically an antibiotic is a substance produced by one microorganism that suppresses growth of another microorganism. The term *antimicrobial* applies to all drugs used to combat microorganisms, including antibiotics and chemically synthesized drugs. Today most antimicrobials, even antibiotics that were once manufactured with cultures of microorganisms, are chemically synthesized. Thus the distinction between antibiotic and antimicrobial is less important. (A box listing antimicrobials can be found at the end of this chapter.)

TYPES OF ANTIMICROBIALS

An antimicrobial can be classified according to the type of microorganism it fights and whether it kills the microorganism or prevents it from replicating and proliferating. The suffix *cidal* usually denotes drugs that kill the microorganism (for example, bactericidal and fungicidal). The suffix *static* usually denotes drugs that inhibit replication but generally do not directly kill the microorganism (for example, bacteriostatic and **fungistatic**).

A drug might have both killing and inhibiting effects depending on the drug concentration attained at the infection site. A low concentration may result in an inhibiting effect, whereas a higher concentration results in death of the organisms. Although all antimicrobials rely on the animal's immune system to help fight infection, drugs that inhibit replication (static drugs) depend more on a functional immune system to defeat the organism. This is the reason people or animals with compromised immune systems (such as people with AIDS, cats with feline immunodeficiency virus infection, and people or animals who receive chemotherapy) usually require drugs that are "cidal" to treat infections.

The type of microorganism against which a drug is effective as well as its mode of action is found in the category description. Examples include the following:

Bactericidal	Kills bacteria
Bacteriostatic	Inhibits bacterial replication
Virucidal	Kills viruses
Protozoistatic	Inhibits protozoal replication
Fungicidal	Kills fungi

Another term sometimes used is **antibacterial.** This is a broad term that includes any drug, synthetic or natural, with either a static or cidal effect on bacteria.

Disinfectants and antiseptics are also antimicrobials. Because they are generally applied outside the body or to the surface of inanimate objects, they are discussed in Chapter 10.

GOALS OF ANTIMICROBIAL THERAPY

The goal of antimicrobial therapy is to kill or disable pathogens (disease-causing microorganisms) without killing the host. Unfortunately, many animals die each year because of side effects or inappropriate administration of antimicrobials. Successful administration of antimicrobials requires the following conditions:

- The microorganism must be susceptible to the antimicrobial drug.
- The antimicrobial must be able to reach the site of infection in high enough concentrations to kill or inhibit the microorganism.
- The animal must be able to tolerate the high concentrations.

Factors such as client compliance, which includes ease of administration and convenient dosage interval and form, and cost also influence drug selection. However, the three conditions listed must be met before any other factors are considered.

The measurement of susceptibility of a bacterial strain to the effects of an antimicrobial is represented by the drug's **minimum inhibitory concentration (MIC)** against that bacterial strain. The MIC represents the lowest concentration of drug at which growth of the bacterium is inhibited (Fig. 9-1). A drug's MIC varies with different bacterial species and strains. For any bacterial strain, the MIC for various antimicrobial drugs may also be different. For example, a strain of *Staphylococcus* bacteria may be very sensitive to the antibiotic amikacin but quite resistant to penicillin. The MIC for amikacin would be fairly low compared with the MIC for penicillin. A dif-

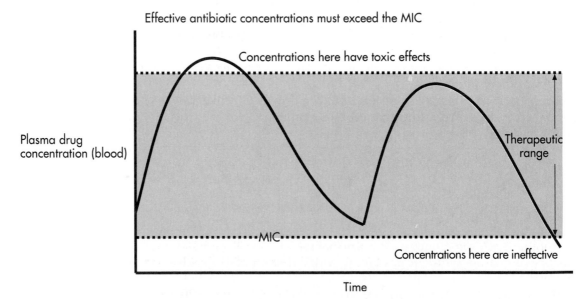

Fig. 9-1 The minimal inhibitory concentration (MIC) is the lowest plasma concentration of an antimicrobial that effectively exerts antimicrobial action. Levels below this are ineffective and levels exceeding the therapeutic range are toxic.

drugs. Thus drugs that target the bacterial cell wall are most effective against actively dividing bacterial colonies.

Effects against the Cell Membrane

Antimicrobials can damage the **bacterial cell membrane** by changing the membrane permeability, making the microorganism "leaky" and allowing antimicrobials to enter the bacterium or vital cytoplasmic components to leave. Unlike drugs that act on the bacterial cell wall, antimicrobials that affect the cell membrane can exert their effect on dividing or static (nondividing) bacteria.

Effects at the Ribosomes

Antimicrobials can inhibit protein synthesis in pathogenic microorganisms such as bacteria and fungi. Cells, including bacteria, manufacture essential proteins from amino acids within the cytoplasm (Fig. 9-3). A strand of messenger RNA carries the genetic code (from the bacterial DNA) for producing essential proteins to the **ribosome,** which is a specialized organelle ("little organ") within the bacterium. Transfer RNA molecules take different amino acids to the ribosome where they are attached together in a sequence determined by the messenger RNA's copied genetic blueprint. The properly linked amino acids produce a functional protein molecule. Some antimicrobials enter the bacterium, combine with the ribosome, and disrupt normal protein production. This results in either a bactericidal or a bacteriostatic effect.

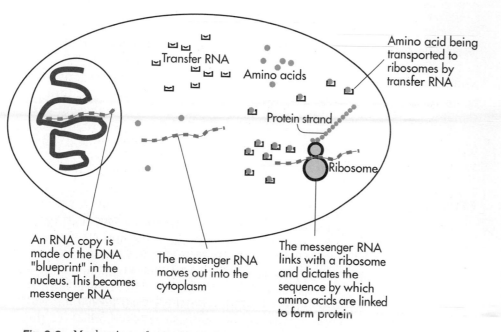

Fig. 9-3 Mechanism of protein synthesis by a cell.

(Figure labels:) Transfer RNA · Amino acids · Amino acid being transported to ribosomes by transfer RNA · Protein strand · Ribosome · An RNA copy is made of the DNA "blueprint" in the nucleus. This becomes messenger RNA · The messenger RNA moves out into the cytoplasm · The messenger RNA links with a ribosome and dictates the sequence by which amino acids are linked to form protein

---

ferent species of bacteria such as *Pseudomonas* might be fairly resistant to amikacin; thus amikacin would have a much higher MIC for *Pseudomonas* bacteria. For some drugs the MIC needed to affect the bacteria in question is so high that such concentrations would be detrimental to the host animal; therefore that drug would not be used against that pathogen.

The veterinary professional must realize that antimicrobials are ineffective if they do not reach the infection site in concentrations high enough to exceed that drug's MIC for the pathogen. For example, if an animal had pneumonia (a bacterial infection in the lungs) and culture and sensitivity testing indicated that the antibiotic neomycin would be effective against those bacteria, neomycin would seem to be the drug of choice. However, neomycin given by mouth is very poorly absorbed from the intestinal tract and never reaches sufficient concentrations in the lungs to affect the bacteria. Thus the drug's ability to reach the target tissue is as important as the sensitivity of the bacteria to that drug.

RESISTANCE OF MICROORGANISMS TO ANTIMICROBIAL THERAPY

Bacteria and other microorganisms have developed the ability to survive in the presence of antimicrobial drugs designed to kill them. This is referred to as **resistance.** Bacteria may be resistant to certain drugs because of genetic changes that were inherited from previous generations of bacteria, or they may acquire resistance as a result of spontaneous mutations of chromosomes or acquisition of an additional piece of DNA called a *plasmid.*

The changes conferred by chromosomes or plasmids provide bacteria with a new mechanism to defeat the effect of antimicrobials that would normally destroy or inactivate the bacteria. The most common example is the ability of bacteria to produce enzymes that render antibiotics (such as penicillins and cephalosporins) useless. Other conferred changes may prevent a drug from attaching to a site on the bacterium where it is intended to work. Bacteria may also develop alternative metabolic pathways that circumvent an antimicrobial's ability to kill the bacteria.

Because bacteria have different resistance characteristics, inappropriate antimicrobial therapy may produce a population of bacteria that is highly resistant (Fig. 9-2). For example, assume that in a population of millions of bacteria, a single bacterium spontaneously becomes resistant. The MIC for antibiotic X to kill this bacterium is now 10 $\mu g/ml$, whereas the MIC for the rest of the bacterial population is only 1 $\mu g/ml$. Normally this would not be a problem because standard doses of antibiotic X achieve concentrations of 15 $\mu g/ml$ at the infection site. However, if the drug is administered improperly (that is, with incorrect dosage or dosage interval or failure to consider physiologic factors) and the resulting concentrations achieved at the infection site are only 7 $\mu g/ml$, the bacteria in the general population are killed but the more resistant bacterium survives and replicates, producing more of the resistant strain of bacteria. Thus antibiotic X is ineffective because inappropriate drug use has induced development of resistant bacteria. Therefore

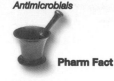

Pharm Fact

An antimicrobial is useless unless it can penetrate the site of infection in amounts sufficient to destroy the infecting microorganisms.

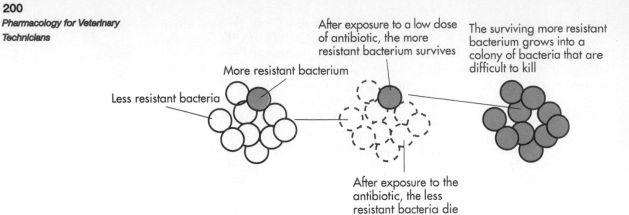

More resistant bacterium

Less resistant bacteria

After exposure to a low dose of antibiotic, the more resistant bacterium survives

The surviving more resistant bacterium grows into a colony of bacteria that are difficult to kill

After exposure to the antibiotic, the less resistant bacteria die

Fig. 9-2 Mechanism by which small doses of an antimicrobial can lead to development of resistant strains of bacteria.

veterinary professionals should follow antimicrobial dosages recommended in package inserts and drug references (that is, a sufficiently large dose given at appropriate intervals for a sufficient time). Following the recommended dosage will reduce the chance for recurrence of the infection in a more resistant form.

Even if the antimicrobial is administered as recommended, bacteria can still develop resistance. In the preceding example the change in the bacterium could have produced resistance requiring an MIC of 1000 μg/ml rather than only 10 μg/ml. Once a bacterium is resistant, the resistant characteristics and mechanism are passed on genetically to daughter cells. In the case of resistance conferred by plasmids, the plasmid itself can be transferred to multiple bacteria via a process called *transduction*. With transduction the plasmids may confer bacterial resistance against multiple antimicrobial agents at one time, resulting in a bacterial colony that is resistant to several antimicrobials.

Veterinary professionals have an obligation to reduce development of microbial resistance to protect the health of the animal and general public. This can be accomplished by following simple principles of antimicrobial administration:

- Administer the appropriate dose at appropriate intervals, for the appropriate time, and in the appropriate manner.
- Educate clients regarding the importance of following the instructions for dispensed medication, including use of the medication until the supply is expended even if the animal's condition has improved after a few days.

CONCERN OVER ANTIMICROBIAL RESIDUES

A **residue** is the prescence of a drug, chemical, or its metabolites in animal tissues or food products, resulting from either administration of that drug or

chemical to an animal, or contamination of food products. Antimicrobial residues in food animals are of growing concern. As discussed in Chapter 3, use of drugs in animals intended for food must be withdrawn a specific number of days before the animal is slaughtered or the food products are able to be sold by the producer. Most antimicrobial residues in food are *not* degraded by cooking or pasteurization.

Exposure to low levels of antimicrobials in food can cause two effects in people: an allergic reaction (hypersensitivity) to the antimicrobial or selection for resistant bacteria in the intestinal tract. For example, a penicillin-sensitive person who consumes meat that contains penicillin residues might have an allergic reaction. Another problem might occur as selection for resistant bacteria in a family who consumes multiple small doses of a drug in a side of beef that contains antimicrobial residues. Consumption of the small doses could cause selection for resistant bacteria in the family members' intestinal tracts, resulting in overgrowth of the resistant bacteria.

Public concern over drug residues has prompted increasingly restrictive legislation regulating drug use in animals intended for food. Unfortunately, the economics of producing livestock for food encourages producers to include low levels of antimicrobials in animal feed to enhance growth and, if antibiotics are used, to shorten withdrawal time to get their animals to market sooner. Both practices, combined with administration of inappropriate quantities of antimicrobials (necessitating a change in withdrawal time that may not be observed), can result in antimicrobial residues in meat, milk, and other food products. Veterinary professionals must take the time to educate food-animal producers on the appropriate use of antimicrobials and withdrawal times, and should label all dispensed medications with clear instructions for proper administration and withdrawal times.

MECHANISMS OF ANTIMICROBIAL ACTION

Antimicrobials work by different mechanisms to kill or inhibit bacteria and other microorganisms. The veterinary technician must have a basic understanding of these mechanisms to select the proper antimicrobial agent and prevent ineffective combinations. Antimicrobials generally exert their effects at five sites in microorganisms: the cell wall, the cell membrane, ribosomes, critical enzymes or metabolites, and nucleic acids.

Effects against the Cell Wall

Antimicrobials can interfere with formation of the **bacterial cell wall.** Normally the bacterial protoplasm draws water into the bacterium via osmosis, producing a tendency to swell. The intact bacterial cell wall keeps the bacterium from bursting, in much the same way that placing a balloon in a rigid container during inflation prevents the balloon from increasing until it bursts. Antimicrobials that interfere with bacterial cell wall formation usually affect it while the wall is forming during bacterial division. Once the bacterial cell wall is constructed, it is not readily affected by antimicrobial

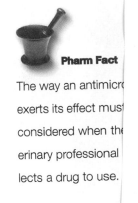

Pharm Fact

The way an antimicro exerts its effect mus considered when th erinary professional lects a drug to use.

Effects against Cell Metabolism

Antimicrobials can interfere with metabolism of pathogenic bacteria by blocking the actions of critical enzymes or binding with essential intermediate compounds the bacteria needs to function. Without these critical components, the bacterium is unable to function properly. Most antimicrobials that work by this mechanism are bacteriostatic unless combined with another antimicrobial or used at higher doses.

Effects against Nucleic Acids

Antimicrobials can impair production of **bacterial nucleic acids** (RNA and DNA). When antimicrobials damage or alter the function of nucleic acids in a pathogenic microorganism such as a bacterium or fungus, the cell usually cannot divide and may be unable to produce critical proteins needed by the cell. Many drugs that attack the pathogen's nucleic acids can also affect mammalian nucleic acids, possibly causing birth defects or death in developing fetuses. Several antifungal drugs work in this manner and thus should not be used in pregnant animals. Exceptions to this dangerous side effect are the quinolone antimicrobials and rifampin, which work at a site on the pathogen's nucleic acid that is not found in mammalian cells, making these drugs much safer.

CLASSES OF ANTIMICROBIALS

Although a myriad of antimicrobials are available for use in veterinary medicine, many drugs share common mechanisms of action, **spectra of antimicrobial activity,** and general considerations for safe and proper administration. By understanding the general mechanisms of action and hazards for each class of antimicrobials, you can better determine whether or not a particular antimicrobial may be used safely and effectively.

PENICILLINS

Penicillins are among the most commonly used antibiotics in veterinary medicine and can usually be recognized by their *cillin* suffix on the drug name. The most frequently used penicillins in veterinary medicine include the natural penicillins G and V; the broad-spectrum aminopenicillins ampicillin, amoxicillin, and hetacillin; the penicillinase-resistant penicillins cloxacillin, dicloxacillin, and oxacillin; and the extended-spectrum penicillins, including among others carbenicillin, ticarcillin, and piperacillin. Several other penicillins are used in human medicine but rarely in veterinary medicine because of cost and lack of FDA approval for use in animals.

Penicillins are generally effective against gram-positive bacteria and varying types of gram-negative bacteria. Penicillins identified as *broad spectrum* or *extended spectrum* are more effective against a wider range of bacteria than the natural penicillins or penicillinase-resistant penicillins.

Mechanism of Action

Penicillins are **bactericidal** and work primarily by interfering with development of the bacterial cell wall, making the bacterium more prone to lysis from osmotic imbalances. Penicillin drugs block bacterial enzymes that are essential for construction of the bacterial cell wall. Different penicillin antibiotics may affect different enzymes, which partially explains the reason one type of penicillin might be effective against a bacterial population whereas another is less effective. Because these enzymes are needed by the bacterium only during cell division when a new cell wall is being produced, penicillins are only effective against an actively dividing colony of bacteria. Thus if a **bacteriostatic** antimicrobial is used in conjunction with penicillin, the bacteriostatic effect prevents division of the bacteria and growth of the colony, decreasing the effectiveness of the penicillin. This is the origin of the myth that all bactericidal and bacteriostatic antimicrobials should not be used together. More accurately, bacteriostatic antimicrobials should not be used or should be used judiciously at the same time as bactericidal drugs that require active bacterial growth and division. Other bactericidal drugs that disrupt cell membranes or interfere with protein synthesis can destroy bacteria, regardless of whether bacterial colony growth has been inhibited by a concurrently administered bacteriostatic drug.

Pharmacokinetics of Penicillins

Penicillins are generally well absorbed from injection sites and the gastrointestinal (GI) tract. Penicillin G should not be given by mouth because it is inactivated by gastric acid and therefore is used only in injectable form. Although oral penicillins are not inactivated by gastric acid, their bioavailability is usually decreased in the presence of food. (Amoxicillin is the notable exception.) Thus owners should be instructed to give an animal orally administered penicillins on an empty stomach.

An advantage of penicillins is that they are well distributed to most tissues in the body. They reach therapeutic concentrations in most tissues, with the exception of the globe of the eye and the brain. However, in situations such as meningitis (inflammation of the meninges covering the brain) where the blood-barrier becomes more permeable, penicillin may enter this compartment but still not reach significant therapeutic concentrations. (Concentrations would still be below the MIC.) Therefore penicillins are not the drug of choice for most central nervous system (CNS) bacterial infections.

Most penicillins are excreted largely unchanged by the kidneys into the urine via filtration, which is a passive diffusion process, and by secretion of drug into the renal tubules, which is an active transport mechanism. Because the penicillin is usually excreted intact and unchanged, it retains bactericidal activity in the urine. Because penicillins are actively secreted into the urine in concentrations usually exceeding the MIC for many bacteria found in the kidneys, bladder (bacterial cystitis), or genitourinary tract, these drugs are commonly used to fight urinary tract infections.

Bacterial Resistance to Penicillins

Each penicillin type is effective against a different bacterial spectrum, which is the range of bacterial types against which a drug is active. Some strains of bacteria such as *Pseudomonas* are very resistant to the penicillin's bactericidal effect, whereas other bacteria are quite susceptible. Therefore knowledge of each penicillin's antibacterial spectrum is important when the veterinary professional selects the most appropriate drug for treating a bacterial infection.

Sometimes a bacterial strain that has been sensitive to a particular penicillin's bactericidal effects develops resistance and is no longer susceptible to the drug. Generally, if a strain of bacteria becomes resistant to one type of penicillin such as amoxicillin, it is also resistant to most other penicillins. This phenomenon is known as **cross-resistance.**

Some bacteria, especially staphylococci, acquire resistance to many penicillins by producing an enzyme that attacks a particular part of the penicillin molecule called the **β-lactam ring,** rendering the drug ineffective. These bacterial enzymes are called **β-lactamases** or **penicillinases** if the enzyme specifically attacks penicillins. (Cephalosporin antimicrobials also have β-lactam rings that are susceptible to β-lactamase).

One group of penicillins is not affected by bacterial β-lactamase enzymes. These β-lactamase–resistant penicillins include oxacillin, dicloxacillin, cloxacillin, and a few expensive products used in human medicine. These penicillins are often used in treatment of bovine mastitis because of the prevalence of β-lactamase–producing staphylococci in many mastitis infections. A disadvantage of these penicillins is their reduced spectrum of activity against many bacterial strains that the more common penicillins can kill. Thus β-lactamase–resistant penicillins are used selectively for infections in which β-lactamase is likely to be produced by the bacteria causing the infection.

Penicillin compounds normally inactivated by β-lactamase can sometimes be chemically combined with another compound to produce a modified or "potentiated" penicillin that is resistant to the β-lactamase enzyme. Clavulanic acid (potassium clavulanate) and sulbactam are added to penicillin drugs such as amoxicillin to produce a potentiated compound that renders bacterial β-lactamase enzymes inactive. For example, clavulanic acid is included with amoxicillin in the product Clavamox.

The molecules of clavulanic acid and sulbactam contain a β-lactam ring. The bacterial β-lactamase attacks the potentiating drug's β-lactam ring, inactivating the enzyme before it destroys the β-lactam ring of the penicillin molecule. The intact penicillin molecule can then exert its bactericidal effect on the bacterial cell wall.

Potentiated drugs tend to be more expensive than their nonpotentiated counterparts. One reason for the higher cost is that tablets of these potentiated drugs are packaged individually because these combination drugs readily absorb moisture from the air. The tablets would decompose if stored freely in a bottle that was opened numerous times.

Many gram-negative bacteria are resistant to penicillin's bactericidal effect because penicillin drugs have difficulty reaching the cell wall components of gram-negative bacteria. Many gram-negative bacteria have an outer mem-

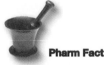

Pharm Fact

Bacteria that develop resistance to one type of penicillin are often resistant to other penicillins.

brane, or capsule, that forms a barrier to most penicillins, protecting the bacterial cell wall during cell development. Lists of bacteria sensitive to penicillins can be found in veterinary microbiology texts.

Precautions for Use of Penicillins

When compared with many other antibiotics, penicillins are very safe drugs. Hypersensitivity reactions (allergic reactions) are the most common adverse reaction to penicillins. Manifestations of hypersensitivity range from a mild skin rash to life-threatening anaphylactic shock. Anaphylactic reactions are more common with injectable penicillin products than with oral products and require aggressive emergency treatment, including administration of epinephrine and corticosteroids. Less severe reactions include skin rashes (urticaria or hives), swelling of the face, swelling of lymph nodes, hematologic changes (eosinophilia, neutropenia), and fever. If an animal exhibits hypersensitivity to one type of penicillin, it is likely to react adversely to other penicillin drugs. The veterinarian must be made aware of any possible adverse reaction to penicillin administration. Such reactions must be clearly marked on the animal's record to prevent future exposures and possibly fatal anaphylactic reactions.

When given orally, penicillins may destroy "beneficial" bacteria residing in the lumen of the intestinal tract, allowing more pathogenic (disease-causing) bacteria, which are generally more penicillin resistant, to proliferate. This condition, called superinfection, or suprainfection, can produce severe diarrhea that can result in death in some species such as guinea pigs, hamsters, and rabbits. Other species in which penicillins must be used with caution include snakes, birds, turtles, and chinchillas.

Because penicillins are readily available to food-animal producers, the importance of observing withdrawal times for penicillins and all other antimicrobials should be emphasized. Milk is frequently tested for the presence of penicillins used to treat or control mastitis in dairy cattle. The veterinary professional has the obligation to the public to educate and inform food-animal producers regarding the appropriate withdrawal times and milk-discard times ("milk out" times) when penicillin products are used.

Considerations for Use of Specific Penicillins

Penicillin G

Penicillin G is a "natural penicillin" that is usually administered via injection because it is largely inactivated by the acidic stomach environment if given orally. Penicillin G is available in three basic forms: an aqueous sodium or potassium form, a form combined with procaine, and a form combined with benzathine. Only the aqueous forms of penicillin G can be given intravenously. (They may also be given subcutaneously and intramuscularly.) Addition of procaine and benzathine to penicillin G delays absorption of the antibiotic from IM injection sites, extending the duration of drug activity. Procaine penicillin G usually provides adequate concentra-

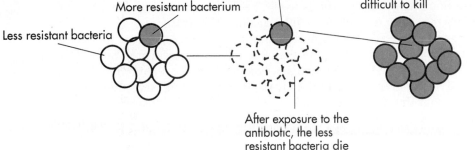

More resistant bacterium

Less resistant bacteria

After exposure to a low dose of antibiotic, the more resistant bacterium survives

The surviving more resistant bacterium grows into a colony of bacteria that are difficult to kill

After exposure to the antibiotic, the less resistant bacteria die

Fig. 9-2 Mechanism by which small doses of an antimicrobial can lead to development of resistant strains of bacteria.

veterinary professionals should follow antimicrobial dosages recommended in package inserts and drug references (that is, a sufficiently large dose given at appropriate intervals for a sufficient time). Following the recommended dosage will reduce the chance for recurrence of the infection in a more resistant form.

Even if the antimicrobial is administered as recommended, bacteria can still develop resistance. In the preceding example the change in the bacterium could have produced resistance requiring an MIC of 1000 μg/ml rather than only 10 μg/ml. Once a bacterium is resistant, the resistant characteristics and mechanism are passed on genetically to daughter cells. In the case of resistance conferred by plasmids, the plasmid itself can be transferred to multiple bacteria via a process called *transduction*. With transduction the plasmids may confer bacterial resistance against multiple antimicrobial agents at one time, resulting in a bacterial colony that is resistant to several antimicrobials.

Veterinary professionals have an obligation to reduce development of microbial resistance to protect the health of the animal and general public. This can be accomplished by following simple principles of antimicrobial administration:

- Administer the appropriate dose at appropriate intervals, for the appropriate time, and in the appropriate manner.
- Educate clients regarding the importance of following the instructions for dispensed medication, including use of the medication until the supply is expended even if the animal's condition has improved after a few days.

CONCERN OVER ANTIMICROBIAL RESIDUES

A **residue** is the prescence of a drug, chemical, or its metabolites in animal tissues or food products, resulting from either administration of that drug or

ferent species of bacteria such as *Pseudomonas* might be fairly resistant to amikacin; thus amikacin would have a much higher MIC for *Pseudomonas* bacteria. For some drugs the MIC needed to affect the bacteria in question is so high that such concentrations would be detrimental to the host animal; therefore that drug would not be used against that pathogen.

The veterinary professional must realize that antimicrobials are ineffective if they do not reach the infection site in concentrations high enough to exceed that drug's MIC for the pathogen. For example, if an animal had pneumonia (a bacterial infection in the lungs) and culture and sensitivity testing indicated that the antibiotic neomycin would be effective against those bacteria, neomycin would seem to be the drug of choice. However, neomycin given by mouth is very poorly absorbed from the intestinal tract and never reaches sufficient concentrations in the lungs to affect the bacteria. Thus the drug's ability to reach the target tissue is as important as the sensitivity of the bacteria to that drug.

Antimicrobials

Pharm Fact

An antimicrobial is useless unless it can penetrate the site of infection in amounts sufficient to destroy the infecting microorganisms.

RESISTANCE OF MICROORGANISMS TO ANTIMICROBIAL THERAPY

Bacteria and other microorganisms have developed the ability to survive in the presence of antimicrobial drugs designed to kill them. This is referred to as **resistance.** Bacteria may be resistant to certain drugs because of genetic changes that were inherited from previous generations of bacteria, or they may acquire resistance as a result of spontaneous mutations of chromosomes or acquisition of an additional piece of DNA called a *plasmid.*

The changes conferred by chromosomes or plasmids provide bacteria with a new mechanism to defeat the effect of antimicrobials that would normally destroy or inactivate the bacteria. The most common example is the ability of bacteria to produce enzymes that render antibiotics (such as penicillins and cephalosporins) useless. Other conferred changes may prevent a drug from attaching to a site on the bacterium where it is intended to work. Bacteria may also develop alternative metabolic pathways that circumvent an antimicrobial's ability to kill the bacteria.

Because bacteria have different resistance characteristics, inappropriate antimicrobial therapy may produce a population of bacteria that is highly resistant (Fig. 9-2). For example, assume that in a population of millions of bacteria, a single bacterium spontaneously becomes resistant. The MIC for antibiotic X to kill this bacterium is now 10 μg/ml, whereas the MIC for the rest of the bacterial population is only 1 μg/ml. Normally this would not be a problem because standard doses of antibiotic X achieve concentrations of 15 μg/ml at the infection site. However, if the drug is administered improperly (that is, with incorrect dosage or dosage interval or failure to consider physiologic factors) and the resulting concentrations achieved at the infection site are only 7 μg/ml, the bacteria in the general population are killed but the more resistant bacterium survives and replicates, producing more of the resistant strain of bacteria. Thus antibiotic X is ineffective because inappropriate drug use has induced development of resistant bacteria. Therefore

chemical to an animal, or contamination of food products. Antimicrobial residues in food animals are of growing concern. As discussed in Chapter 3, use of drugs in animals intended for food must be withdrawn a specific number of days before the animal is slaughtered or the food products are able to be sold by the producer. Most antimicrobial residues in food are *not* degraded by cooking or pasteurization.

Exposure to low levels of antimicrobials in food can cause two effects in people: an allergic reaction (hypersensitivity) to the antimicrobial or selection for resistant bacteria in the intestinal tract. For example, a penicillin-sensitive person who consumes meat that contains penicillin residues might have an allergic reaction. Another problem might occur as selection for resistant bacteria in a family who consumes multiple small doses of a drug in a side of beef that contains antimicrobial residues. Consumption of the small doses could cause selection for resistant bacteria in the family members' intestinal tracts, resulting in overgrowth of the resistant bacteria.

Public concern over drug residues has prompted increasingly restrictive legislation regulating drug use in animals intended for food. Unfortunately, the economics of producing livestock for food encourages producers to include low levels of antimicrobials in animal feed to enhance growth and, if antibiotics are used, to shorten withdrawal time to get their animals to market sooner. Both practices, combined with administration of inappropriate quantities of antimicrobials (necessitating a change in withdrawal time that may not be observed), can result in antimicrobial residues in meat, milk, and other food products. Veterinary professionals must take the time to educate food-animal producers on the appropriate use of antimicrobials and withdrawal times, and should label all dispensed medications with clear instructions for proper administration and withdrawal times.

MECHANISMS OF ANTIMICROBIAL ACTION

Antimicrobials work by different mechanisms to kill or inhibit bacteria and other microorganisms. The veterinary technician must have a basic understanding of these mechanisms to select the proper antimicrobial agent and prevent ineffective combinations. Antimicrobials generally exert their effects at five sites in microorganisms: the cell wall, the cell membrane, ribosomes, critical enzymes or metabolites, and nucleic acids.

Effects against the Cell Wall

Antimicrobials can interfere with formation of the **bacterial cell wall.** Normally the bacterial protoplasm draws water into the bacterium via osmosis, producing a tendency to swell. The intact bacterial cell wall keeps the bacterium from bursting, in much the same way that placing a balloon in a rigid container during inflation prevents the balloon from increasing until it bursts. Antimicrobials that interfere with bacterial cell wall formation usually affect it while the wall is forming during bacterial division. Once the bacterial cell wall is constructed, it is not readily affected by antimicrobial

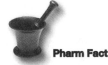

Pharm Fact

The way an antimicrobial exerts its effect must be considered when the veterinary professional selects a drug to use.

drugs. Thus drugs that target the bacterial cell wall are most effective against actively dividing bacterial colonies.

Effects against the Cell Membrane

Antimicrobials can damage the **bacterial cell membrane** by changing the membrane permeability, making the microorganism "leaky" and allowing antimicrobials to enter the bacterium or vital cytoplasmic components to leave. Unlike drugs that act on the bacterial cell wall, antimicrobials that affect the cell membrane can exert their effect on dividing or static (nondividing) bacteria.

Effects at the Ribosomes

Antimicrobials can inhibit protein synthesis in pathogenic microorganisms such as bacteria and fungi. Cells, including bacteria, manufacture essential proteins from amino acids within the cytoplasm (Fig. 9-3). A strand of messenger RNA carries the genetic code (from the bacterial DNA) for producing essential proteins to the **ribosome,** which is a specialized organelle ("little organ") within the bacterium. Transfer RNA molecules take different amino acids to the ribosome where they are attached together in a sequence determined by the messenger RNA's copied genetic blueprint. The properly linked amino acids produce a functional protein molecule. Some antimicrobials enter the bacterium, combine with the ribosome, and disrupt normal protein production. This results in either a bactericidal or a bacteriostatic effect.

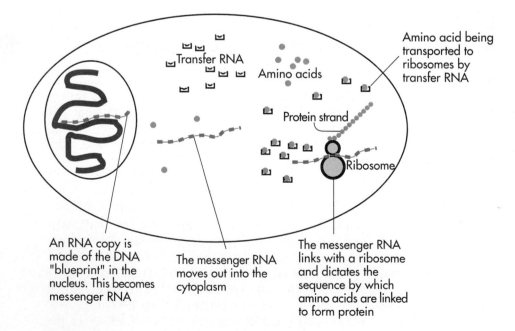

Fig. 9-3 Mechanism of protein synthesis by a cell.

tions for 48 hours, and benzathine penicillins produce effective blood concentrations for 5 days. A disadvantage of the procaine and benzathine forms is that peak plasma concentrations are not as high as those attained with the sodium or potassium form of the drug. This can result in therapeutic failure if peak drug concentrations do not exceed the bacteria's MIC for penicillin G (Fig. 9-4).

Penicillin V

Penicillin V is usually administered orally because it is relatively stable in the acidic environment of the stomach. Because the presence of food decreases the rate and extent of drug absorption, penicillin V should be given 1 hour

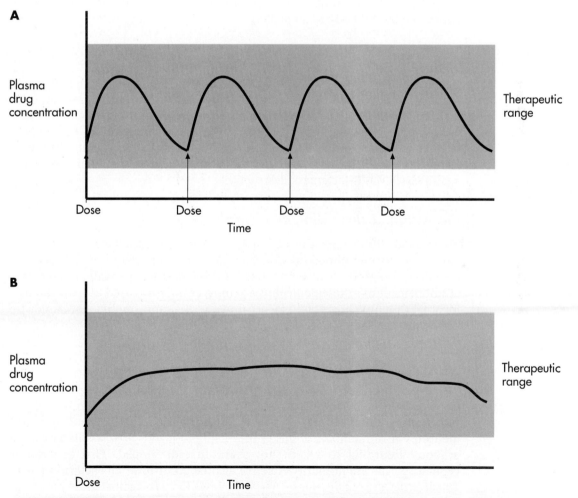

Fig. 9-4 Fluctuation of plasma drug concentrations produced by standard parenteral formulations and extended-absorption formulations of penicillin. **A,** Penicillin concentrations after parenteral administration. **B,** Penicillin concentrations when combined with procaine or benzathine.

before or 2 hours after a meal; this general rule applies to any drugs for which food interferes with absorption. If the powdered form of penicillin V is used, the reconstituted suspension and solution must be refrigerated and the unused portion discarded after 14 days.

Ampicillin

This commonly used veterinary product shares many characteristics with the other aminopenicillins amoxicillin and hetacillin. Veterinary products are available in oral (capsules and liquid suspension) and injectable forms. Ampicillin generally has a broader spectrum of antibacterial activity than penicillin G or V. Although ampicillin is probably used less frequently than amoxicillin in small animal medicine, ampicillin still provides a relatively broad spectrum of antibacterial activity at a reasonable cost. Hetacillin is converted by the body to ampicillin.

Amoxicillin

Because this aminopenicillin is more readily absorbed than ampicillin and amoxicillin is available as convenient coated tablets for easier oral administration, amoxicillin has largely supplanted ampicillin for dispensing in small animal practice. Although amoxicillin by itself is susceptible to destruction by β-lactamase, it is also available in combination with clavulanic acid (veterinary product Clavamox and human product Augmentin), which protects against bacterial β-lactamase destruction.

Cloxacillin, dicloxacillin, and oxacillin

These penicillins share the distinction of being naturally resistant to β-lactamase. As mentioned previously, their overall spectrum of antibacterial activity is slightly less than that of the natural penicillins and the aminopenicillins. These penicillins are most commonly used to treat staphylococcal osteomyelitis, staphylococcal pyoderma, and staphylococcal mastitis (by intramammary infusion).

CEPHALOSPORINS

Cephalosporins are β-lactam antimicrobials that have a mechanism of action similar to that of the penicillins. The *ceph* or *cef* prefix in the drug name identifies most members of this group. Cephalosporins are classified by generations according to when they were first developed. First-generation cephalosporins are primarily effective against gram-positive bacteria such as *Streptococcus* and *Staphylococcus*. They are less effective against gram-negative bacteria than the second- or third-generation cephalosporins.

Almost all third-generation cephalosporins are injectable, which is a disadvantage if these drugs are used initially to treat an infection in a hospitalized animal because they cannot be dispensed to pet owners for continued use at home. Generally the newer cephalosporins (of later generations) have a similar spectrum of activity as earlier generations against gram-positive bacteria, but their activity against gram-negative bacteria exceeds that of the first-generation cephalosporins. Susceptibility of bacteria to cephalosporins varies enough to require the veterinary professional to perform culture and sensitivity testing to help select the proper drug.

Many different cephalosporin drugs are available; however, most are human products and many are too expensive to be used as the drug of first choice in most animal infections. Veterinary products include cefadroxil (first generation, Cefa-Tabs), cephapirin (first generation, Cefa-Lak and Cefa-Dri intramammary infusions), and ceftiofur (third generation, Naxcel injectable). Human products used in veterinary medicine include cephalothin (first generation, Keflin), cephalexin (first generation, Keflex), cefoxitin (second generation, Metoxin), and cefotaxime (third generation, Claforan).

Mechanism of Action

Cephalosporins are β-lactam antibiotics with bactericidal mechanisms similar to those of penicillins. The cephalosporins inhibit synthesis of a key component of bacterial cell walls, which prevents the cell wall from maintaining the bacterium's osmotic balance and causes the bacterium to lyse easily with osmotic changes. Like penicillins, cephalosporins are most effective against rapidly dividing bacterial colonies.

Because cephalosporin molecules have a β-lactam ring, they are susceptible to β-lactamase enzymes produced by bacteria. Some β-lactamase enzymes may render cephalosporins ineffective without adversely affecting penicillin drugs. These bacterial β-lactamases are sometimes referred to as **cephalosporinases.**

Pharmacokinetics of Cephalosporins

First-generation cephalosporins are well absorbed from the GI tract. Various cephalosporins differ in the extent their absorption is affected by the presence of food. Therefore the veterinary professional should consult the drug package insert or drug references to properly advise clients regarding the way to give the medication. Like penicillins, cephalosporins do not readily pass through the blood-brain barrier and therefore are not the drug of choice to treat bacterial infections of the CNS. β-Lactam antibiotics generally pass through the placental membranes of pregnant females to enter fetal tissues and can be found in the animal's milk after systemic administration.

Some cephalosporins are metabolized by the liver and then excreted via the kidneys. Other members of this group are renally excreted in their original form. The concentrations of cephalosporins in urine can be high because the drugs are usually excreted by filtration and active secretion into the renal tubules.

Precautions for Use of Cephalosporins

Cephalosporins, like penicillins, are considered safe antimicrobials. Also similar to penicillins is the potential for hypersensitivity reactions. However, the incidence of hypersensitivity reactions to cephalosporins is lower than that caused by penicillins. Cephalosporins should not be used in animals with a known sensitivity to penicillins because of the possibility of cross-reactivity. Hypersensitivity reactions can cause fever, rashes, eosinophilia, and anaphylaxis.

Many cephalosporins cause pain if injected intramuscularly; some can cause local inflammation, swelling, and tissue necrosis when administered perivascularly (outside the blood vessel). The veterinary professional should study the warnings and adverse effects listed on the package insert and closely follow guidelines for administration before giving the first dose. The veterinary professional should not assume that what is safe for one cephalosporin is safe for all cephalosporins.

Superinfection caused by overgrowth of pathogenic bacteria may be associated with oral administration of first-generation cephalosporins. In addition, orally administered cephalosporins may cause anorexia, vomiting, and diarrhea. Because cephalosporins are most effective against a population of bacteria that is rapidly dividing, simultaneous use of bacteriostatic antibiotics such as chloramphenicol may reduce the efficacy of cephalosporins.

Cephalosporins reportedly can produce **nephrotoxicosis** (kidney damage), although this effect is rare when they are used at recommended doses in animals with normal renal function. It has been reported that the use of other nephrotoxic drugs such as aminoglycoside antibiotics (gentamicin, amikacin, and neomycin) and amphotericin B in conjunction with cephalosporins increases the risk of nephrotoxicosis. However, the risk of nephrotoxicosis with cephalosporin use has only been documented with cephaloridine, a cephalosporin that is no longer marketed. However, caution should be exercised when two potentially nephrotoxic drugs are used concurrently.

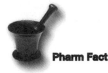

Pharm Fact

The efficacy of cephalosporins may be reduced if they are used concurrently with bacteriostatic drugs.

BACITRACINS

Bacitracins are a group of polypeptide antibiotics, of which bacitracin A is the major component. Bacitracin is a common ingredient in topical antibiotic creams and ointments and is often combined with polymyxin B and neomycin to provide a wide spectrum of antibacterial activity. Bacitracin resembles penicillin and cephalosporins in its ability to disrupt the bacterial cell wall. However, its mechanism of action is different and the drug molecule does not contain a β-lactam ring; hence bacitracin is not susceptible to β-lactamase.

Bacitracin is toxic to the kidneys. However, because it is used primarily as a topical drug and is poorly absorbed through intact skin, the drug does not enter the body in significant amounts. Bacitracin is also added to the water or feed of poultry to help control certain intestinal pathogens. Bacitracin is hydrophilic and therefore is poorly absorbed from the intestinal tract, reducing the likelihood of nephrotoxicity.

AMINOGLYCOSIDES

Aminoglycosides are a powerful group of antimicrobials used in veterinary medicine to combat a variety of serious bacterial infections. Safe use of these antimicrobials requires understanding of their toxic mechanisms. Aminoglycosides used in veterinary medicine include gentamicin, amikacin, neomycin, streptomycin, dihydrostreptomycin, apramycin, kanamycin, and tobramycin. With the exception of amikacin, aminoglycosides can be identified by the *micin* or *mycin* suffix in the chemical or nonproprietary name. Many trade or proprietary names of tetracyclines also use the *mycin* suffix; drugs with these trade names should not be confused with aminoglycosides.

Mechanism of Action

Aminoglycosides are bactericidal through their action on the bacteria's ribosomal production of essential proteins. Because the ribosome is located within the bacterial cytoplasm, aminoglycosides must be transported through the bacterial cell membrane to exert their effects. Aminoglycosides are actively transported into the bacterium via an oxygen-dependent mechanism. For this reason, aminoglycosides are highly effective against many **aerobic** bacteria, which require oxygen to survive, but ineffective against most **anaerobic** bacteria, which do not require oxygen. Once taken up by the aerobic bacterium, the aminoglycoside combines with the ribosome and prevents normal synthesis of protein from amino acids.

Although some cross-resistance occurs between members of the aminoglycoside family, it is not as common as with the penicillins. For example, some strains of *Pseudomonas* bacteria are resistant to gentamicin but sensitive to amikacin. Bacterial resistance is attributable to destructive enzymes produced by the bacteria or inability of the aminoglycoside to cross the cell wall or cell membrane.

Pharmacokinetics of Aminoglycosides

Aminoglycosides are potentially nephrotoxic (toxic to the kidney) and **ototoxic** (toxic to the inner ear) even at "normal" doses. Therefore anyone who administers these drugs or monitors their effects in an animal should be aware of the way these drugs act in the body.

Aminoglycosides are hydrophilic at most physiologic pHs, and therefore are usually administered parenterally (by injection) because absorption after oral administration would be limited. The few aminoglycosides that are used orally are intended to remain in the intestinal tract and are not absorbed to any significant extent. Neonates, animals with intestinal hypomotility (slow gut movement), and animals with hemorrhagic or necrotic intestinal disease absorb greater amounts of aminoglycosides administered orally and thus are at greater risk of systemic side effects.

Although aminoglycosides are not well absorbed across intact skin, they are well absorbed through denuded or abraded skin, or when used to irrigate

Pharm Fact

Aminoglycosides must be used cautiously because of their potential to cause nephrotoxicity and ototoxicity.

and surgical sites. When the drug is placed in the uterus or bladder, most of it remains at the site and little is absorbed through the membrane surfaces.

When administered parenterally and absorbed, aminoglycosides remain mostly in the extracellular fluid. The hydrophilic aminoglycoside molecules do not penetrate the blood-brain barrier or the globe of the eye to any significant degree. Because they are found in high concentrations in the bronchial secretions, aminoglycosides are often used to treat cases of pneumonia in which part of the infection is located within the lumen of the bronchioles.

The volume of distribution for aminoglycosides is often much larger in neonates and young animals than in adult animals because bodies of young animals generally contain a larger ratio of extracellular water to fat. For this reason, if 50 mg of amikacin were administered to a 10-lb puppy and 50 mg to a 10-lb adult dog, the puppy would likely have lower drug concentrations in its body because the drug would be diluted in a proportionally larger volume of extracellular fluid.

The kidneys and inner ears accumulate aminoglycosides via an active transport process. This accumulation is thought to contribute to the nephrotoxicity and ototoxicity produced by large or frequent doses of aminoglycosides. Aminoglycosides cross the placenta readily and can produce nephrotoxicity and ototoxicity in a pregnant animal and its developing fetus.

Aminoglycosides are eliminated almost exclusively via glomerular filtration in the kidneys. Because the molecules are hydrophilic, minimal drug resorption occurs in the loop of Henle and most of the drug is excreted in the urine. This efficient elimination helps explain the short half-life of aminoglycosides (usually 1 to 2 hours depending on the species) in animals with normal renal function. Because these drugs are almost exclusively eliminated by the kidneys, any decrease in renal function from old age, dehydration, shock, or kidney disease can slow elimination and increase half-life, prolong high plasma drug concentrations, and increase the risk of nephrotoxicity or ototoxicity.

Precautions for Use of Aminoglycosides

The veterinary professional should evaluate the risk of nephrotoxicity or ototoxicity in any animal receiving aminoglycosides. As mentioned previously, cells of the inner ear and kidney actively take up aminoglycosides, which has a toxic effect on these cells. The drug can only leave those cells by passive diffusion, so the dosage interval (time between doses) must be increased to allow aminoglycoside plasma concentrations to decrease enough to set up a concentration gradient that permits drug movement out of the cells and into the plasma. If the drug were to be given by continuous IV infusion or too frequently (for example, every 4 hours instead of every 12 hours), plasma and extracellular fluid concentrations would not decrease sufficiently to permit this concentration gradient to develop.

If aminoglycosides are to be used in patients with marginal kidney function, renal function must be closely monitored with blood urea nitrogen

(BUN), serum creatinine, and urine specific gravity measurements. An early sign of aminoglycoside nephrotoxicity is the appearance of casts or protein in the urine. In the absence of aminoglycoside plasma concentration measurements, daily urinalyses of high-risk patients may provide indications of impending nephrotoxicity. By the time the BUN and creatinine levels rise, nephrotoxicity has already occurred. Nephrotoxicity may be reversible if the drug is withdrawn or the dosage is significantly altered before extensive renal tubular necrosis has occurred.

For most other antimicrobials, delayed elimination resulting from renal or hepatic problems requires dose reduction. However, when aminoglycosides are used in animals with reduced renal function, the same dose is used but the interval between injections is increased. When the dosage interval is extended, plasma concentrations of aminoglycoside decrease enough to prevent toxicity (Fig. 9-5). The degree of renal dysfunction and measurements of plasma drug concentrations dictate the dosage interval increase and whether a dosage increase is also needed. Recent research has indicated that using a single daily dose of aminoglycosides, even in animals with normal renal function, may still provide significant bactericidal activity while reducing the risk for nephrotoxicity by extending the dose interval.

Aminoglycoside use resulting in ototoxicity can cause deafness in treated animals. Although deafness is not a serious disability in most domestic animals, it can pose a significant problem in certain animals. Dogs trained to assist hearing-impaired people require a considerable investment of time, expense, and emotion, all of which would be lost if a dog became deaf as a result of inappropriate aminoglycoside administration. Because ototoxicity also often affects balance (that is, the vestibular system of the inner ear), service and working dogs can be rendered completely ineffective if unable to maintain their balance. Cats are apparently very sensitive to the vestibular toxic effects of aminoglycosides and may show circling, fall over, and/or experience repetitive, rapid eye movements (nystagmus) as a result of inappropriate aminoglycoside administration. The benefits of aminoglycoside administration must be weighed carefully against the potential risks in these types of animals.

Neomycin appears to have the greatest potential for inducing nephrotoxicity in animals and people if it is systemically absorbed. However, it is rarely injected and is poorly absorbed from the intestinal tract, thus limiting its nephrotoxic risk under normal circumstances. Nephrotoxicity from gentamicin use has been reported in many species, including exotic animals, wildlife, and birds.

Veterinary professionals must be aware that the combined use of parenterally administered and topically applied aminoglycosides on injured skin (for example, from degloving injuries, burns, severe abrasions, thermal or chemical burns, sloughed skin) can allow toxic concentrations of the drug to be absorbed.

Aminoglycosides should either not be used or should be used with extreme caution in combination with other potentially nephrotoxic or ototoxic drugs. Cephalosporins are thought to increase the risk of nephrotoxicity when used with aminoglycosides; however, this interaction has only been reported with cephaloridine, a cephalosporin no longer marketed, and

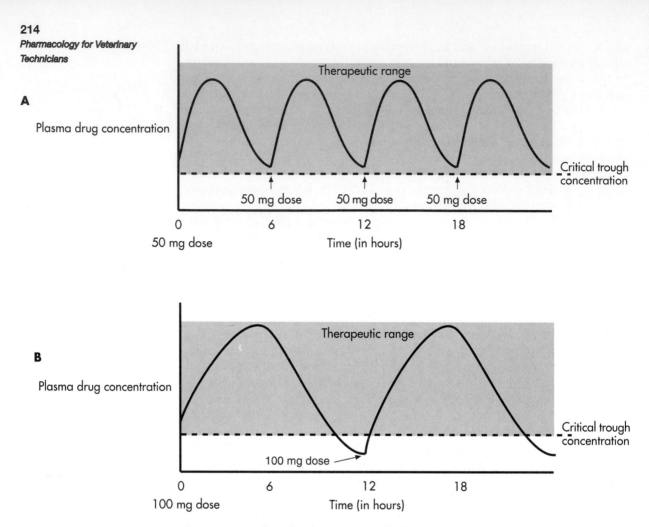

A

Plasma drug concentration

Therapeutic range

Critical trough concentration

50 mg dose   50 mg dose   50 mg dose

0   6   12   18

50 mg dose   Time (in hours)

B

Plasma drug concentration

Therapeutic range

Critical trough concentration

100 mg dose

0   6   12   18

100 mg dose   Time (in hours)

Fig. 9-5 Extending the dosage interval allows the plasma drug concentration to fall below a critical level. **A,** 50 mg of aminoglycoside given q6h: trough concentration does not decrease low enough to prevent nephrotoxicity. **B,** Same daily dose with 100 mg of aminoglycoside given q12h: trough concentration is low enough to decrease risk of nephrotoxicity.

cephalothin (Keflin), a human drug occasionally used in veterinary medicine.

Although aminoglycosides are very effective against many bacteria, cellular debris (such as pus) can render them ineffective. Cellular debris is comprised of ruptured cells and cell contents, including the nucleic acids of ribosomes. As stated previously, aminoglycosides attach to the nucleic acids of ribosomes in bacteria to produce their bactericidal effect. If an aminoglycoside enters an infection site that contains a significant amount of cellular debris, the drug tends to bind to the nucleic acids in the cellular debris and therefore less drug is absorbed into the bacteria. Thus pyogenic (pus producing) infections, such as abscesses or topical infections with necrotic tissue, must be cleaned or flushed thoroughly to remove cellular debris before application of aminoglycosides can be instituted.

Gentamicin, amikacin, kanamycin, and tobramycin should not be stored in the same syringe or bottle with penicillins because these β-lactam drugs chemically inactivate the aminoglycoside over hours to days. However, penicillins and aminoglycosides are often used together to treat severe infections because they affect different bacteria sites and their spectra of activity against bacterial strains are complementary. When monitoring aminoglycoside plasma concentrations in an animal that has been treated both with penicillins and aminoglycosides, the serum sample collected for aminoglycoside analysis should be processed quickly or frozen to prevent artificially low plasma concentrations of aminoglycoside caused by penicillins in the serum.

QUINOLONES

Quinolones are bactericidal antimicrobials that are gaining favor for a variety of uses in veterinary medicine. Three newer products being used are enrofloxacin, ciprofloxacin, and sarafloxacin, which are sometimes referred to as *fluoroquinolones*. An older quinolone, nalidixic acid, and another human fluoroquinolone, norfloxacin, are not used in veterinary medicine to any significant extent.

Enrofloxacin (Baytril) is a veterinary drug approved for use in dogs and more recently cats. Sarafloxacin (Saraflox) was the first quinolone approved for use in food animals (poultry only). Enrofloxacin has been used as an extra-label drug to treat neonatal diseases in swine and cattle when other antimicrobials were ineffective. Ciprofloxacin is only approved for use in people, and any animal use is unapproved. These three quinolones, which are most commonly used in veterinary medicine, have similar spectra of antibacterial activity and are considered equivalent therapeutic drugs.

Mechanism of Action

In bacteria the DNA molecule must be tightly coiled to be properly stored within the bacterial cell. An enzyme called *DNA gyrase*, facilitates this "supercoiling" process. Quinolone antimicrobials interfere with DNA gyrase, preventing bacterial DNA supercoiling and subsequently disrupting DNA function; this rapidly kills the bacterium. Quinolones do not disrupt the mammalian cell function because the bacterial and mammalian DNA gyrases are different.

The fluoroquinolones are effective against common gram-negative and gram-positive bacteria found in skin, respiratory, and urinary infections, including β-lactamase–producing *Staphylococcus, Pseudomonas, Klebsiella, Escherichia coli,* and *Salmonella* species. However, these quinolones have varying effects on *Streptococcus* species, which are a widely occuring gram-positive bacterial specie, and are not recommended for use in streptococcal infections. Quinolones in general are ineffective against most anaerobic bacteria and should not be used to treat anaerobic infections.

Pharmacokinetics of Quinolones

The veterinary product Baytril (enrofloxacin) is available in injectable and oral tablet forms. Saraflox (sarafloxacin) is marketed as a water-soluble, orally administered powder and in an injectable form. These drugs are more efficiently absorbed from the intestinal tract of dogs and cats than of adult horses. Although calves can adequately absorb orally administered enrofloxacin, bioavailability is less than 20% after oral administration in mature ruminants. Unlike some penicillins, enrofloxacin absorption after oral administration is not significantly affected by food; food only slightly delays the onset of absorption.

An advantage of enrofloxacin and ciprofloxacin compared with other antimicrobials is that they accumulate in high concentrations in the kidneys, liver, lungs, bone, joint fluid, aqueous humor of the eyeball, and respiratory tissues. Thus quinolones are often used to treat severe infections of the skin (pyoderma), respiratory tract, and urinary tract. Because enrofloxacin is able to accumulate in the prostate, an organ few antimicrobials are able to penetrate in significant concentrations, it is one of the few antimicrobials that effectively treats prostate infections.

Ciprofloxacin and to a lesser degree enrofloxacin are both metabolized by the liver, producing a variety of metabolites. It is interesting to note that one of the metabolites of enrofloxacin is ciprofloxacin. Both the unchanged (not metabolized) and metabolized forms of quinolones are excreted via the kidney and liver. Because there are two routes of elimination for these drugs, reduced kidney function may not require a significant change in the dosage of enrofloxacin or ciprofloxacin. However, it is probably prudent to slightly reduce the daily dose in animals with severe renal disease to prevent drug accumulation in the body.

Precautions for Use of Quinolones

Although quinolones are considered very safe drugs, they can adversely affect developing joint cartilage. During periods of rapid growth in dogs, quinolones may cause bubblelike lesions in the joint cartilage. Although these reported changes occurred after administration of 5 times the normal dose, the manufacturer states that enrofloxacin is contraindicated in small- and medium-sized dogs between the ages of 2 and 8 months. The veterinary professional must remember that large-breed dogs have periods of rapid cartilage and bone development that extend well beyond 8 months; therefore use of quinolones is contraindicated for a longer period in these animals than in smaller breeds. Because quinolones can affect fetal cartilage development, it is better to avoid using them in pregnant animals unless no other antimicrobials are effective. Although enrofloxacin has been used in horses (but is unapproved), the drug should not be used in young horses and should be used with caution in older horses because of the potential of cartilage damage.

Because ciprofloxacin reportedly causes crystalluria (urine crystal formation) in humans, animals treated with enrofloxacin or ciprofloxacin should have sufficient water to maintain proper hydration, ensure normal renal perfusion, and prevent precipitation of drug crystals.

There is some evidence to support the warning against using quinolones in animals that are prone to seizures. In instances described as rare or infrequent, use of quinolones has precipitated seizure activity in animals predisposed to seizures. Therefore the benefits of enrofloxacin or ciprofloxacin use should be weighed against the possibility of producing seizures before using either of these antibiotics in epileptic animals.

The veterinary professional should be aware that enrofloxacin is often used as the initial choice for treating infections; many of these infections would respond to treatment with more traditional drugs, such as penicillins or sulfonamides. Indiscriminate use of enrofloxacin for routine infections could lead to development of bacterial resistance, thus reducing the drug's effectiveness in severe infections in which quinolones are often more effective than penicillins or sulfa drugs. Veterinary professionals should use new or more potent antimicrobials carefully and somewhat restrictively to delay the inevitable onset of bacterial resistance.

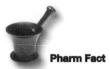

Pharm Fact

Indiscriminate use of new, potent antimicrobials can hasten development of resistant strains of microorganisms.

Regulatory controversy

After approving sarafloxacin for use in poultry, the FDA's Center for Veterinary Medicine announced that it would more closely monitor and enforce use of fluoroquinolones for label indications only. This would make enrofloxacin or sarafloxacin use in neonatal swine or cattle illegal. As other new fluoroquinolones are approved for use in veterinary medicine, it is likely that regulations governing fluoroquinolone use will be more strictly enforced.

TETRACYCLINES

Tetracyclines are a group of bacteriostatic antimicrobials that have been used in veterinary medicine for many years, especially in food-animal production. Therefore many microorganisms are resistant to most of the tetracyclines, forcing veterinarians to use other antimicrobials. Although overall use of tetracyclines has decreased in the past 10 years, tetracyclines are usually the drugs most commonly used for rickettsial diseases (Rocky Mountain spotted fever in humans; ehrlichiosis and salmon poisoning in dogs, hemobartonellosis in dogs and cats), *Mycoplasma* pneumonia, chlamydial infections (especially those manifested as ocular disease in cats), psittacosis in birds, and borreliosis (Lyme disease). Tetracyclines have also been prescribed, with variable results, to help control tear staining (epiphora) on dogs' faces.

Tetracycline drugs can usually be recognized in the written form by the *-cycline* suffix of the nonproprietary name. Tetracycline and oxytetracycline have similar spectra of antibacterial activity and actions in the body. The newer and more lipophilic doxycycline and minocycline are human drugs that are being used more frequently in animals (unapproved use) because of their longer half-life, broader spectrum of antibacterial action, and better penetration of tissues than the older tetracyclines.

Mechanism of Action

Tetracyclines bind to bacterial ribosomes and prevent transfer RNA from linking to the ribosome, thereby disrupting protein synthesis. In contrast to the aminoglycosides, which also bind to ribosomes and disrupt protein synthesis in a slightly different way, tetracyclines inhibit bacterial cellular function and division, but do not cause immediate bacterial destruction. Because tetracyclines are usually bacteriostatic, they depend on a functional immune system to help them overcome a microbial invasion.

The reason for part of the antibacterial action of tetracyclines is that bacteria appear to actively take up tetracycline and concentrate it within the bacterial cell. Mammalian cells generally do not concentrate tetracyclines, thereby avoiding some of their toxic effects. However, at higher dosages, tetracyclines can also affect protein synthesis in mammalian cells.

Pharmacokinetics of Tetracyclines

Members of the tetracycline family vary in their absorption from the GI tract. Generally, doxycycline and minocycline are absorbed much better than oxytetracycline or tetracycline. In addition, tetracycline and oxytetracycline are readily **chelated** (bound to and precipitated out of solution) by mineral ions with two positive charges such as calcium (Ca^{++}), magnesium (Mg^{++}), iron (Fe^{++}), and copper (Cu^{++}).

If oxytetracycline or tetracycline is administered by mouth with a meal that includes dairy products such as milk or cheese or other foods high in divalent cations (ions with two positive charges) or trivalent cations (three positive charges), much of the drug is chelated in the gut and is not absorbed. In addition to milk and cheese, other common items that can chelate tetracyclines include iron supplements, oral antacids (Mg^{++}), or antidiarrheal products that contain kaolin, pectin (Kaopectate), or bismuth subsalicylate (Pepto-Bismol). In contrast to oxytetracycline or tetracycline, doxycycline's absorption is only reduced by about 20% in the presence of most of these products, which is not clinically significant in most cases.

Oxytetracycline is the most commonly used injectable tetracycline because of its good absorption from IM injection sites. In contrast to oxytetracycline, tetracycline is erratically absorbed from IM injection sites and therefore produces more reliable concentrations when administered by mouth. Oxytetracycline injectable is also commonly marketed in a longer-acting form as LA-200, which is normally administered every 2 or 3 days.

Once absorbed into the systemic circulation, tetracyclines are distributed to most tissues and can reach significant concentrations in saliva and bronchial secretions. Because tetracycline and oxytetracycline are hydrophilic, they do not achieve significant concentrations in the CNS; doxycycline and minocycline more readily cross the blood-brain barrier. Because of their lipophilic nature, doxycycline and minocycline also penetrate both the globe of the eye and the prostate gland better than oxytetracycline or tetracycline. Doxycycline is preferred over tetracycline and oxytetracycline for treatment of CNS signs associated with borreliosis (Lyme disease) in people.

Tetracyclines and oxytetracycline are excreted via filtration through the kidneys mostly unchanged. Because this is an important elimination pathway for these two drugs, any change in kidney function such as renal disease or decreased renal perfusion may allow accumulation of drug in the body unless the dose is decreased. These two drugs are also excreted by the liver into the intestine in bile, where they may be chelated by intestinal contents and be excreted with the feces. Any tetracycline or oxytetracycline not chelated may be resorbed back into the body, a process known as *enterohepatic circulation* (movement from the intestine to the liver and back). Unlike the renal excretion of oxytetracycline and tetracycline, doxycycline is largely excreted into the intestine. Because it does not depend on glomerular filtration for elimination, the dose of doxycycline does not necessarily have to be reduced in animals with impaired kidney function.

Precautions for Use of Tetracyclines

The major problems with tetracyclines relate to their binding with calcium and other divalent cations. Tetracycline and oxytetracycline are chelated with the minerals of developing tooth enamel, imparting a yellow, mottled discoloration if given while teeth are developing. Therefore the veterinary professional should be careful not to administer tetracycline during the first few months of an animal's life. Although doxycycline can cause the same effect, it is less likely to cause the discoloration than the more water-soluble oxytetracycline or tetracycline.

In addition to tooth enamel, tetracyclines combine with the calcium in bones and can impair bone development in young animals at higher concentrations. Because tetracyclines can cross the placental barrier readily and affect fetal bone growth, these drugs should not be given to pregnant animals during the last half of gestation unless the benefits outweigh the risk of possible adverse effects on the fetus.

As with other broad-spectrum antimicrobials, the tetracyclines when administered orally can produce superinfections from overgrowth of pathogenic bacteria in the gut. In ruminants, high oral doses can kill off significant numbers of normal ruminal flora, resulting in ruminoreticular stasis (rumen inactivity). In dogs, even if superinfections do not occur, diarrhea, vomiting and anorexia are common. Cats tolerate tetracyclines even less and may show fever, depression, or abdominal pain. Doxycycline is not adversely affected to any significant degree by the presence of food in the intestines, and the presence of food tends to decrease some of these GI side effects. For these reasons, animals with GI upset from oral doxycycline administration may be able to better tolerate the drug if it is given with a small meal that is low in Ca^{++} or other divalent or trivalent cations.

Intravenous injections of relatively small doses of doxycycline in horses have resulted in cardiac arrhythmias, collapse, and death. These signs have been observed in other species receiving rapid IV injections of normal doses, but horses appear to be especially susceptible to these effects. The proposed mechanism for this reaction is chelation of Ca^{++}, which reduces the Ca^{++} needed for proper cardiac muscle function. Until further research is done, parenteral administration of doxycycline is not recommended in horses.

Veterinary professionals should be aware of some important drug interactions with tetracyclines. The inhalant anesthetic methoxyflurane can produce nephrotoxicity through metabolism to fluoride ions, which are toxic to kidney cells. Of the tetracycline drugs, only oxytetracycline and tetracycline appear to enhance this nephrotoxic effect and therefore should not be used in animals anesthetized with methoxyflurane.

Because tetracycline drugs are bacteriostatic, they may interfere with the efficacy of penicillins and cephalosporins, which require an actively dividing bacterial population to exert their antibacterial action. Although some sources cite a similar impairment of aminoglycosides by tetracyclines, the clinical significance of this interaction is questionable.

Expired tetracycline and oxytetracycline can decompose to form a nephrotoxic compound. This compound damages the cells of the kidneys proximal convoluted tubule, resulting in **Fanconi's syndrome,** a condition in which resorption of glucose from the glomerular filtrate is impaired, resulting in glucosuria (glucose in the urine). Unlike diabetes mellitus, where glucosuria is associated with high blood glucose concentrations, in Fanconi's syndrome glucose concentrations are normal.

SULFONAMIDES AND POTENTIATED SULFONAMIDES

Sulfonamides (sulfa drugs) were the first antimicrobials used on a widespread basis in human and veterinary medicine. Because they have been in use for many years, many strains of bacteria have become resistant to them. To increase the efficacy of sulfonamides and convert them from bacteriostatic to bactericidal drugs, they are sometimes combined with other compounds such as trimethoprim and ormetoprim to potentiate (increase) their antibacterial effects.

Some of the more common sulfonamides used in veterinary medicine include sulfadimethoxine (combined with ormetoprim in the veterinary drug Primor), sulfadiazine (combined with trimethoprim in the veterinary drug Tribrissen), sulfamethoxazole (combined with trimethoprim in the human drug Septra), sulfachlorpyridazine (used in livestock and poultry), and sulfasalazine (used for its antiinflammatory effect in inflammatory bowel disease). Other sulfonamides are used to a limited extent in veterinary medicine as a result of the prevalence of resistant bacteria and the availability of cost-effective alternatives.

Sulfonamides are sometimes described as *enteric* or *systemic* sulfas. An enteric sulfa such as sulfasalazine is designed to remain in the intestinal tract after oral administration and is not absorbed into the body. The site of action of an enteric sulfa is within the bowel lumen. Systemic sulfas are absorbed from the intestinal tract and are used to treat infections in tissues other than the bowels.

Mechanism of Action

To survive, bacteria must synthesize folic acid and then convert it to other folate compounds for use by the bacterium. Sulfonamides inactivate the enzymes involved in synthesis of folic acid; trimethoprim and ormetoprim interfere with conversion of folic acid to other essential folate compounds. This helps explain the reason sulfas and trimethoprim and ormetoprim separately are bacteriostatic, but when combined into potentiated sulfas become bactericidal.

Potentiated sulfas used in veterinary medicine have a fairly broad spectrum of antibacterial activity, including many gram-positive organisms such as streptococci, staphylococci, and *Nocardia*. Although sulfas and potentiated sulfas are not very effective against gram-negative organisms, they are the drugs of choice for treatment of some protozoal infections, including *Coccidia* and *Toxoplasma* organisms.

Unlike other sulfonamides, sulfasalazine is not commonly used for its antimicrobial effect; rather, it is used for its antiinflammatory effect on the colon. When sulfasalazine is given orally, less than one-third of the drug is absorbed. The remainder stays in the bowel lumen, where it passes into the colon and is transformed by colonic bacteria into another sulfonamide (sulfapyridine) and an aspirin-like antiinflammatory drug (aminosalicylic acid). As discussed in Chapter 4, the salicylate inhibits prostaglandin formation, decreasing inflammation and hypersecretion associated with inflammatory bowel disease.

Pharmacokinetics of Sulfonamides

With the exception of the enteric sulfonamide sulfasalazine, sulfonamides and their potentiated forms are well absorbed from the GI tract of monogastric (single-stomach) animals. In ruminants the trimethoprim component of potentiated sulfas may be trapped in the rumen after oral administration and degraded to some degree, thereby reducing the amount of trimethoprim absorbed. Generally, sulfonamides are well distributed throughout the body, including pleural fluid, peritoneal fluid, synovial fluid, and ocular fluid. Concentrations in these fluids, including the cerebrospinal fluid (CSF) during meningitis, can achieve 50% to 80% of the plasma concentration. Sulfonamides cross the placenta and can attain concentrations that are therapeutic or toxic to the fetus. Sulfonamides can also pass into the milk of nursing females.

Sulfa drugs vary in the degree to which they are excreted intact in the urine or metabolized by the liver before renal excretion. Several sulfonamides are both filtered by the glomerulus and actively secreted into the renal tubules, achieving significant concentrations in the urine. This is one of the reasons sulfonamides are used for urinary tract infections.

In the potentiated compounds, the sulfonamide component and the potentiating compound usually have different half-lives of elimination and different patterns of distribution. Thus it is difficult to predict the amount of each component that will reach the infection site and the length of time it will remain at the site. Trimethoprim is fairly quickly eliminated from the plasma; however, it may remain within some tissues for a longer time than

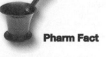

Pharm Fact

Sulfonamides alone are bacteriostatic, while potentiated sulfonamides exert bactericidal action.

its short half-life would indicate. The pharmacokinetics of ormetoprim in domestic animals have not been well described.

Clinically these pharmacokinetic differences are important because the sulfonamides and their potentiating compounds (trimethoprim and ormetoprim) by themselves are bacteriostatic. Only if both compounds penetrate the infection site together, producing concentrations above the MIC for the bacterial species involved, is the bactericidal effect achieved. This may be the reason some clinicians administer trimethoprim-sulfonamide products twice daily, although once-daily use is recommended.

Precautions for Use of Sulfonamides

A disadvantage of some sulfonamides or their metabolites is that they may precipitate out in the kidney if there is insufficient fluid volume (dehydration) or if the urine becomes acidic. The resulting **crystalluria** (crystals in the urine) can damage the renal tubules. The older sulfonamides and sulfadiazine are more prone to precipitation (crystallization) than the newer compounds. Because an alkaline pH keeps sulfonamides from precipitating as readily, and because herbivores generally have alkaline urine, crystallization is not as much a concern in herbivores as in carnivores with their more acidic urine. Precipitation and crystallization can be prevented by water intake that is sufficient to maintain urine production and by preventing overdosing of sulfonamides.

Because most sulfonamides are metabolized by the liver to some extent, many manufacturers advise caution in using these drugs in animals with hepatic disease. The kidneys are also important for elimination of metabolized and intact sulfonamides, so similar precautions should be observed in animals with reduced kidney function.

One of the more common reactions to sulfonamides in dogs is decreased tear production, resulting in keratoconjunctivitis sicca, which is more commonly called KCS, or "dry eye". Dogs with sulfonamide-induced KCS will suddenly begin to accumulate mucoid or crusty matter around the eye, show signs of ocular discomfort by rubbing the face or pawing at the eyes, and develop a dull corneal surface. A veterinarian should examine dogs with these signs immediately to determine if tear production is reduced. In the past many cases of sulfonamide-induced keratoconjunctivitis sicca could not be reversed. A cyclosporine ophthalmic ointment (Optimmune) is now available that will restore production of near normal levels of tears. However, affected dogs must be treated with cyclosporine for the rest of their lives.

Other reactions associated with sulfonamides include skin reactions, which are manifested as pruritus (itching), swelling of the face, and hives; hypersensitivity reactions in large-breed dogs; and liver dysfunction.

Unlike the systemically absorbed sulfonamides, sulfasalazine, the enteric sulfa, poses a risk to cats because they cannot well tolerate salicylates. As mentioned previously, sulfasalazine is metabolized by GI bacteria to sulfapyridine and aminosalicylic acid. If the salicylate compound is absorbed in sufficient amounts to overwhelm the cat's ability to metabolize the drug, it can produce toxicity. Therefore sulfasalazine must be used cautiously in cats and animals with aspirin (salicylate) hypersensitivity.

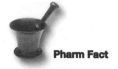

Pharm Fact

The use of sulfonamides can result in keratoconjunctivitis sicca, or "dry eye."

Regardless of which sulfonamide is used, veterinary professionals should know the signs of an adverse reaction to sulfonamides and advise animal owners of possible side effects to prevent the serious complications caused by an adverse reaction.

OTHER ANTIMICROBIALS USED IN VETERINARY MEDICINE

Lincosamides

Lincosamide antibiotics include lincomycin and clindamycin (Antirobe). These drugs are bacterial protein inhibitors and can be bacteriostatic or bactericidal, depending on the concentrations attained at the infection site. The lincosamides are generally effective against many gram-positive aerobic cocci. Clindamycin has good efficacy against many pathogenic anaerobes. For this reason clindamycin and lincomycin (to a lesser extent) are indicated for use in deep pyodermas (skin infections), abscesses, dental infections, bite wounds, and osteomyelitis caused by *Staphylococcus aureus*. Bacterial cross-resistance is likely between lincosamide antibiotics.

Because lincosamides are generally metabolized in the liver and then excreted in the urine or bile, severe liver or renal disease can prolong the half-life of elimination and necessitate reducing the dose to prevent toxicity.

Lincomycin is approved for use in a variety of species, including dogs, cats, swine, and poultry, but clindamycin is only approved for use in dogs. Lincosamides in general are contraindicated for use in rabbits, hamsters, guinea pigs, horses, and ruminants because in these species they can cause serious GI effects, resulting in death. Even in approved species, vomiting, diarrhea, and bloody diarrhea may occur. Lincosamides can pass into the milk of lactating animals, which may cause nursing puppies and kittens to develop diarrhea.

Information on clindamycin as a treatment for toxoplasmosis in cats has been published. However, a preliminary study of cats experimentally infected with toxoplasmosis indicated that a larger-than-expected number of the cats, who were treated with clindamycin, died suddenly. Until clindamycin use is further investigated, veterinary professionals should consider clindamycin as contraindicated for use in cats with active toxoplasmosis.

Simultaneous use of kaolin antidiarrheal preparations such as Kaopectate and lincomycin can reduce absorption of the lincosamide up to 90%. If the two compounds must be used in an animal, they should be given 2 hours apart, preferably with the lincomycin being given 2 hours before the antidiarrheal drug. Resorption of clindamycin is not affected as greatly by concurrent administration of kaolin.

Macrolides

The macrolide antibiotics erythromycin and tylosin (Tylan) are approved for use in a variety of companion and food animals, including dogs, cats, swine, sheep, cattle, and poultry. Although tylosin is approved for use in dogs and cats, its primary use is in livestock. Both drugs are bacteriostatic and work by inhibiting bacterial protein synthesis. They share similar spectra of antibacterial activity and bacterial cross-resistance.

Although erythromycin and tylosin are well distributed to most body tissues (including the prostate gland) and fluids, they do not penetrate the CNS or cerebrospinal fluid very well. Macrolide antibiotics are primarily excreted unchanged in the bile, with a small portion (less than 5% for erythromycin and slightly more for tylosin) being eliminated via the kidney. Erythromycin is fairly safe to use in animals with compromised renal function without significantly reducing the dose.

Although erythromycin is indicated for treatment of selected infections in foals *(Rhodococcus equi),* oral use of erythromycin in adult horses is controversial because it may produce fatal diarrhea. For a similar reason, use of oral erythromycin in ruminants and oral tylosin in horses is contraindicated. Although oral erythromycin should not be used in ruminants, injectable erythromycin is sometimes effective against stubborn respiratory infections in ruminants.

Because lincosamides and erythromycin compete for the same site on the bacterial ribosome, this competitive antagonism may decrease the efficacy of the individual drugs if they are used simultaneously.

Tilmicosin (Micotil) is a macrolide approved for subcutaneous (SC) administration for treatment of bovine respiratory diseases. The drug concentrates well in lung tissues and is especially effective against the organisms that cause bovine respiratory disease complex. The drug is very irritating if given intramuscularly and can cause death if given intravenously. Horses, swine, and primates (and presumably humans) are much more sensitive to the toxic effects of tilmicosin, which include tachycardia (rapid heart rate) and arrhythmias. Because tilmicosin can be dangerous in humans, veterinary professionals should be especially careful to prevent accidental injection into humans and to prevent contact of the drug with the eyes. Several cases of accidental injections were reported in 1994, none of which resulted in any severe reactions. However, a physician should be contacted immediately in cases of accidental human injection or contact with the eyes.

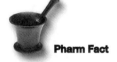

Pharm Fact

Horses and pigs are much more sensitive than cattle to the toxic effects of tilmicosin.

Metronidazole

Metronidazole (Flagyl) is a bactericidal antimicrobial that is also effective against protozoa that cause intestinal disease, such as *Giardia* (giardiasis) organisms, *Entamoeba histolytica* (amebiasis), *Trichomonas* (trichomoniasis) organisms, and *Balantidium coli* (balantidiasis). Although there is no approved veterinary form of metronidazole, human formulations are used for treatment of protozoal infections of the large bowel in dogs and cats, and enteric bacterial infections caused by anaerobic bacteria in horses, dogs, and cats. Because metronidazole has been used successfully in common domestic species, it is also being used to treat anaerobic infections in avian and reptilian species.

The exact mechanism of action of metronidazole is not known, but in bacteria it is thought to disrupt synthesis of DNA and nucleic acids. This mechanism may or may not be involved with birth defects in laboratory animals treated with metronidazole. Although there have been no reports of similar teratogenic (birth defect) effects in dogs, cats, or horses, the drug should be avoided if possible in pregnant animals, especially during the first few weeks of gestation.

Metronidazole has been reported to produce some neurologic side effects, including loss of balance, head tilt, nystagmus (rapid, repeated horizontal, vertical, or circular eye movement), disorientation, and even tremors and seizures. These effects are observed more frequently in animals receiving an overdose; however, they have also been observed in animals treated with recommended doses for long periods of time.

Nitrofurans

The nitrofurans are a large group of antimicrobials, of which nitrofurantoin (Furandantin) is most commonly used in veterinary medicine. Nitrofurantoin is bacteriostatic or bactericidal, depending on concentrations attained at the infection site. This drug is eliminated by the body so rapidly that it usually does not attain therapeutically significant concentrations in tissues. However, approximately half of the drug administered is filtered unchanged through the glomerulus and actively secreted into the renal tubule, and therefore it is used to treat infections of the lower urinary tract (that is, in the bladder and urethra) in dogs, cats, and occasionally horses. The drug is administered orally and is well absorbed but is rapidly eliminated into the urine. To prolong nitrofurantoin retention in the body, the drug has been formulated in a macrocrystalline form (Macrodantin) that is slowly absorbed from the GI tract.

GI side effects are fairly common with nitrofurantoin; however, delayed absorption of the macrocrystalline form is thought to reduce GI upset. Because this drug relies heavily on renal excretion, it is contraindicated for use in animals with renal disease or decreased kidney function.

Chloramphenicol and Florfenicol

Chloramphenicol is an antimicrobial that is bacteriostatic at low concentrations but may become bactericidal at higher dosages. It works by binding to ribosomes in sensitive bacteria and disrupting bacterial protein synthesis. However, chloramphenicol can also disrupt mitochondrial function in bone marrow cells of mammals, and has produced fatal aplastic anemia in humans. For this reason, chloramphenicol use in food animals is *totally* banned.

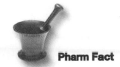

Pharm Fact

Chloramphenicol use in food animals is against FDA regulations.

In the past chloramphenicol has been used to treat small animals because of its ability to penetrate tissues and fluids, including the prostate gland, globe of the eye, and CNS fluids and its effectiveness against rickettsiae. Because some new antimicrobials have greater antibacterial activity and fewer side effects, chloramphenicol is less commonly used in small animal practice.

In dogs, most of a chloramphenicol dose is metabolized by glucuronide conjugation, and very little drug is excreted unchanged into the urine. Because cats poorly metabolize chloramphenicol in the liver, more of the drug is excreted intact via the kidneys. Therefore adequate renal function is a more important consideration for chloramphenicol use in cats than in dogs. The reduced metabolism and slower rate of elimination in cats are the reasons that chloramphenicol doses for cats are significantly lower than those for dogs. Neonates (especially neonatal kittens) can easily develop chloramphenicol toxicosis because of their poor hepatic function. In addition, chloramphenicol can be passed in the milk of lactating animals and subsequently ingested by the nursing offspring. Therefore lactating animals should not be given chloramphenicol.

Chloramphenicol can inhibit hepatic biotransformation of drugs such as phenobarbital, pentobarbital, primidone, and phenytoin (that is, all anticonvulsants and/or anesthetic barbiturates). Concurrent use of any of these drugs with chloramphenicol necessitates a reduction in dose of the anticonvulsants and barbiturates. Chloramphenicol is bacteriostatic at most dosages used in veterinary medicine; therefore it interferes with the bactericidal effects of penicillins, which require an actively growing bacterial population to exert their effect. Chloramphenicol binds to the same site on the ribosome as tylosin, erythromycin, lincomycin, and clindamycin, and may reduce the efficacy of these drugs if used simultaneously. However, the clinical effect of this antagonism has not been established in veterinary patients.

As mentioned, chloramphenicol can disrupt division of mammalian bone marrow cells, resulting in suppression of bone marrow cell formation **(myelosuppression)** and subsequent nonregenerative anemia, lymphopenia, and neutropenia. Therefore when handing chloramphenicol powder in capsules or tablets or while mixing the powder into a suspension, veterinary technicians must avoid repeated contact with or inhalation of the powder. Precautions include washing hands after handling capsules or tablets, avoiding inhalation of chloramphenicol powder, and using care when breaking chloramphenicol tablets or opening capsules.

Florfenicol (Nuflor) is a new antibiotic related to chloramphenicol but with some significant differences that enable this drug to be safely used in cattle for bovine respiratory diseases such as shipping fever or pneumonia. Like chloramphenicol, florfenicol is bacteriostatic, disrupts protein synthesis at the bacterial ribosomes, and penetrates tissues fairly well. Unlike chloramphenicol, florfenicol is approved for use in cattle and, according to the manufacturer's literature, lacks the chemical component that makes chloramphenicol toxic to the human bone marrow. Florfenicol is only approved for IM injection administered as 2 injections 48 hours apart. The drug has a 28-day withdrawal time. Because insufficient data is available regarding florfenicol's effect on bovine reproduction, pregnancy, and lactation, the drug should not be used in cattle of breeding age. The veterinary technician should thoroughly read the drug information on this and any new drug before use.

Rifampin

Rifampin is a bactericidal or bacteriostatic antimicrobial belonging to the class of antimicrobials known as rifamycins. It is primarily used with or without erythromycin for treatment of *Corynebacterium (Rhodococcus) equi* infections in young foals, and sometimes in conjunction with antifungal agents for treatment of aspergillosis or histoplasmosis in dogs and cats.

Rifampin suppresses formation of the RNA chain by inhibiting an RNA polymerase needed for RNA synthesis. Like quinolones, rifampin only affects bacterial RNA polymerase and does not disrupt the function of mammalian RNA polymerases.

Rifampin is a potent inducer, or accelerator, of hepatic microsomal enzyme function responsible for metabolism of some other drugs. Rifampin accelerates metabolism of those drugs, with subsequent shortened half-lives and lower plasma concentrations. Some of these drugs include heart medications such as propranolol and quinidine, chloramphenicol, benzodiazepine tranquilizers such as diazepam and zolazepam—Telazol, barbiturates such as phenobarbital and pentobarbital, and corticosteroids such as prednisone and dexamethasone.

Rifampin imparts a reddish-orange color to urine, tears, sweat, and saliva. Owners of animals being treated with rifampin should be informed of this change so they are not unduly alarmed.

ANTIFUNGALS

This group of antimicrobial drugs is effective against many of the fungal organisms that cause superficial mycoses (fungal skin infections) such as ringworm, and the deep or systemic mycoses (fungal infections within the body) such as histoplasmosis, blastomycosis, cryptococcosis, coccidioidomycosis, candidiasis, sporotrichosis, and aspergillosis. Because most antifungal drugs have potentially severe side effects, veterinary technicians must be aware of the correct procedures for safe handling, administration, storage, and disposal of antifungals.

Amphotericin B and Nystatin

Amphotericin B and nystatin belong to the same general group of antifungals and have similar antifungal spectra. (They are effective against most of the deep mycoses listed above.) However, the two drugs are used in very different ways. Amphotericin is administered parenterally for treatment of deep or systemic mycotic infections, and nystatin, because of its toxicity to tissues, is used only to treat *Candida* infections (candidiasis) on the skin, mucous membranes (for example, the mouth and vagina), and lining of the intestinal tract in dogs, cats, and birds. Both drugs are poorly absorbed from the GI tract. Amphotericin B is given intravenously to reach areas of deep mycotic infection. Because of its toxic effect on internal tissues, nystatin is applied topically to the skin, used as a lavage or flushing solution for oral or vaginal fungal infections, and given orally for candidiasis involving the intestinal tract.

Both drugs act by binding to a specific site on the fungal cell membrane, causing damage and allowing critical cellular components to leak from the fungal cell. This effect can be fungicidal or fungistatic, depending on the concentration of drug achieved at the fungal infection site. When injected intravenously, amphotericin B cannot penetrate many tissues, including muscle, bone, body fluids (pleural fluid, pericardial fluid, peritoneal fluid, joint fluid), or the CNS, but it remains for an extended time in the tissues it does penetrate. Humans treated with this drug excrete amphotericin for weeks after conclusion of treatment, reflecting the saturation of tissues with the drug and subsequent diffusion of the drug back into the systemic circulation. This accumulation in tissues also explains the reason amphotericin is administered every other day or 3 times a week.

Because nystatin is not injected parenterally and is poorly absorbed from sites of application such as the skin, mouth, vagina, and GI tract, side effects are usually limited to vomiting and anorexia associated with oral administration. Amphotericin, however, can cause several serious side effects, including nephrotoxicosis, fever, anorexia, and nausea. Most canine patients show some degree of nephrotoxicosis after amphotericin B administration; therefore evaluation of renal function (including BUN, creatinine, and urinalysis) must be done before treatment with amphotericin B so the degree of renal damage can be evaluated after the treatment. Unfortunately, renal damage caused by amphotericin B is frequently irreversible. In an attempt to decrease the risk of nephrotoxicity, some veterinary professionals have used mannitol (osmotic diuretic), IV infusion of concentrated saline solutions, and IV infusion of large volumes of fluids to maintain renal perfusion and urine production. These treatments are not consistently successful in preventing nephrotoxicosis caused by use of amphotericin B.

Ketoconazole and Itraconazole

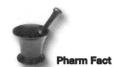

Pharm Fact

The antifungals ketoconazole and itraconazole produce fewer adverse effects than amphotericin B.

Ketoconazole and itraconazole are imidazole antifungals. Nearly all deep or systemic mycoses in animals are treated with these drugs or with amphotericin B. Ketoconazole and its newer relative, itraconazole, both cause leakage in the fungal cell membrane like amphotericin and nystatin, but this effect occurs at a different site and the onset of fungistatic or fungicidal activity is usually delayed 5 to 10 days. This drawback is balanced by the fewer side effects of the imidazoles as compared with amphotericin B. Of the two imidazoles, itraconazole has fewer side effects than ketoconazole and is apparently safe for use in cats.

Ketoconazole, and to a much lesser extent itraconazole, should be used with caution in breeding dogs because ketoconazole decreases steroid production in dogs and thus may reduce concentrations of testosterone and glucocorticoids (cortisol). Dogs given large doses of ketoconazole may require supplementation with corticosteroid drugs to compensate for reduced production of endogenous glucocorticoids. Testosterone and cortisol levels rebound after ketoconazole is withdrawn. Interestingly, cats are much more resistant to this effect than dogs.

Ketoconazole has caused death in embryonic rats and may be associated with mummified (dead) fetuses in dogs. Although ketoconazole is not absolutely contraindicated in pregnant dogs, the potential benefits of ketoconazole treatment should be weighed against the possible adverse effect on developing fetuses. Itraconazole has not been studied enough in veterinary patients to determine its effects on fetuses; it too should be used with caution in pregnant dogs.

Griseofulvin

Griseofulvin is a fungistatic drug used primarily to treat infections from *Trichophyton*, *Microsporum*, and *Epidermophyton* dermatophytes, all of which are superficial fungi, or literally "skin plants" found on dogs, cats, and horses. These fungi usually infect the skin, hair, nails, and claws, causing the condition known as *ringworm*. Griseofulvin is available as the veterinary product Fulvicin for oral use as a powder (for horses) or tablets. To be absorbed from the GI tract, the particles of griseofulvin must be very small. Therefore griseofulvin products are produced in "microsize" and "ultramicrosize" formulations. The ultramicrosize formulation is better absorbed than the microsize formulation. Therefore the dosage is adjusted according to the form of griseofulvin being administered.

Griseofulvin is metabolized by the liver and conjugated with glucuronide. Cats are slow to conjugate any drugs with glucuronide, so they eliminate griseofulvin slowly. The slow rate of elimination predisposes cats to accumulate a toxic level of the drug. For this reason, doses of griseofulvin for cats are lower than for dogs.

Griseofulvin is reportedly teratogenic in cats, producing cleft palates and other skeletal, skull, and nervous system defects in kittens of queens treated during gestation. Therefore griseofulvin is contraindicated for use in pregnant animals. More common side effects of orally administered griseofulvin

Antimicrobial Drug Categories and Names

Penicillins

Natural penicillins
   Penicillin G
   Penicillin V
Aminopenicillins
   Ampicillin
   Amoxicillin
   Hetacillin
Penicillinase-resistant
   Cloxacillin
   Dicloxacillin
   Oxacillin
Extended-spectrum
   Carbenicillin
   Ticarcillin
   Piperacillin

Penicillin adjuncts

Clavulanic acid
Sulbactam
Benzathine
Procaine

Cephalosporins

First-generation
   Cefadroxil (Cefa-Tabs)
   Cephapirin (Cefa-Lak)
   Cephalexin (Keflex)
   Cephalothin (Keflin)
Second-generation
   Cefoxitin (Mefoxin)
Third-generation
   Ceftiofur (Naxcel)
   Cefotaxime (Claforan)

Bacitracin

Aminoglycosides

Amikacin
Gentamicin
Kanamycin
Neomycin
Tobramycin

Continued

Antimicrobial Drug Categories and Names—cont'd

Quinolones

Ciprofloxacin
Enrofloxacin (Baytril)
Sarafloxacin (Saraflox)

Tetracyclines

Tetracycline
Oxytetracycline (LA-200)
Doxycycline
Minocycline

Sulfonamides

Sulfadiazine (Tribrissen)
Sulfadimethoxine (Primor)
Sulfamethoxazole
Sulfachlorpyridazine
Sulfasalazine

Sulfonamide potentiating compounds

Trimethoprim
Ormetoprim

Other antimicrobials

Lincosamides
  Lincomycin
  Clindamycin (Antirobe)
Macrolides
  Erythromycin
  Tylosin (Tylan)
  Tilmicosin (Micotil)
Metronidazole (Flagyl)
Nitrofurans-nitrofurantoin (Furadantin)
Chloramphenicol
Florfenicol
Rifampin
Antifungals
  Amphotericin B
  Nystatin
  Ketoconazole
  Itraconazole
  Griseofulvin (Fulvicin)

are anorexia, vomiting, and diarrhea. Although more severe effects such as anemia and leukopenia have been reported, these are rare at normal dosages. Griseofulvin should be used with caution in cats and especially in kittens because of the increased sensitivity of these animals to this drug.

Recommended Reading

Appel MJ, Jacobson RH: Canine lyme disease. In Bonagura JD, editor: *Kirk's current veterinary therapy XII*, Philadelphia, 1995, WB Saunders.

Boothe DM: GI pharmacology update, *Vet Prev* 1(2):2, 1994.

Collins BR: Antimicrobial drug use in rabbits, rodents, and other small mammals. Proceedings of the Miles Antimicrobial Therapy in Caged Birds and Exotic Pets Symposium, Orlando, Fla, Jan 1995.

Frank LA: Clinical pharmacology of rifampin, *JAVMA* 192(1):114, July 1990.

Jacobson ER: Use of antimicrobial therapy in reptiles. Proceedings of the Miles Antimicrobial Therapy in Caged Birds and Exotic Pets Symposium, Orlando, Fla, Jan 1995.

Legendre AM: Antimycotic drug therapy. In Bonagura JD, editor: *Kirk's current veterinary therapy XII*, Philadelphia, 1995, WB Saunders.

Legendre AM: Itraconazole. Proceedings of the North American Veterinary Conference, Orlando, Fla, Jan 1996.

Lumeij JT: Psittacine antimicrobial therapy. Proceedings of the Miles Antimicrobial Therapy in Caged Birds and Exotic Pets Symposium, Orlando, Fla, Jan 1995.

Orsini JA, Perkons S: The fluoroquinolones: clinical applications in veterinary medicine, *Compend Cont Educ* 14(11): 1491, Nov 1992.

Papich MG: Clinical pharmacology and selection of antimicrobial drugs. Proceedings of the SmithKline Beecham Symposium *Managing microbes: a systems approach to antimicrobial usage,* Orlando, Fla, Jan 1995.

Snyder PS: Oral third generation cephalosporins. Proceedings of the North American Veterinary Conference, Orlando, Fla, Jan 1996.

Vaden SL, Papich MG: Empiric antibiotic therapy. In Bonagura JD, editor: *Kirk's current veterinary therapy XII,* Philadelphia, 1995, WB Saunders.

Walker RD: Antimicrobial chemotherapy. In Robinson NE, editor: *Current therapy in equine medicine 3,* Philadelphia, 1992, WB Saunders.

Review Questions

1. What is the difference between bactericidal and bacteriostatic antimicrobials? Which type should be used in animals with impaired immune function such as with certain viral diseases?

2. A brochure for a new antibiotic states that it attains concentrations of 50 μg/ml when given at a dosage of 100 mg/kg, whereas a competing drug attains concentrations of 30 μg/ml when given at 100 mg/kg. Why is this information essentially worthless?

3. Explain how failure to administer the full prescribed course of antibiotics could create a resistant strain of bacteria.

4. A farmer complains that government regulations prevent him from immediately selling livestock after he gives them antibiotics. He feels that the processes of pasteurizing and cooking kill the bacteria and thereby break down any drug residues. As your clinic's veterinary technician, how would you respond to the farmer?

5. The doctor at your clinic comments that penicillins are not very effective against "sleeping" bacteria because bacteria that are not dividing and proliferating are not killed by penicillin. What is the significance of this comment?

6. Are antimicrobials that affect DNA safe for use in people and animals? Explain your answer.

7. Penicillins are generally safe, but they occasionally cause death in a treated animal. How does this happen?

8. Tetracycline and penicillins have slightly different spectra of antibacterial activity (with considerable overlap). It would seem that using them together would be much more effective than using either drug alone. Why is this not the case?

9. The general rule for bacteriostatic and bactericidal antibiotics is that they should never be used together. In what circumstances is this not true?

10. A dog develops facial swelling after an injection of penicillin G. Would amoxicillin be a safe alternative drug to use in this dog?

11. Why are bacteria, especially staphylococci, resistant to penicillins?

12. Which penicillins are naturally resistant to bacterial enzyme degradation? Why are these drugs not routinely used in place of penicillin G or amoxicillin?

13. Why is clavulanic acid included with amoxicillin in the product Clavamox? Why are tablets of clavulanate-amoxicillin individually wrapped?

14. As your clinic's veterinary technician, you have been giving a mare IM injections of penicillin G for 3 days, and the animal is developing soreness at the injection sites. You consider adding the penicillin G to molasses and giving it to the mare by mouth. What would be the result?

15. Why are hetacillin and ampicillin really the "same drug"?

16. One drug is listed as a "first-generation cephalosporin" and another is listed as a "third-generation cephalosporin." What is the difference between the two? Which drug is more likely to be dispensed to a client for home treatment of an animal?

17. How do β-lactamase, penicillinase, and cephalosporinase differ?

18. Bacitracin is very nephrotoxic and yet is widely used. Why does bacitracin not cause more kidney damage in animals and people than is reported?

19. Why are aminoglycosides like amikacin and gentamicin not very effective in treating infection of deep puncture wounds?

20. Like penicillin, amikacin is bactericidal. Does amikacin, like penicillin, require an actively dividing bacterial population? Is the action of amikacin inhibited by simultaneous administration of a bacteriostatic antimicrobial?

21. What two organs are most affected by aminoglycoside toxicosis?

22. How can an animal develop nephrotoxicosis after topical administration of a gentamicin preparation to an open wound?

23. Why is the dosage of gentamicin or amikacin for older animals often different from that for younger animals? Is liver function a consideration with use of gentamicin or amikacin? How is the dosage altered for older animals?

24. What signs would be expected in a cat with ototoxicity caused by aminoglycoside use?

25. Why are aminoglycosides not very effective in treating abscesses or infections in areas with much pus or cellular debris?

26. What is a simple way to detect early signs of renal damage caused by aminoglycoside use?

27. Why are quinolone drugs, which attack DNA, not mutagenic (that is, producing mutations) or teratogenic (that is, producing birth defects), as are other drugs that attack bacterial DNA?

28. Why is enrofloxacin (Baytril) effective in prostate infections when so many other antimicrobials are not?

29. In what circumstances are quinolones contraindicated in companion animals?

30. A veterinarian gives enrofloxacin to neonatal pups with severe bacterial pneumonia. Is use of enrofloxacin likely to cause joint damage in these animals?

31. Why should enrofloxacin not be used routinely for initial treatment of most infections?

32. What effect has the approval of quinolones for use in food animals had on the extra-label use of quinolones?

33. What is the drug of choice for treatment of each of the following: borreliosis (Lyme disease); Rocky Mountain spotted fever; chlamydial infections of the eye in cats; hemobartonellosis?

34. How do doxycycline and minocycline differ from oxytetracycline and tetracycline?

35. Why should tetracycline capsules not be taken with milk or used in young animals that are nursing?

36. What are the precautions for use of oxytetracycline or tetracycline in puppies and kittens?

37. Why is diarrhea a fairly common side effect of orally administered tetracyclines?

38. How can expired tetracycline cause kidney damage?

39. Are sulfonamides bactericidal or bacteriostatic?

40. Why are some sulfonamides described as *enteric sulfonamides* and others as *systemic sulfonamides?*

41. Why are sulfonamides used so commonly to treat bacterial infections of the urinary tract?

42. Why is it important for an animal receiving sulfonamides to consume sufficient water every day?

43. The package insert for a commonly used veterinary sulfonamide cautions the reader to watch for signs of keratoconjunctivitis sicca. What is this condition and what are the signs associated with it? What is the treatment for drug-induced keratoconjunctivitis sicca?

44. Why is the lincosamide antibiotic clindamycin possibly contraindicated for treatment of cats with toxoplasmosis?

45. Erythromycin is an excellent oral antibiotic for treatment of certain bacterial infections in foals. Why is oral erythromycin contraindicated in adult horses? Can the drug be safely used in adult horses if given by another route of administration? Can tylosin (Tylan) be safely given via oral administration to adult horses?

46. Tilmicosin (Micotil) was developed for SC administration in treating bovine respiratory diseases. It poses some risk to the human operator and so should not be administered with automatic syringes. What adverse effect can accidental self-injection of tilmicosin cause in people?

47. What antimicrobial is indicated for treatment of infection with *Giardia,* a protozoal contaminant of water sources?

48. Nitrofurans rarely achieve significant concentrations in tissues but are often used for treatment of bacterial cystitis (infection of the urinary bladder). How can this be explained?

49. Which antibiotic, once widely used in small and large animals, is now completely banned from use in food animals? Why was the ban instituted?

50. For what types of problems is rifampin used? For what species has rifampin been approved? About what side effect of rifampin should owners be cautioned?

51. What organ is almost always adversely affected by amphotericin B during treatment of deep mycoses? Can anything be done to reduce the effect on this organ?

52. What drugs have largely replaced amphotericin B and nystatin for treatment of some deep mycoses? What are the advantages and disadvantages of these newer drugs?

53. What is griseofulvin used to treat? In what species does griseofulvin have teratogenic effects?

Disinfectants and Antiseptics

Key Terms

alcohol
antiseptic
bactericidal
biguanides
coagulum
disinfectant
enveloped virus
fungicidal
germicide
halogen
microbicidal
microbiostatic
nosocomial infection
phenols
protozoacidal
quaternary ammonium
   compounds
sanitizer
scrub
solution
spore form
sporicidal
sterilizer
tincture
unenveloped (naked)
   virus
vegetative form
virucidal

Terminology Describing Disinfecting
   Agents
Appropriate Use of Disinfecting Agents
Selecting an Appropriate Disinfecting
   Agent

Types of Disinfecting Agents
   Phenols
   Alcohols
   Quaternary ammonium compounds
   Chlorine compounds
   Iodine compounds and iodophors
   Biguanides
   Other disinfecting agents

Learning Objectives

*After studying this chapter,
the veterinary technician should know the following:*

Terminology used to describe disinfecting agents
The way disinfecting agents are used
The way to select an appropriate disinfecting agent
Types of disinfecting agents and their clinical applications

Disinfection is the destruction of pathogenic microorganisms. Disinfection is important in maintaining the health of all animals whether they are on a farm, in a veterinary hospital, in a research facility, or in a breeding colony. However, disinfection is often taken for granted. Disinfecting agents are often chosen because of a practice's long-term use or an appealing price or sales pitch. This haphazard method of selecting disinfecting agents can lead to contamination of clean or sterile areas and subsequent spread of pathogenic microorganisms. Therefore technicians should be aware of the limitations of all disinfecting agents used in their facility and know when these limitations are likely to be encountered during use.

Disinfection of hospital equipment and premises is especially important because of the natural selection for resistant strains that occurs when populations of microorganisms are exposed to low concentrations of antimicrobial chemicals (see Chapter 9). **Nosocomial infections,** which are any infections acquired during a period of hospitalization, are especially difficult to control because of the resistance of the organisms involved. Common sites of nosocomial infections are the urinary tract (associated with urinary catheters), respiratory tract (associated with endotracheal tubes), surgical sites, wounds, and intravenous (IV) catheter insertion sites. Improper use of disinfecting agents can cause an otherwise healthy animal to acquire an infection during its stay in the veterinary hospital. (A box listing disinfecting agents can be found at the end of this chapter.)

TERMINOLOGY DESCRIBING DISINFECTING AGENTS

The terminology used to describe disinfecting agents can be confusing. In addition to the scientific terms, many vague terms are frequently used by the general public. The veterinary technician must understand the terms used to describe disinfectants to make rational decisions about the appropriate use of the proper agent.

Antiseptics are chemical agents that kill or prevent the growth of microorganisms on living tissues. **Disinfectants** are chemical agents that kill or prevent growth of microorganisms on inanimate objects such as surgical equipment, floors, and tabletops.

Antiseptics and disinfectants may also be described as *sanitizers* or *sterilizers*. The difference refers to the degree of microbial destruction achieved. **Sanitizers** are chemical agents that reduce the number of microorganisms to a "safe" level without eliminating all microorganisms. **Sterilizers** are chemicals or other agents that destroy all microorganisms.

Many household cleaning products are advertised as **germicides.** A germicide is any chemical agent that kills microorganisms. Because microorganisms include viruses, bacteria, protozoa, and fungi, the term *germicide* is very nonspecific and therefore should not be used by veterinary professionals.

The veterinary professional should know against which organisms the antiseptic or disinfectant is effective (Table 10-1). **Bactericidal** chemicals kill bacteria, **virucidal** chemicals kill viruses, **fungicidal** chemicals kill fungi, **protozoacidal** chemicals kill protozoa, and **sporicidal** chemicals kill microbial spores.

Unlike some antimicrobials, disinfectants are usually **microbicidal** rather than **microbiostatic.** Inanimate objects do not have an immune system;

Table 10-1   *Relative Efficacy of Disinfectants and Antiseptics*

	Chlorhexidine	Quaternary ammonium compounds	Alcohol	Iodophor	Chlorine	Phenols
Bactericidal	3+	2+	2+	3+	2+	2+
Lipid enveloped virucidal	3+	2+	2+	2+	3+	1+
Nonenveloped virucidal	2+	1+	—	2+	3+	—
Sporicidal	—	—	—	1+	1+	—
Effective in presence of soap	1+	—	2+	2+	2+	2+
Effective in hard water	1+	1+	1+*	2+	2+	1+
Effective in organic material	3+	1+	1+	—	—	—

Ratings are relative indicators. Effectiveness depends on concentration of compound used.
+, Relative efficacy. The higher the number, the greater the efficacy.
—, Not effective
*Do not dilute.

therefore disinfectants used should be able to completely eliminate all microorganisms. Bacteria and fungi can exist in two forms: an actively growing **vegetative form** or a more static **spore form.** Bacterial spores are especially resistant to many disinfectants and antiseptics. Therefore sporicidal disinfectants should be used if bacterial spores are likely to be encountered, especially those of *Bacillus, Clostridium,* or *Pseudomonas* organisms.

APPROPRIATE USE OF DISINFECTING AGENTS

Although appropriate use of disinfecting agents may seem to require little more than common sense, the basic tenets of proper disinfection are often ignored. The results are inadequate reduction of populations of pathogenic microorganisms and the potential for spread of disease.

Following are the characteristics of the ideal disinfecting agent:

Broad-spectrum antimicrobial activity—A single disinfectant that could destroy all viruses, bacteria, and other pathogens would be ideal. Realistically, the chemicals used in most disinfectants often leave certain groups of pathogens untouched. Therefore the veterinary professional should know the various disinfectant's spectra of antimicrobial activity to select the appropriate one for use against the microorganisms most likely to be inhabiting the site of application.

Nonirritating and nontoxic to animal and human tissue—Many disinfecting agents are irritating and/or toxic, especially those with a broad spectrum of antimicrobial activity. Several disinfecting agents can cause toxicity if accidentally ingested, and some are dangerous if too much is applied to the skin or mucous membranes. Even approved antiseptics can be cytotoxic (cell killing) if applied in inappropriate concentrations or to open wounds. Therefore technicians should be aware of the potential dangers that disinfectants pose to themselves and animals under their care.

Easily applied to inanimate objects and causes no corrosion or stains—Concentrated hydrochloric acid could certainly destroy the microorganisms on the surface of a surgery table. However, the corrosive action of the acid would damage the table surface and create minute crevices in which contaminants and microorganisms could accumulate. Some antiseptic or disinfecting agents contain dyes that stain porous or easily marked surfaces.

Stable and not easily inactivated after application—Most disinfecting agents take several seconds or minutes to reduce the population of microorganisms to safe levels. If the agent is inactivated by cellular debris, blood, or other organic materials, it cannot sufficiently reduce the number of microorganisms. The same is true if the antiseptic is inactivated by alcohol such as might be applied to skin before surgery. Inactivation of disinfectants and antiseptics commonly results from inappropriate application. In addition to remaining active in the environment, a disinfecting agent should not lose its potency or effectiveness while in storage for an extended time.

Inexpensive—Because disinfecting agents are used to such a great extent in veterinary medicine, these agents must be economical and affordable. Although this is an important consideration in selecting a disinfectant, it should not be the most important criterion.

The ideal disinfectant or antiseptic has yet to be discovered. Each disinfecting agent currently in use in veterinary medicine lacks one or more of the ideal characteristics listed. However, by being aware of the deficiencies of any given disinfectant and matching its strengths with the given task, technicians can select the appropriate agent.

SELECTING AN APPROPRIATE DISINFECTING AGENT

Three factors should be considered before selecting a particular disinfectant for a given application:

- The type of microorganism the agent must eliminate (bacteria, viruses, fungi, or vegetative or spore forms)
- The environment in which the disinfectant will be used (living tissue versus inanimate object or presence or absence of dirt or debris)
- The characteristics of the disinfectant (corrosiveness, cost, and antimicrobial spectrum)

Technicians should know whether the pathogens of greatest concern in a given situation are viruses, bacteria, fungi, protozoa, or a combination. Technicians should also consider whether spores, especially bacterial spores, are likely to be encountered. If a virus is likely to be present, technicians should know the general susceptibility of that virus to disinfecting agents. Some viruses, such as feline infectious peritonitis (FIP) virus, feline

Pharm Fact

The positive and negative characteristics of a disinfecting agent should be matched to the purpose of its application.

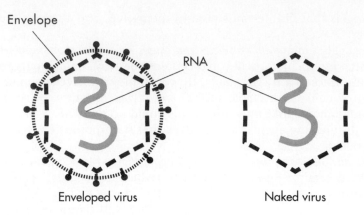

Fig. 10-1 Enveloped and nonenveloped (naked) virus particles.

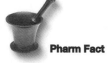

leukemia virus (FeLV), and canine distemper virus, are surrounded by a lipid envelope. This envelope is fairly easily destroyed by many disinfectants, rendering the virus harmless and unable to infect cells. Thus **enveloped viruses** are much easier to kill with disinfecting agents than **unenveloped (naked) viruses** such as feline distemper virus or parvoviruses (Fig. 10-1). Knowledge of a microorganism's inherent resistance or susceptibility to disinfecting agents is an important consideration in selection of an appropriate disinfectant.

The environment in which the disinfecting agent is used influences its efficacy. Some otherwise excellent agents may be inactivated by dirt or organic material such as pus, blood, and cellular debris, necessitating a thorough cleaning of the site before application of the agent.

Thorough cleansing of the site or surface is always prudent; however, technicians should know which disinfectants function poorly if cleansing is not properly performed. Some disinfectants are inactivated by soap or heavily mineralized ("hard") water. In these situations, special attention must be paid to rinsing and preparation of the site after initial cleansing. Without knowledge of these special limitations, the veterinary technician could select a disinfectant of little value in a particular circumstance.

Given the limitations of the products available, the type of microorganism most likely to be encountered, and environmental considerations, veterinary technicians should become familiar with the range of veterinary products available so that money is not wasted on an agent that will be ineffective.

TYPES OF DISINFECTING AGENTS

Phenols

Phenols are used as mouthwashes, scrub soaps, and surface disinfectants. Phenols are also the main disinfecting agent found in many household disinfectants such as Lysol, pine oil, and similar cleansers. Phenolic compounds are very effective against gram-positive bacteria but generally ineffective against gram-negative bacteria, viruses, fungi, or spores. Phenols are not as easily inactivated by organic material as detergents, quaternary ammonium compounds, and chlorine solutions. However, because phenols have a slower onset of action than povidone-iodine or chlorhexidine, they are less commonly used as antiseptics for preparing surgical sites.

Hexachlorophene is a phenolic surgical scrub that has decreased in popularity because of its suspected neurotoxicity (damage to the nervous system) and teratogenic effects (birth defects) in pregnant nurses who performed hexachlorophene scrubs regularly. (NOTE: Do not confuse hexachlorophene with chlorhexidine, which is a commonly used disinfectant and antiseptic that is *not* a phenolic compound.)

When applied to denuded or thin skin, hexachlorophene is more readily absorbed into the body and more likely to have a systematic toxic effect. Although phenols are generally safe, prolonged contact with concentrated solutions may damage the skin. For example, bird perches disinfected with phenols may cause lesions on the feet of birds. Dermal ulceration has been reported in reptiles kept in cages that are consistently disinfected with phenols. Dogs may develop skin lesions when runs are cleaned with phenols and not adequately rinsed.

Because many other effective antiseptics and disinfectants are available, use of phenols has declined in veterinary hospitals and research institutions. Nevertheless phenols are still used, and technicians should be very familiar with the safety concerns and spectrum of antimicrobial activity associated with each phenol product used in their facility.

Alcohols

Alcohols such as 70% ethyl alcohol and 50% or 70% isopropyl alcohol are among the most common antiseptics applied to skin. Solutions of 70% alcohol are used to disinfect surgical sites, injection sites, and rectal thermometers.

Advantages of alcohol include its low cost, general lack of toxicity when applied topically, and bactericidal activity against gram-positive and gram-negative bacteria. However, technicians should be aware that alcohol is ineffective against bacterial spores. In addition, alcohol must be applied in sufficient quantities and remain in contact with the site for several seconds to be effective against bacteria (several minutes for fungi). Therefore a cursory swipe with an alcohol-soaked swab on an animal's skin, especially if the skin is encrusted with dirt or feces, does little to disinfect an injection site.

Only enveloped viruses are susceptible to the virucidal effects of alcohol. Because alcohol does not penetrate dirt or feces, technicians should be aware of the potential for transmission of enteric (intestinal) viruses such as parvovirus if fecal debris is not adequately removed from a rectal thermometer or fecal loop. A rectal thermometer contaminated with feces is *not* disinfected merely by soaking it in an alcohol bath.

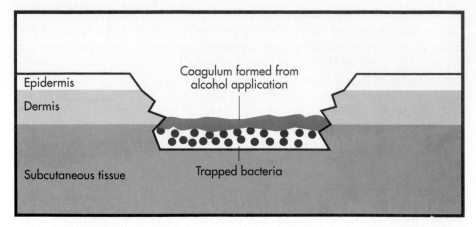

Fig. 10-2   Application of alcohol to an open wound can create a coagulum, trapping bacteria beneath it.

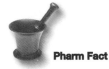

Unlike some other antiseptics, alcohol should not be applied to open wounds because it causes pain and may also facilitate survival of pathogens. Open wounds usually contain a serum exudate that is rich in protein. Alcohol denatures the structure of this protein, causing it to form a superficial barrier, or **coagulum** (Fig. 10-2). This coagulum may seal in or protect underlying bacteria, thereby preventing topical disinfectants from reaching the organisms. The infection could then spread to underlying tissues.

Repeated application of alcohol to intact skin, whether as an antiseptic or a vehicle for other compounds such as insecticides in flea products, removes some of the skin's lipid component, resulting in drying. Animals may develop dry skin, pruritus (itchiness), or flaky skin after repeated alcohol application.

Alcohols are generally effective if dirt and organic material are removed from the skin before application, the microorganisms present are susceptible to alcohol, and the alcohol is applied in enough quantity to keep the area moist for a sufficient time. Otherwise disinfection is incomplete and contamination by microorganisms persists.

Quaternary Ammonium Compounds

Quaternary ammonium compounds are used frequently in veterinary medicine to disinfect the surfaces of inanimate objects. Many household disinfectants contain dilute quaternary ammonium compounds. These household products should be differentiated from industrial products, which tend to be highly concentrated and could present a risk to veterinary technicians who are unaware of the difference in concentrations. One commonly used quaternary ammonium compound used in veterinary medicine is benzalkonium chloride.

Quaternary ammonium compounds are effective against a wide variety of gram-negative and gram-positive bacteria, but they are ineffective against bacterial spores and have poor efficacy against fungi. Although quaternary ammonium compounds can destroy enveloped viruses, they are ineffective against unenveloped viruses such as parvovirus. They act rapidly at the site of application and normally are not irritating to the skin or corrosive to metals.

Quaternary ammonium compounds bind to organic materials, rendering them less effective against many pathogenic microorganisms within or under such debris. Thus thorough cleansing of a site before application of a quaternary ammonium compound is essential for adequate reduction of microbial populations.

Because quaternary ammonium compounds are inactivated by detergents and soaps, the application site must be rinsed to remove soap or detergent residue before the disinfectant is applied. Finally, hard water reduces the antimicrobial activity of quaternary ammonium compounds. Cleansing, rinsing, and drying the site before application of the quaternary ammonium compound helps prevent the reduced efficacy associated with soaps and hard water.

Although quaternary ammonium compounds are generally low in toxicity and nonirritating to skin, prolonged contact may irritate epithelial surfaces. Use of these compounds in aviaries or other avian confinement operations without proper rinsing has resulted in damage to the mouth, toes, eyes, and respiratory tract of the birds that are kept in these confines. A similar situation could occur in dogs and cats if a highly concentrated industrial quaternary ammonium compound is applied but not adequately rinsed from the corners of cages or horizontal surfaces with poor drainage. Contact irritation can usually be avoided by following the same rules outlined previously for proper application of phenolic compounds.

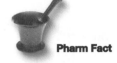

Pharm Fact

Quaternary ammonium compounds should never be in contact with tissues for an extended time.

Chlorine Compounds

Chlorine compounds belong to a larger group of compounds known as **halogens.** Chlorine kills both enveloped and unenveloped viruses. Chlorine compounds are the disinfectants most commonly used to kill parvovirus organisms. Chlorine is also effective against fungi, algae, and vegetative forms of bacteria. Like many other disinfectants, chlorine is not effective against bacterial spores.

Chlorine disinfectants are most commonly available as sodium hypochlorite (Clorox). It is inexpensive and easily obtained. As might be expected, fabric that comes in contact with high concentrations of chlorine compounds can result in bleaching and deterioration of the fabric. Chlorine is also corrosive to most metals except high-quality stainless steel. Repeated chlorine application can result in pitted or damaged metal tabletops.

The pungent vapor of chlorine compounds can irritate the eyes and other exposed mucous membranes if the compounds are used in a poorly ventilated area. Failure to rinse a chlorine-disinfected surface may result in skin irritation if an animal is in contact with it for more than a few minutes. Although chlorine is the most commonly used disinfectant for fighting enteric viruses such as parvovirus, it is largely inactivated by organic material such as feces, blood, and pus. Therefore the site should be thoroughly cleansed before application of chlorine compounds. In addition, the chlorine solution should remain in contact with the site for several minutes to ensure destruction of pathogens.

"Color-fast bleaches" contain concentrated hydrogen peroxide but no chlorine. Despite its effervescent foaming when applied to a wound, hydrogen peroxide has minimal bactericidal activity and is often cytotoxic.

Iodine Compounds and Iodophors

Iodine compounds and iodophors are most commonly used as topical antiseptics before surgical procedures or for disinfection of tissue. Iodine compounds are also classified as halogens. An iodophor is a combination of iodine and a carrier molecule that releases the iodine over time, prolonging the antimicrobial activity. The most common iodophor is iodine complexed with polyvinylpyrrolidone, a combination more commonly known as *povidoneiodine.* When combined with a detergent, iodophors are often referred to as *surgical scrubs.* Iodine or iodophor solutions, or tinctures, do not contain detergent. Aqueous solutions, which are water based, and tincture of iodine, which is an alcohol solution, both have higher concentrations of free iodine available for microbicidal activity; however, both preparations are much more irritating and cytotoxic than the iodophor (povidone-iodine) form.

Iodine and iodophors are bactericidal, virucidal, protozoacidal, and fungicidal. For example, these topical agents are very effective against the dermatophytes that cause ringworm. Iodophors are also effective against bacterial spores if the solution remains moist and in contact with the site for more than 15 minutes. A disadvantage of iodophors is that they are partially inactivated by organic material but not to the degree that chlorines are. This inactivation is the reason that several applications of surgical iodophor are recommended before adequate disinfection can be attained.

Iodophor compounds are generally not irritating when properly used. The technician must distinguish between an iodophor **scrub** and an iodophor **solution,** or **tincture,** when applying an iodophor. In certain situations such as an abscess cavity, the foaming action of the detergent contained in the scrub may not be desirable. Conversely, the detergent plays an important role in cleansing the skin before surgery.

Although less corrosive than chlorine compounds, iodine compounds can also be corrosive to metal if left in contact for an extended time. In addition, high concentrations of iodine can be very irritating to tissues. Some iodine and iodophor preparations are available in concentrated forms; therefore technicians should always check the container label to see whether dilution of the product is required before applying it to living tissue.

Some iodophor pastes turn from dark brown to yellow as the iodophor molecule releases iodine. Iodophors sometimes stain clothing and linen a dark blue color as the iodine reacts with starch in the fabric, but this discoloration can be easily removed with washing. Iodophors stain the skin yellow when applied. This may be helpful when a patient is being prepared for surgery because the areas of application are readily visible.

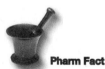

Pharm Fact

It is important to differentiate between iodine scrubs and iodine solutions.

Biguanides

Chlorhexidine, a member of a class of antiseptics known as **biguanides,** is one of the most commonly used disinfectant and antiseptic compounds in veterinary medicine. Chlorhexidine is used for a variety of purposes, including cleaning cages, treating teat infections in cattle, and maintaining oral hygiene in companion animals. Its wide range of uses is likely related to its low tissue irritation and its virucidal, bactericidal (both gram-positive and gram-negative), and fungicidal properties.

Chlorhexidine is less inactivated by organic material than the halogen compounds, but thorough cleansing of the application site is still recommended. Because chlorhexidine binds to the outer surface of the skin, it has some residual activity for up to 24 hours if left in contact with the site. Hard water may reduce some of the activity of chlorhexidine. Mixing saline solutions with chlorhexidine may cause precipitation, thereby inactivating the product.

The veterinary technician should be careful when applying chlorhexidine to open wounds because many concentrations of chlorhexidine are toxic to fibroblasts (cells involved with the healing process). Ototoxicity has been reported from instillation of chlorhexidine into the middle ear. However, subsequent studies have failed to produce the same ototoxic effects. Regardless, a technician should not be overly zealous in applying chlorhexidine or any antiseptic to open wounds or healing tissue.

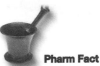

Pharm Fact

Hard water or saline solution can reduce the effectiveness of chlorhexidine.

Other Disinfecting Agents

Peroxides and oxidants are sometimes used to debride (remove) dead, injured, or necrotic tissue and kill bacteria. Hydrogen peroxide kills anaerobic bacteria residing in wounds, releasing oxygen when it reacts with cellular debris and devitalized tissue. Although the foaming action of oxidizing agents in wounds is dramatic, these compounds are not virucidal and may actually damage tissue that is healthy or marginally viable.

Glutaraldehyde has a wide spectrum of activity against bacteria, viruses, fungi, and bacterial spores. It is not inactivated by organic debris and is effective in the presence of hard water. Glutaraldehydes are not widely used in veterinary medicine because of their cost, short shelf life (that is, the time during which they retain their activity), and toxicity to tissues.

Acetic acid is sometimes used as a 0.25% solution to kill *Pseudomonas* organisms as well as a variety of other gram-positive and gram-negative bacteria.

Disinfecting Agent Categories and Names

Phenols
Hexachlorophene

Alcohols
Ethyl alcohol
Isopropyl alcohol

Quaternary ammonium compounds
Benzalkonium chloride

Chlorine compounds
Sodium hypochlorite

Iodine compounds and iodophors
Povidone-iodine

Biguanides
Chlorhexidine

Other disinfecting agents
Hydrogen peroxide
Glutaraldehyde
Acetic acid

Recommended Reading

Clem MF: Sterilization and antiseptics. In Auer JA, editor: *Equine surgery,* Philadelphia, 1992, WB Saunders.

Lemarie RJ, Hosgood G: Antiseptics and disinfectants in small animal practice, *Compend Cont Educ* 17(11):1339, 1995.

Lozier SM: Topical wound therapy. In Harari J, editor: *Surgical complications and wound healing in small animal practice,* Philadelphia, 1993, WB Saunders.

Phillips MA, Vasseur PB, Gregory CR: Chlorhexidine diacetate versus povidone-iodine for pre-operative preparation of the skin, *JAAHA* 27:105, 1991.

Rochar MC, Mann FA, Berg JN: Evaluation of a one-step surgical preparation technique in dogs, *JAVMA* 203(3):392, 1993.

Swaim SF, Riddel KP, Geiger DL: Evaluation of surgical scrub and antiseptic solutions for surgical preparation of canine paws, *JAVMA* 198(11):1941, 1991.

Review Questions

1. A pharmaceutical sales representative is offering a new sanitizer that destroys all microorganisms, including bacteria and viruses. He claims that it is good to use on dog runs contaminated with parvovirus and as a presurgical scrub. What is your initial impression of the product? What questions should you ask about the product?
2. A product is labeled as a germicide. What does this mean?
3. An advertisement describes a product as virucidal, sporicidal, bactericidal, and protozoicidal. The product is also fairly inexpensive. What information should you obtain before you purchase it to use as a skin antiseptic?
4. Why is it not very effective to disinfect a dog run by spraying away the fecal material with a hose to which a bottle of disinfectant is attached?
5. Considering iodine's high efficacy as an antiseptic, why do many surgeons prefer at least three iodine scrubs when preparing a surgical site?

6. Why are there so many different types of virucidal compounds if they all destroy viruses?

7. You discover several old containers of hexachlorophene scrub that have been stored for years. Is this scrub likely to still be effective? Is there any danger in using this outdated scrub?

8. Is chlorhexidine the same as hexachlorophene?

9. A dog with a bad "road burn" (skin badly abraded or avulsed) is anesthetized so that some lacerations may be sutured and cleaned. The doctor wants you to clean the affected area. You must decide whether to use alcohol or another antiseptic. What are some considerations with using alcohol on this type of open wound?

10. Are contaminated rectal thermometers sterilized by storage in an alcohol bath?

11. In what class of disinfectants is benzalkonium chloride? What is its spectrum of antimicrobial activity?

12. In recent weeks, dogs kept in the runs in your clinic have been excessively licking their feet and ventral abdominal area; the skin in these areas is red and inflamed. What is a likely cause of this problem?

13. Why does the doctor caution you about leaving the chlorine disinfectant on the surgery table too long?

14. Why does the doctor remind you to leave the kennel fan on when disinfecting the runs with liquid laundry bleach (Clorox)?

15. There is a sale on color-fast bleach. Should you stock up on it for use as a disinfectant?

16. The doctor wants to flush an open wound with an iodine compound. Which is more appropriate for this purpose, iodophor scrub or iodophor solution?

17. Some advertisements refer to their product as an *iodine-based* disinfectant, whereas others refer to their product as an *iodophor*. What is the difference?

18. With regard to inactivation by organic material, how does chlorhexidine compare with iodine and chlorine?

19. The veterinarian wants to dilute a stock chlorhexidine solution to flush an infected ear. You must decide whether to use sterile saline or distilled water. Which is a more appropriate diluent?

Antiparasitics

Key Terms

acetylcholine
acetylcholinesterase
adulticide
anthelmintic
anticestodal
antinematodal
antiprotozoal
antitrematodal
coccidiostat
delayed neurotoxicity
   syndrome
gamma amino butyric
   acid (GABA)
glutamate
insect development
   inhibitor
insect growth regulator
juvenile hormone mimic
microfilaricide
muscarinic receptor
nicotinic receptor
proglottid
selective toxicity
SLUDDE
vermicide
vermifuge

Principles of Antiparasitic Use
Internal Antiparasitics
Terminology Used to Describe Internal
   Antiparasitics
Antinematodals
   Piperazines
   Benzimidazoles
   Organophosphates
   Ivermectin
   Pyrantel
   Febantel
   Other antinematodal drugs
Anticestodals
   Praziquantel
   Epsiprantel

Antiparasitics Used in Heartworm
   Treatment
Antiprotozoals
   Amprolium
External Antiparasitics
Chlorinated Hydrocarbons
   Lindane
Organophosphates and Carbamates
Pyrethrins and Pyrethroids
Amitraz
Imidacloprid
Fipronil
Insect Growth Regulators
Insect Repellents
Other External Antiparasitics

Learning Objectives

After studying this chapter,
the veterinary technician should know the following:

The terminology used to describe antiparasitics

The way antiparasitics are used

The way to select an appropriate antiparasitic

Types of antiparasitics and their clinical applications

Precautions for using antiparasitics

Drugs and chemicals for use against intestinal parasites, fleas, ticks, and other internal or external parasites constitute the widest array of products available to veterinary professionals and the general public. These compounds include nonprescription products found in grocery stores and products dispensed daily from veterinary hospitals and clinics. (A box listing antiparasitic drugs can be found at the end of this chapter.)

Flea sprays, deworming medications, and other antiparasitic drugs are often dispensed with little consideration of the drugs' effects. The veterinary professional must remember that these chemicals have been carefully formulated to kill the parasite without killing the host. A disruption in the balance of safety and efficacy may result in incomplete destruction of the parasites or toxicity to the treated animal.

Following are characteristics of an ideal antiparasitic drug:

- **Selective toxicity:** The chemical should be very toxic to the parasite, but should have little effect on the host's tissue and person(s) applying or administering the product.
- *Does not induce resistance in the target parasite:* Similar to the way bacteria can develop resistance to antimicrobials, many external and internal parasites can develop resistance to certain parasiticides. The ideal compound would not induce such resistance and thus would avoid selection for a "superparasite" that could not be killed by common antiparasitics.
- *Economical:* An economical yet effective product is most desirable for treatment of parasitism. Because it is a business, economics is most critical in parasite control in livestock production. While of some concern, economics plays a comparatively smaller role in equine or small animal parasite control.
- *Effective and easy to apply:* Ideally, internal antiparasitic drugs should kill all the adult parasites as well as any migrating larvae or immature forms with a single treatment. Likewise, external antiparasitics should be effective with one treatment and convenient to reapply because fleas, flies, lice, and mites usually cannot be totally eradicated from the environment, and reinfestation is likely to occur.

Other desirable characteristics include a fragrant odor (external antiparasitics) and environmental safety. No single product incorporates all of these ideal features. Therefore veterinary professionals should know the specific needs of the animal and client, the environment in which the product will be used, and the characteristics of the antiparasitic product to make a rational, economical, and safe recommendation.

PRINCIPLES OF ANTIPARASITIC USE

With proper use of an antiparasitic, most of the drug reaches the location of the parasite. If the parasite is free-living within the lumen of the intestinal tract, an orally administered antiparasitic need not be absorbed systemically to be effective. In contrast, if the parasite's life cycle includes a stage of arrested development (slowed metabolism) or larvae migration throughout the body and the drug only kills the adult worms within the intestinal tract, a single treatment will not eliminate the problem. Although the adult worms are eliminated, larvae eventually migrate to the intestinal tract and mature to new adult worms. Therefore the veterinary professional must understand the features of the parasite's life cycle. One of the major reasons for failure of antiparasitic treatment is misunderstanding the limitations of the activity of the antiparasitic compound against various stages of the parasite's life cycle.

In the past, potent compounds including mercury, arsenic, and strychnine were used to treat intestinal parasitism. If these toxic compounds were not absorbed by the host's body to any great extent, they killed the intestinal parasite without producing significant toxic effects in the animal host. However, because these toxic compounds were not absorbed, they did not kill any migrating phases of the life cycle; if they had, they most likely would have killed the parasite and host. Today numerous safe and effective intestinal antiparasitics are available and veterinary professionals as well as the general public no longer have to depend on more toxic chemicals used in the past.

Client education is essential for successful treatment of internal or external parasites. For example, clients must understand the reasons for additional control efforts that are required on their part, including collection and disposal of feces, repeated treatments, and treatment of other animals. Simply instructing clients to perform certain control procedures without explaining the underlying reason may not convince them to comply. Clients should also understand that any medication given must be administered or applied according to the dosage instructions; that is, in the recommended amount, in the appropriate way, and at the appropriate time(s).

As a general rule, internal and external antiparasitic agents should be used with caution in old, young, debilitated, or pregnant animals. Certain antiparasitics also have additional high-risk groups of animals; for example, Collies are a high-risk group with use of ivermectin. Because of the idiosyncrasies of each antiparasitic drug, the veterinary professional should consult the drug package insert or a veterinary drug reference before administering or applying antiparasitics to prevent inappropriate use of a compound in a high-risk animal.

INTERNAL ANTIPARASITICS

A walk down any drugstore or supermarket pet-product aisle will reveal that products for treating worms in dogs and cats constitute a big business. This is also true of antiparasitic products available at feed stores, farming implement stores, and tack shops. Because many of the products available to veterinarians are also available to the general public, veterinary professionals are asked many questions concerning safe use of these nonprescription or over-the-counter (OTC) products.

TERMINOLOGY USED TO DESCRIBE INTERNAL ANTIPARASITICS

Various terms are used to describe internal antiparasitics. Veterinary technicians should be familiar with these terms to better understand the effects and limitations of a particular product.

Anthelmintic is a general term used to describe compounds that kill various types of internal parasites such as helminths, or worms. A **vermicide** is

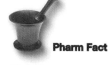

Pharm Fact

All antiparasitics should be used with caution in very young, old, debilitated, or pregnant animals.

an anthelmintic that kills the worm, as opposed to a **vermifuge,** which only paralyzes the worm and often results in passage of live worms in the stool.

Antinematodal compounds treat infections of nematodes, or "round-worms". Nematodes include hookworms, ascarids, whipworms, and strongyles. However, a particular antinematodal drug may not kill every type of roundworm. Therefore veterinary technicians should be familiar with the spectrum of antiparasitic activity for each of the products they dispense.

Anticestodal compounds treat infections of cestodes, which are tapeworms or segmented "flatworms". Similar to antinematodals, a particular anticestodal drug may not be effective against all species of tapeworms commonly encountered in veterinary practice. Therefore the veterinary technician should carefully read the package insert to determine the drug's spectrum of anticestodal activity.

Antitrematodal compounds treat infection of trematodes, which are flukes or unsegmented flatworms including *Paragonimus, Fasciola,* and *Dicrocoelium* parasites.

Antiprotozoal compounds treat infection of protozoa, which are single-celled organisms including *Coccidia, Giardia,* and *Toxoplasma* organisms. **Coccidiostats** are drugs that specifically inhibit the growth of coccidia. Many antiprotozoal compounds are also antimicrobials (for example, sulfonamide drugs).

ANTINEMATODALS

Piperazines

Piperazine is a vermicide that has been used for many years and is the active ingredient in most of the "once-a-month" deworming medications sold in grocery stores and pet shops. Piperazine is very safe but is only effective against ascarids. Many veterinary clients believe there is no reason to have the veterinarian microscopically examine fecal samples from their animal because they have dewormed the pet with an OTC piperazine product. The veterinary technician should inform the client that piperazines do not kill hookworms, tapeworms, whipworms, or protozoa (coccidia) that commonly infect dogs and cats. Piperazine is also a vermifuge. If it is given to a puppy with a heavy ascarid infection, a wriggling mass of live roundworms may be passed with the stool.

Benzimidazoles

The benzimidazoles include some of the most commonly used antiparasitic drugs on the market. Drugs in this class of anthelmintics can usually be recognized when written out by the *-azole* suffix of the chemical name. The benzimidazoles include fenbendazole (Panacur), mebendazole (Telmin, Telmintic), thiabendazole (Equizole, Tresaderm Otic), oxibendazole (Anthelcide EQ, Filaribits-Plus), albendazole, oxfendazole, and cambendazole. Most of these products are formulated as pastes and solutions for use in control of equine intestinal parasites. Most also have applications in cattle, other food animals, and companion animals. Characteristics that distinguish one benzimidazole from another are noted below.

Thiabendazole is the prototype (representative) benzimidazole and has a wide range of activity against ascarids and strongyles. The drug is safe when used at recommended dosages and rarely causes significant side effects, although dying parasites may produce some signs. In addition to its antiparasitic activity, thiabendazole is unique in that it also has some antiinflammatory and antifungal activity. For this reason thiabendazole is sometimes added to otic (ear) medications (for example, Tresaderm Otic) and topical products.

Oxibendazole has long been used as an equine dewormer. More recently it has been combined with diethylcarbamazine (Filaribits-Plus) for daily use in preventing heartworm and hookworm infections in dogs. This combination also removes whipworms and ascarids from the intestine. While oxibendazole and piperazine are apparently safe for use in horses, this combination of drugs has reportedly caused liver dysfunction (periportal hepatitis) in dogs treated daily. The manufacturer warns that dogs treated daily should be monitored for liver disease, especially those with previous liver problems or concurrently receiving other hepatotoxic drugs.

Mebendazole is formulated as a granular powder for use in controlling internal parasites in dogs and horses. In dogs the spectrum of antiparasitic activity of this drug includes roundworms, hookworms, whipworms, and the tapeworm *Taenia pisiformis*. Mebendazole is not effective against the tapeworm *Dipylidium caninum*. Like oxibendazole, mebendazole may cause liver damage in dogs. Although this adverse effect is uncommon, animals with previous liver problems, previous reactions to other benzimidazoles, or receiving repeated doses of mebendazole should be closely monitored for signs of liver disease.

Fenbendazole (Panacur) is a popular anthelmintic used in small animals, food animals, and horses. It has a wide spectrum of activity against nematodes and a variety of other parasites. Like mebendazole, fenbendazole is effective against only certain species of tapeworms and should not be used as a general cestocide unless the particular species of tapeworm has been identified. Vomiting is occasionally noted in dogs and cats given this medication, but the liver problems associated with some of the other benzimidazoles have not been reported with fenbendazole. The drug must be given for 3 consecutive days for maximal efficacy because a single dose of fenbendazole does not destroy all of the worms in dogs and cats.

Organophosphates

Organophosphates are used as internal antiparasitics (Task, Combot), as well as external antiparasitics to combat fleas, ticks, and flies. Organophosphates are one of the few compounds that are effective against bots in horses. As discussed in more detail in the section on external antiparasitics, organophosphates are neurotoxic. Although they have the potential to produce neurologic effects in treated animals, when properly used they are effective with little evidence of side effects. Internal and external use of organophosphates combined with exposure to organophosphates spread around the garden or lawn can produce cumulative effects, resulting in nervous system toxicity in treated animals.

Similar to the benzimidazoles, organophosphates constitute a fairly large group of compounds with similar actions and side effects. The organophosphates most commonly used internally are dichlorvos and trichlorfon. The manufacturers' recommendations should be closely followed, and treated animals should be monitored for signs of adverse reactions such as gastrointestinal (GI) disturbances, colic in horses, excessive salivation, and changes in stool consistency.

Organophosphate antiparasitics should not be used in animals with heartworm infection *(Dirofilaria immitis)*. Use of these drugs in dogs with heartworm can produce severe reactions, including dyspnea, collapse, and sudden death. More information concerning the mechanism of action and toxicity of organophosphates is included in the section on external antiparasitics.

Pharm Fact

Organophosphates should not be used in dogs infected with heartworms.

Ivermectin

Ivermectin (Ivomec, Eqvalan, Heartgard-30, Heartgard-30 Plus, Heartgard for cats) is an antiparasitic drug that belongs to the class known as *avermectins*. It is widely used in almost every species treated by veterinarians. Ivermectin kills parasites by enhancing the effects of inhibitory neurotransmitters, **glutamate,** and, to a lesser degree, **gamma amino butyric (GABA).** GABA was thought to be the primary inhibitory neurotransmitter affected by ivermectin; however, more recent evidence has focused on glutamate and its inhibition of the central nervous system (CNS).

Ivermectin is safe when properly used, but in certain situations it can cause illness. For example, ivermectin can cause massive death of *Onchocerca* parasites in the skin of horses, which can produce swelling and severe pruritus (itchiness). This reaction can be reduced by giving corticosteroids before and for several days after ivermectin administration. Cattle can experience an allergic reaction to migrating cattle grubs *(Hypoderma bovis)* that die as a result of ivermectin administration. Cattle grubs may migrate through the host's nervous system, GI tract, and other vital areas. Unlike the reaction to death of *Onchocerca* parasites in the skin of horses, which is manifest as a cutaneous reaction, the signs associated with death of cattle grubs after ivermectin use reflect the location of the grubs and the subsequent inflammation and swelling.

Ivermectin can produce adverse reactions in Collies and Collie crossbreeds. These reactions and general ivermectin use in dogs are discussed in the section on heartworm treatment.

Pyrantel

Anthelmintics containing pyrantel (Strongid, Nemex, Banminth, Imathal) are very safe. They are marketed as pyrantel pamoate and a more water-soluble salt, pyrantel tartrate. Although pyrantel products are labeled for use only in dogs, horses, and swine, they are used in most species treated by veterinarians. Pyrantel mimics the action of the neurotransmitter **acetyl-choline,** causing initial stimulation and then paralysis of nicotinic receptors on muscles, thus killing the parasite by paralysis. The drug also inhibits **acetylcholinesterase,** which further enhances the acetylcholine effect. Because of its mechanism of action, this drug should be used with caution in animals exposed to organophosphate insecticides or other parasiticides that block acetylcholinesterase and enhance acetylcholine effects.

The pleasant taste of liquid pyrantel pamoate facilitates medication of animals by the veterinary professional or the client. Although not approved for use in cats, pyrantel pamoate is preferred by some parasitologists for treatment of feline hookworms. In addition to the forms of pyrantel used by veterinarians, OTC pyrantel products are also available. Liquid suspensions of pyrantel should be thoroughly shaken and mixed before administration because the drug particles quickly settle to the bottom of the bottle. Failure to thoroughly mix the suspension before each dose can result in underdosing when using the low concentrations at the top of the bottle, or overdosing when using the high concentrations at the bottom of the bottle.

Pyrantel pamoate has been incorporated into a number of veterinary products to extend their spectra of activity. Heartgard-30 Plus combines the heartworm preventive ivermectin with pyrantel, and Drontal-Plus combines the antinematodal activity of pyrantel and febantel with the anticestodal (tapeworm-killing) activity of praziquantel. Morantel tartrate (Nematel) is very similar to pyrantel and has similar effects, uses, and precautions.

Febantel

Febantel is marketed in a palatable paste formulation for horses or in combination with the anticestodal drug praziquantel (Drontal tablets, Vercom paste) for dogs and cats. Febantel by itself is safe for use in horses for ascarids, strongyles, and pinworms. Studies show that single doses of up to 40 times the recommended dosage failed to produce significant adverse effects in horses. The combination products have a more narrow safety range.

Other Antinematodal Drugs

Various other antinematodal drugs are available. Levamisole is primarily used in food animals and horses. Like pyrantel, levamisole produces a cholinergic response by stimulating nicotinic acetylcholine receptors. This parasympathetic stimulation may cause salivation, frothing at the mouth, vomiting, and diarrhea, especially in dogs. Before introduction of ivermectin and other **microfilaricides** (drugs used to kill circulating heartworm microfilariae), levamisole was used as a microfilaricide in dogs. In addition to GI signs, dogs treated with levamisole often exhibit sedation, ataxia, panting, shaking, or other signs attributable to the CNS. Some of these CNS signs may appear in other species to a lesser degree.

Phenothiazine dewormers have been used to treat horses for various nematode infections. Phenothiazine toxicity has been reported in horses receiving phenothiazine deworming agents. Dogs and small ruminants appear to be very sensitive to these compounds.

ANTICESTODALS

Praziquantel

Praziquantel is marketed in injectable and tablet forms for use in dogs and cats (Droncit tablets), and in combination with other antiparasitics. The advantages of praziquantel are its efficacy with a single dose and its activity against a wide range of anticestodes, including *Echinococcus* species.

Unlike some of the older anticestodal drugs (taeniacides), praziquantel reduces the tapeworm's resistance to digestion by the host's intestinal tract. Vermifuges may detach tapeworm segments from the worm's body but do not detach the head, which lodges itself in the bowel wall. After praziquantel administration, the entire worm disintegrates, including the head that is buried in the bowel wall. Owners usually do not see tapeworm segments **(proglottids)** passing after administration of praziquantel because the worm disintegrates. Vomiting is an occasional side effect of praziquantel use in dogs and cats. However, this drug is otherwise safe when used as recommended.

Although a single dose of praziquantel is effective, elimination of the tapeworm *Dipylidium caninum* requires elimination of fleas from the host and the immediate environment because fleas are involved in that tapeworm's life cycle. Failure to prevent flea infestation is likely to result in reinfection with this tapeworm.

While praziquantel is effective against the adult tapeworms, it is not ovicidal (capable of destroying the tapeworm eggs). Therefore after administration of the drug and death of the parasite, microscopic tapeworm eggs may pass in the feces for a period of time. Because accidental ingestion of tapeworm eggs by humans poses a potential public health hazard, the veterinary professional should instruct the pet owner to follow proper hygiene procedures (washing hands) after cleaning a cat litter box or disposing of feces that might be contaminated with tapeworm eggs.

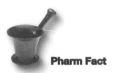

Pharm Fact

Tapeworm segments are usually not seen in the feces after treatment with praziquantel.

Epsiprantel

Epsiprantel (Cestex) is an oral anticestodal that is effective against *Taenia* and *Dipylidium* tapeworms but the manufacturer does not list it as effective against *Echinococcus* species. Unlike praziquantel, epsiprantel is not absorbed to any significant degree from the GI tract. This lack of absorption minimizes the risk of systemic side effects. Like praziquantel, epsiprantel causes digestion of the entire tapeworm within the bowel, so there is little evidence of the tapeworm in the stool.

ANTIPARASITICS USED IN HEARTWORM TREATMENT

Heartworm *(Dirofilaria immitis)* infection in dogs continues to be a problem in Canada and most parts of the United States. As veterinary parasitologists gain a better understanding of the heartworm life cycle, pharmaceutical manufacturers will produce new drugs, and the American Heartworm Society will recommend new protocols. The reader should consult the Recommended Reading lists at the end of this chapter for sources of information on heartworm infection.

Adult heartworms live within the right ventricle of the heart and surrounding large blood vessels. An **adulticide** is a drug used to kill mature (adult) heartworms. Female adult heartworms produce young called *microfilariae,* which circulate in the bloodstream of infected dogs and are taken up by mosquitoes when they feed on an infected dog's blood. Microfilaricides are drugs used to kill the circulating microfilariae produced by the adult heartworms.

After the microfilariae have been ingested by a mosquito, they undergo changes to become infective third-stage larvae. These infective larvae migrate to the head and mouthparts of the mosquito, from which they enter another dog's body the next time the mosquito feeds. The infective larvae migrate through the dog's body and eventually reach the right ventricle, where they mature to adults. Heartworm preventives are drugs given to kill these infective larvae.

For many years the only drug approved for treatment of adult heartworms was thiacetarsamide sodium (Caparsolate). In 1996, melarsomine dihydrochloride (Immiticide) was approved as an adulticide. In contrast to thiacetarsamide, which can only be given intravenously, melarsomine is administered via deep IM injection. Thiacetarsamide and melarsomine are organic arsenical compounds that kill adult heartworms but do not significantly affect circulating microfilariae. Melarsomine is more effective against immature adult worms ("fifth-stage larvae") than thiacetarsamide, and has fewer side effects and contraindications than thiacetarsamide.

Thiacetarsamide is an arsenical that is metabolized by the liver and excreted via the liver (about two-thirds of a dose) and the kidneys. Therefore animals with compromised liver function, renal disease, or cardiovascular disease should not be given thiacetarsamide until their condition is stabilized to some degree. Adverse reactions to thiacetarsamide include vomiting, which is fairly common, tubular casts in the urine (if there is renal injury), hepatotoxicity, which is less common, and tissue necrosis after perivascular injection (see below). Vomiting or urine casts by themselves are not reasons to stop thiacetarsamide therapy. However, anorexia, vomiting, or diarrhea associated with lethargy, bilirubinuria, melena (digested blood in the stool), or icterus (jaundice) strongly suggest hepatotoxicity, and drug administration should be stopped to prevent a fatal reaction. Generally, treatment that is stopped because of these signs should not be attempted again for at least 3 or 4 weeks.

Thiacetarsamide has a very narrow therapeutic range, and the dose needed to kill the adult heartworms is only slightly less than that producing adverse reactions in or death of the host. For this reason, doses of thiacetarsamide must be carefully calculated. An accidental overdose is likely to result in toxicity or death. No antidote is currently available for thiacetarsamide.

Thiacetarsamide is generally administered twice daily for 2 days (4 doses total) by IV injection. The drug is very irritating to the tissues of the skin, and perivascular injection (outside the vein) can result in marked swelling, pain, and sloughing of the skin at the injection site. If it is suspected that some of the drug has leaked or has been injected outside the vein, the perivascular area should be immediately infiltrated with saline mixed with dexamethasone, and dimethyl sulfoxide should be applied topically.

Melarsomine may replace thiacetarsamide because of its lower toxicity, greater effectiveness, and simpler treatment regimen (that is, 2 IM injections q24h versus 4 IV thiacetarsamide injections q12h). The drug should be injected only in the epaxial muscles, which are located dorsally, on either side of the spinal column. Specifically the drug should be injected into the epaxial muscles between the third and fifth lumbar vertebrae, 1 to 2 inches lateral to the dorsal spinous process, which marks the center of the spinal column. Dogs that weigh less than 10 kg (22 lb.) should be injected with a 23-gauge, 1-inch needle, and larger dogs with a 22-gauge, 1.5-inch needle. The longer needles are required to place the drug deep within the belly of the epaxial muscles. The small gauge needle (has narrow needle diameter) helps prevent drug leakage from the injection site.

The manufacturer claims that doses as high as 2.5 times the recommended dose of melarsomine are well tolerated by animals. A similarly increased dose of thiacetarsamide would produce severe toxicity. Animals receiving an inadvertent overdose of melarsomine can be treated with BAL (British Anti-Lewisite or dimercaprol), one of the standard antidotes for heavy-metal poisoning such as from arsenic or lead. In tests conducted on dogs before approval of melarsomine, about one third of the treated dogs had reactions at the injection site, indicated by pain, swelling, and tenderness within the muscle mass. No skin swelling, sloughing, or severe redness was noted in any of these dogs.

Neither thiacetarsamide nor melarsomine is indicated in animals with Class-4 heartworm disease, in which large numbers of heartworms are found not only in the right ventricle but also in the right atrium and the venae cavae. These animals with this "caval syndrome" usually require surgical removal of the adult heartworms. Class-3 heartworm disease, which is characterized by fatigue, dyspnea, severe right heart changes on radiographs, and right heart failure, can be treated with melarsomine in a modified dosage, which involves giving 1 dose of melarsomine, resting the animal for 1 month, and then giving the regular set of 2 injections.

In the weeks following adulticide treatment with either drug, the dead adult heartworms degenerate, forming emboli that can travel along the pulmonary arteries to lodge in the smallest arterioles in the lung, where they can initiate an inflammatory reaction. During this postadulticide period the animal must not be allowed to exercise or become excited because of the potential for increased blood flow (and turbulence) through the heart and lungs, resulting in an increase of emboli bombarding the lungs. Aspirin and glucocorticoids are sometimes used to combat emboli-induced pulmonary inflammation. Use of glucocorticoids is still controversial; some specialists claim that administration of glucocorticoids soon after adulticide treatment may decrease the efficacy of thiacetarsamide against the adult heartworms.

Antiparasitics

Pharm Fact

Melarsomine may replace thiacetarsamide in adulticide heartworm therapy because of its lower toxicity, greater efficacy, and ease of use.

After the animal has been allowed 3 to 4 weeks to recover from adulticide treatment and embolic pulmonary inflammation, a microfilaricide can be administered to eliminate circulating heartworm microfilariae. It has become standard practice to use a single dose of ivermectin (for example, 1% Ivomec injectable, approved for use in livestock) as the microfilaricide of choice. The ivermectin solution is administered by mouth rather than by injection, using a tuberculin syringe to accurately measure the correct dose. (Forms of ivermectin injectable for large animals are quite concentrated.) Milbemycin oxime (Interceptor), a drug very similar to ivermectin, has also been used as a microfilaricide. In the future, dosages are likely to be proposed for use of milbemycin as a microfilaricide.

Ivermectin and milbemycin kill parasites by increasing the effect of the inhibitory neurotransmitter glutamate. Previously, it was believed that the inhibitory neurotransmitter GABA played the major role; more recent evidence indicates that GABA is less important than glutamate. Like parasites, mammals have sites on which ivermectin and milbemycin act; theoretically, mammals should be susceptible to the same paralytic effect experienced by parasites. The difference is that in mammals the receptor sites to these drugs are in the CNS and are protected by the blood-brain barrier (see Chapter 3). Because ivermectin and milbemycin poorly penetrate the CNS, there is little chance for the drug to reach their sites of action in any considerable concentration; hence mammals are generally protected against the drugs' toxic effects. Collies and Collie crossbreeds are the exceptions. The blood-brain barrier of these dogs is more permeable to ivermectin (and theoretically to milbemycin), allowing the drug access to receptor sites and causing general inhibition of the central nervous system.

Signs associated with ivermectin toxicity appear 2 to 4 hours after oral administration and sooner after injection. Signs reflect loss of motor control (that is, inability to maintain posture, crossed limbs, ataxia), loss of vision and visual reflexes (that is, no menace response, pupils fixed and dilated), and coma. Depressed respiration and bradycardia may also be noted. There is no specific antidote for ivermectin toxicosis, but supportive therapy such as with glucocorticoids, IV fluids, and parenteral nutrition and intensive care to prevent pressure sores for days to weeks may help the animal with ivermectin toxicity to survive. Less severe toxic reactions or signs in other breeds usually resolve within 6 to 8 hours.

In one study, Collies receiving 20 times the recommended heartworm preventive dosage of milbemycin showed depression, ataxia, salivation, and mydriasis (dilated pupils). These signs resolved within 48 hours after milbemycin administration. These same Collies had previously exhibited similar signs from a correspondingly large dose of ivermectin, suggesting similar patterns of toxicity for the two drugs. One advantage of milbemycin is that it is not yet available in large animal (concentrated) dosage forms (livestock injectable, equine pastes); therefore it is less likely that Collies or other susceptible breeds would inadvertently come in contact with a highly concentrated dose as sometimes occurs with ivermectin.

Animals treated for microfilaremia (circulating microfilariae) with ivermectin should be observed for a few hours for adverse effects and then released. The blood should be examined microscopically for circulating microfilariae 3 weeks later, and a second dose of ivermectin should be given if microfilariae are still present.

After microfilariae have been cleared from the blood, the animal can begin receiving heartworm preventive to prevent reinfection. Heartworm preventives are available in two basic forms: those given daily and those given monthly. Diethylcarbamazine (DEC), which is marketed as Caricide, Nemacide, and Filaribits, among others, is given daily during seasons when an animal could be bitten by a mosquito and for 2 months thereafter. Failure to give the drug daily allows any infective larvae injected by a mosquito to mature to young adult heartworms.

Adverse reactions to diethylcarbamazine are rare, unless the animal has circulating microfilariae from an existing heartworm infection. In approximately 5% of heartworm-infected dogs that are given DEC, the adverse reaction occurs within 20 minutes of diethylcarbamazine administration and is initially manifested as GI signs or depression, which quickly progress to prostration, shock, dyspnea, and possibly death within 1 or 2 hours. Treatment is supportive and includes IV fluids and glucocorticoids. Veterinary professionals should test dogs over 6 months of age for circulating microfilariae before administering diethylcarbamazine as heartworm preventive.

Because ivermectin (Heartgard-30) and milbemycin (Interceptor) are given only once a month, these drugs have captured a significant percentage of the heartworm preventive market. The dose of ivermectin for prevention of heartworm infection, which is 0.006 mg/kg, is much lower than that used for microfilaricidal activity, which is 0.05 mg/kg. Thus the likelihood of a Collie breed experiencing an adverse reaction to ivermectin used as a heartworm preventive is minimal. Nevertheless the manufacturer recommends observing the animal for 8 hours after administration of the preventive dose of ivermectin. When used at the higher microfilaricidal dose, ivermectin may produce a shock-like anaphylactic reaction similar to that observed with diethylcarbamazine, presumably from dying microfilariae. Heartgard-30 Plus includes the antinematodal drug pyrantel with ivermectin.

A formulation of ivermectin (Heartgard for Cats) is now approved as a preventive for use in cats. The product comes in chewable cubes that are packaged in two forms for use in cats less than 5 lbs and for cats greater than 5 lbs. Like the canine Heartgard, the medication is administered once a month. It is recommended that the Heartgard be crumbled into food or given to the cat in small pieces to facilitate dissolution of the cube and absorption of the drug. Heartworm testing is recommended before the cat is started on Heartgard. If the test results are positive for heartworms, the drug can be used to prevent further infection. The drug appears to be safe in cats even at three times the recommended dose.

Milbemycin oxime (Interceptor) was introduced in 1991 as a monthly canine heartworm preventive that also eliminates adult hookworms, ascarids *(Toxocara canis),* and whipworm. Like ivermectin, milbemycin oxime kills migrating microfilariae at any stage of development. At higher doses, milbemycin may also cause a mild shock-like syndrome in some dogs with circulating microfilariae. Studies in Collies have shown the drug to be safe at up to 20 times the recommended dose. Milbemycin has also shown some promise in treatment of demodectic mange that is resistant to other treatments.

ANTIPROTOZOALS

Antiprotozoals are most commonly used against coccidia, *Giardia*, and other protozoa. They include sulfonamide antimicrobials such as sulfadimethoxine (Albon, Bactrovet), metronidazole, benzimidazole anthelmintics (fenbendazole, albendazole, and mebendazole), and amprolium (Corid). The benzimidazoles were discussed previously and the sulfonamides and metronidazole are discussed in Chapter 9.

Amprolium

Amprolium is an antiprotozoal used in calves and avian species. It is structurally similar to thiamin but does not possess thiamin's intrinsic vitamin activity. Thus when the parasite absorbs amprolium, competitive antagonism between amprolium and thiamin occurs and thiamin activity is inhibited. The parasite dies from thiamin deficiency. Use of amprolium in large doses for extended periods can also result in thiamin deficiency in the host animal.

EXTERNAL ANTIPARASITICS

External antiparasitics are used to control flies, grubs, and lice on livestock, flies (bots and maggots) on horses, and fleas, ticks, and mange mites on companion animals. In controlling these external parasites, diseases spread by arthropod vectors (such as Lyme disease, bubonic plague, and Rocky Mountain spotted fever) are decreased. Because many of these compounds are insecticides (chemicals that kill arthropods or insects) and are very toxic, veterinary technicians must be familiar with their side effects, adverse reactions, and contraindications as well as the potential problems associated with misapplication.

Insecticides and external antiparasitics are available in many formulations. For example, flea products are marketed as collars, powders, dips, aerosol sprays, pump sprays, baths, foggers, foams, pour-ons, drop-ons, and even roll-ons. Most of these formulations are designed to appeal to the companion animal owner. Insecticides and external antiparasitics for livestock are designed for ease of application to groups of animals; hence they are incorporated into rubbing bars and dust bags. Animals coming in contact with the apparatus receive a dusting of the chemical that kills or repels insects. Other formulations for livestock include pour-on products that are absorbed through the skin, dips, impregnated ear tags from which insecticide diffuses into the body, and feed additives. Products for companion animal can be applied in a carefully controlled dose to each animal, whereas some of the products formulated for food animals can easily be overdosed or underdosed.

Because new flea and tick products are constantly introduced to the market, the veterinary professional may find it difficult to keep up with all the different products available. Therefore veterinary professionals must know the insecticidal compounds likely to be found in external antiparasitics so they can make informed decisions about when to use certain products.

CHLORINATED HYDROCARBONS

Chlorinated hydrocarbons constitute one of the oldest groups of synthetic insecticides. DDT and some other insecticides in this group have been withdrawn from the market because they are readily absorbed into the body and are very resistant to biodegradation. (That is, they remain for years in the environment). Chlorinated hydrocarbons that are applied to animals or plants to control insects are eventually washed away and accumulate in streams or lakes. The high lipid solubility of these compounds allows them to become deposited in the fat of fish. This may not cause adverse reactions in the fish; however, the animals that feed on the contaminated fish begin to accumulate the insecticide as they continue to eat more fish. Like the fish, the predator also accumulates the insecticide in its fat. If this predator is normally eaten by another animal farther up the food chain, the effect of the accumulating insecticide becomes magnified in the higher orders of predator species. In addition, the effect of the insecticide becomes magnified as it moves to higher orders of predator species. When this effect culminates near the top of the food chain in such species as hawks, eagles, large carnivores (bears), and people, the results can be devastating. The decline of the bald eagle population was traced to fragile egg shells (low viability) as a result of this biological magnification of DDT. People who use chlorinated hydrocarbons must be certified to apply them because of the environmental threat from these insecticides. Therefore these products have reduced usefulness in veterinary medicine.

Lindane

The only chlorinated hydrocarbon currently used in veterinary medicine is lindane, which is incorporated in some dog shampoos. Lindane is easily absorbed through the skin and can produce harmful side effects if absorbed in sufficient quantities. Therefore owners should wear waterproof gloves, an apron, and boots when bathing an animal with lindane shampoo. Veterinary professionals should dispose of empty bottles and even the bath water containing lindane residues in accordance with state pesticide or Environmental Protection Agency (EPA) policies. The EPA has stated, "Improper disposal of excess pesticide, spray mixture, or rinsate is a violation of Federal law."

Lindane should never be used on cats, puppies less than 3 weeks old, lactating animals, or animals that will be used for meat or other food products. With all of the restrictions on lindane and similar chlorinated hydrocarbons and the availability of products that are safer for people and the environment, it is likely that these products will eventually disappear from the market.

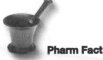

Pharm Fact

The veterinary professional must carefully dispose of chlorinated hydrocarbons, which accumulate in the environment.

ORGANOPHOSPHATES AND CARBAMATES

Organophosphates and carbamates, which are two different types of insecticides, are usually grouped together because of their similar mechanisms of action, effects of insects, and toxic effects. Unlike the chlorinated hydrocarbons, organophosphates and carbamates decompose readily in the environment and do not pose a significant threat to wildlife. These products are among the most widely used of the potent insecticides. In addition to veterinary applications, they also have several agricultural applications, including use on crops, garden plants, and nursery trees.

Organophosphates and carbamates are general names for this broad class of insecticides. Manufacturers modify the basic organophosphate molecule to produce new products. They usually give the new chemical a generic name and a trade name. For example, chlorpyrifos is a very common organophosphate marketed under the trade name of Dursban. Because of this, the labels of flea and tick products may not include the words *organophosphate* and *chlorpyrifos,* but may list only the trade names. Therefore veterinary technicians should be familiar with the names of the different organophosphates and their trade names.

Most products that contain organophosphates or carbamates have a label stating that the product contains a cholinesterase inhibitor. Thus the precautions and warnings on the label may indicate the type of insecticide, even if the specific (main) ingredient is not familiar.

Two other common trade names of organophosphates are Supona and Vapona. Carbamate insecticides can be recognized by the words carbamate or methylcarbamate in the ingredient list, the chemical names carbaryl and propoxur, or the trade names Sevin (carbaryl) and Baygon (propoxur). Some of the references at the end of this chapter may help the veterinary technician to identify the type of insecticide in a given product.

Organophosphates and carbamates work in similar ways. As shown in Fig. 11-1, they bind to acetylcholinesterase, which is the enzyme that normally breaks down the neurotransmitter acetylcholine to terminate its action at the receptor site. With acetylcholinesterase inhibition, acetylcholine molecules continue to stimulate receptor sites. There are two classes of acetylcholine receptors: **muscarinic receptors** and **nicotinic receptors.** The clinical signs associated with organophosphate or carbamate toxicity depend on which acetylcholine receptor is stimulated the most.

Stimulation of muscarinic receptors produces signs of toxicity related to parasympathetic nervous system stimulation. These classic signs of organophosphate toxicosis can be remembered by the acronym **SLUDDE: S**alivation, **L**acrimation (tearing), **U**rination, **D**efecation, **D**yspnea, and **E**mesis. Bradycardia and a weak pulse may also suggest overstimulation of the parasympathetic nervous system.

One of the most characteristic signs of organophosphate or carbamate toxicity is miosis (pinpoint pupils). Miosis may not be present with toxicity caused by every organophosphate because certain organophosphates produce this sign more than others. When miosis does appear with other SLUDDE signs, it is highly suggestive of organophosphate or carbamate toxicity.

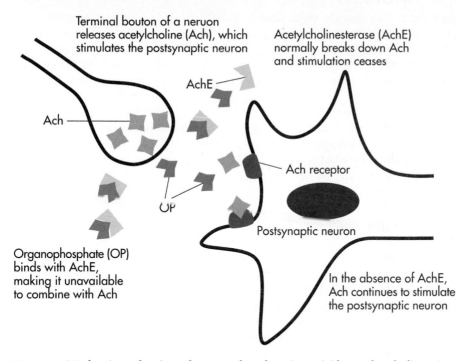

Terminal bouton of a neruon releases acetylcholine (Ach), which stimulates the postsynaptic neuron

Acetylcholinesterase (AchE) normally breaks down Ach and stimulation ceases

AchE

Ach

Ach receptor

OP

Postsynaptic neuron

Organophosphate (OP) binds with AchE, making it unavailable to combine with Ach

In the absence of AchE, Ach continues to stimulate the postsynaptic neuron

Fig. 11-1 Mechanism of action of organophosphate insecticides at the cholinergic synapse.

Although SLUDDE and miosis are the classic signs of organophosphate toxicity associated with muscarinic stimulation, some organophosphates such as chlorpyrifos may have these signs obscured by signs attributable to stimulation of nicotinic receptors. In these cases the nicotinic receptors, which are primarily located where nerves contact muscles, initially produce muscle tremors that progress to paralysis (ataxia, loss of motor control). In cats, onset of signs of chlorpyrifos toxicity is usually delayed. Affected cats show the expected tremors and ataxia associated with nicotinic receptor stimulation, but they may also exhibit seizures, anorexia, and depression. Rather than constricted pupils such as with classic organophosphate toxicity, animals poisoned by chlorpyrifos often have mydriasis (dilated pupils). These signs may persist for 2 to 4 weeks.

Treatment of acute organophosphate toxicity consists of removing any insecticide remaining on the animal and blocking the parasympathetic effects with atropine, which blocks the muscarinic receptors so they cannot be stimulated, or with pralidoxime (2-PAM), which separates the organophosphate from the acetylcholinesterase molecule, thereby freeing the enzyme molecule to work again.

In addition to acute organophosphate toxicosis, a **delayed neurotoxicity syndrome** has been reported in people, cats, dogs, and some livestock. This syndrome usually occurs 1 or 2 weeks after short-term exposure to large doses of some organophosphates. The animal becomes ataxic in the hind legs, may buckle over, and has difficulty maintaining posture. This state may progress to complete paralysis of the hind limbs. Metabolism of certain organophosphates produces a metabolite that is toxic to the myelin sheath covering the nerves. This damage may result in death of the neuron and impaired function of the muscles innervated by that neuron. The effect has been likened to "chemical transection" of the nerve. Affected cattle may show weakness, depression, droopy ears, and bloat. Fortunately, this syndrome is fairly rare. Treatment is supportive and symptomatic.

Because organophosphates and carbamates work by a similar mechanism, they should not be used simultaneously or with other products that increase acetylcholine activity or decrease acetylcholinesterase activity. Many cases of organophosphate toxicity result from failure to observe this precaution.

An animal might be predisposed to toxicity in situations where an overanxious dog owner dips the dog in chlorpyrifos, powders the dog's bed with methylcarbamate, fogs the house with dichlorvos, sprays the yard with a concentrated insect spray such as malathion, and gives the dog a cythioate tablet. Just one of these treatments would be safe, and the dog might be able to tolerate use of two or three products simultaneously. However, each application exposes the animal to increasing amounts of organophosphates and carbamates and decreases acetylcholinesterase levels. Owners may forget that the rose dust they applied to their plants or the aphid spray they used around the garden is also an organophosphate. If the animal is in contact with these areas, it can receive an additional dose of organophosphate.

Organophosphates and carbamates should be used cautiously in Persian cats, sick cats, Whippets, Greyhounds, and certain exotic breeds of cattle because of these species' increased susceptibility to toxic reactions. As a general rule these insecticides should not be used on animals recovering from surgery, sick animals, pregnant animals, or animals that might otherwise be considered stressed. Because organophosphates and carbamates increase activity of the parasympathetic nervous system, the respiratory tree often produces greater amounts of mucus and respiratory secretions and some degree of bronchoconstriction. Thus organophosphates and carbamates should not be used in animals with respiratory disease. The same is true for animals with GI disease because organophosphates increase GI activity and secretions.

Technicians should have knowledge of the oral organophosphate cythioate (Proban). This insecticide is given by mouth, absorbed from the GI tract, and distributed to body tissues. When a flea bites the treated animal, it takes in blood and tissue fluid containing the insecticide and dies. The efficacy of this product depends on a sufficient amount of organophosphate in the animal's body fluids to kill the insect. Cythioate does *not* prevent the flea from biting the animal. Therefore animals with sensitivity to flea saliva (flea-bite hypersensitivity) will still have hypersensitivity reactions until all of the fleas in the environment and on the dog are eliminated. Although cythioate is labeled for use every 3 days, blood concentrations sufficient to kill fleas are probably maintained for only the first 12 hours after administration. Thus fleas biting the animal on the second or third day after treatment may survive.

Other products with the prefix *Pro-* in the trade name are not necessarily organophosphates. For example, Pro-Spot is an organophosphate (fen-

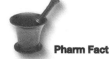

Pharm Fact

Organophosphates should be used cautiously in Persian cats, sick cats, Whippets, and Greyhounds.

thion), but Pro-Powder is a pyrethrin, and Pro-Kill is a rotenone insecticide.

Pour-on and other topical organophosphates (Spot-on, Pro-Spot, Tiguvon) are designed for application in small amounts, with the intent that they will be absorbed and distributed throughout the tissue fluid. The veterinary professional or animal owner should follow special precautions when using these products because of the potential for absorption of the insecticide through the skin. The person applying these products should wear gloves to prevent accidental exposure. There have also been reports of clients dipping their dogs or cats in the pour-on cattle products resulting in a fatal toxicity in the pet. Clients and veterinary personnel must be aware that pour-on products are formulated for specific species and are very concentrated, and only a small amount is needed for each treatment.

Because of this potential for toxicity, veterinary professionals should be very familiar with the organophosphate or carbamate product they are using and thoroughly educate the client who applies the product at home or on the farm.

PYRETHRINS AND PYRETHROIDS

Pyrethrins and pyrethroids (synthetic pyrethrins) constitute the largest group of insecticides marketed for use against external parasites and as common household insect sprays. Unlike organophosphate and carbamate insecticides, pyrethrins and pyrethroids are usually safe. Pyrethrins are natural insecticides derived from chrysanthemum flowers. They produce a quick "knockdown" effect, as evidenced by the way flies drop or fleas fall from an animal sprayed with pyrethrins. However, the killing activity of pyrethrins is not as marked as the stunning effect, and the immobilized flies or fleas may recover after several minutes.

Pyrethroids are synthetic versions of pyrethrin, with the pyrethrin molecule modified to enhance the insecticidal effect. When the chemical name is written out, most pyrethroids can be recognized by the *-thrin* suffix. Pyrethroid drugs include resmethrin, allethrin, permethrin, tetramethrin, bioallethrin, and fenvalerate.

Pyrethrins and pyrethroids have very selective toxicity. A very small dose is toxic to insects, whereas a much larger dose is necessary to produce any adverse effects in animals. Although pyrethrins are very safe for mammals, fish unfortunately readily absorb pyrethrin insecticides through their skin and can easily become poisoned and die. Therefore pyrethrin and pyrethroid use around streams, lakes, decorative ponds, fish farms, and aquaculture establishments must be carefully controlled.

Because of their general safety, pyrethrins and pyrethroids can be used in conjunction with organophosphate and carbamate products without increasing the risk of toxicity. Unlike the chlorinated hydrocarbons, pyrethrins and pyrethroids break down fairly rapidly in the environment.

Synergists are added to the pyrethrin products to enhance their insecticidal effect. The synergist most commonly used with pyrethrins is piperonyl butoxide. This synergist is generally safe, but it may cause neurotoxicity in cats licking their treated hair coat. Because pyrethroids have sufficient insecticidal activity, they are not often combined with a synergist.

Veterinary technicians should be aware of certain features of pyrethroids. Resmethrin is degraded by ultraviolet light, leaving an odor like stale urine. Permethrin and fenvalerate adhere to synthetic fibers such as those found in nylon or synthetic carpets, which causes these insecticides to lose their residual activity or become completely inactivated. Permethrin has been incorporated into some external antiparasitic protocols because of its effectiveness in killing and repelling ticks as well as fleas. This combination is appealing to the public because of awareness of tick-borne diseases such as Lyme disease (borreliosis) and Rocky Mountain spotted fever.

Because manufacturers of some pyrethroids have claims of considerable residual effect with use of their drug, the veterinary professional should consult product literature and drug references to determine if residual activity is degraded by changes in application, exposure to water or bathing the animal, or exposure to sunlight. The veterinary professional should carefully read information provided by the insecticide manufacturer before accepting as fact any claims of residual activity.

AMITRAZ

Amitraz, a diamide insecticide, was one of the first effective agents available for treatment of demodectic mange in dogs. Since its introduction, amitraz has been incorporated into other insecticidal products. Amitraz is toxic to cats and rabbits and should not be used in those species. Demodectic mange in dogs is treated with the liquid form, available as a dip or sponge-on bath product (Mitaban). Again, gloves should be worn during application of this product to decrease contact with skin. With the normal dipping procedure, animals may show sedation and incoordination (reflecting CNS depression) for 24 to 72 hours after treatment.

Because they are wet after treatment, some animals develop hypothermia if left in a cool place or metal cage without padding. Technicians should monitor body temperature during recovery. Pruritus (itching) often occurs for several days after treatment and is usually caused by death of the mites and the subsequent foreign body allergic reaction.

Amitraz is also available as Preventic, which is a tick collar for dogs, and as Taktic, which is available as a topical liquid or as a collar for use in cattle. Amitraz can be very toxic if ingested by animals or people. Ingestion of Taktic collars has produced severe toxicity in dogs. Therefore veterinary technicians should caution pet owners or livestock producers that collars and discarded segments of collars should be disposed of properly so they are out of reach of children and animals.

Application of Taktic has been advocated for some nonresponsive cases of demodectic mange in dogs. This is an extra-label (unapproved) use. Because such use could potentially cause toxicity in treated dogs, owners must be well informed of the expected outcomes and the potential risks of this treatment. Amitraz toxicosis is treated with supportive therapy and multiple doses of yohimbine, the α_2 receptor antagonist.

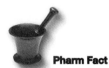

Pharm Fact

Amitraz can be very toxic if ingested.

IMIDACLOPRID

Imidacloprid (Advantage) is a new chloronicotinyl nitroguanidine insecticide used topically to kill adult fleas. Like organophosphates, carbamates, and pyrethroids, imidacloprid is an insect neurotoxin. Unlike these other compounds, however, imidacloprid blocks the receptor site for acetylcholine neurotransmitter molecules, thereby blocking transmission of the impulse across the synapse. Also unlike most organophosphate flea products, imidacloprid is marketed for use in both dogs and cats.

Imidacloprid is applied to the back of the neck in cats or between the shoulder blades in dogs (and over the rump area of large dogs). The drug is disseminated across the skin by the animal's movement. Imidacloprid is poorly absorbed through the skin and kills adult fleas on contact. The manufacturer claims 4 weeks of residual activity in cats, with a slightly longer residual effect in dogs. The compound appears to be safe, according to studies conducted for approval by the FDA. Because its mechanism of action is descibed as specific for the insect nervous system, imidacloprid has a wide safety margin.

FIPRONIL

Fipronil (Frontline) is another new flea and tick control product for use in dogs and cats. Fipronil resembles ivermectin in its insecticidal activity more than the organophosphates or pyrethroids. The drug obstructs the chloride channels of the insect's neuronal cells. Because chloride influx into the neuron normally inhibits neuronal firing, obstructing the chloride channel allows overstimulation of the insect's nervous system and subsequent death. The receptors in insects for this compound are different enough from mammals to reduce the chloride channel-blocking effect in veterinary patients.

Frontline is being marketed as a measured-dose spray product (Frontline spray) and as a concentrated topically applied liquid (Frontline Top Spot). The spray product is somewhat unusual in that the fipronil is applied at a dose of 3ml/kg body weight. The spray container itself is calibrated to administer a fairly precise amount of insecticide to allow accurate dosing. The residual effect of fipronil in efficacy trials indicated a residual insecticidal effect of at least 30 days, even if the animal is bathed; the residual effect is even longer in some animals. The topical liquid product is applied on the back between the shoulder blades and works its way over the rest of the body surface by the animal's movements. Thus Frontline is being marketed as a spray and topical liquid that only require once-a-month applications.

The manufacturer claims that fipronil is unlikely to produce toxicity via oral ingestion if an animal licks the application site. The reason is that fipronil binds with the dermis, hair follicles, and sebaceous glands. A disadvantage of fipronil in its present spray formulation is that, like many sprays, the active ingredient is dissolved in an alcohol base. Alcohol dries the skin, causes salivation if the site is licked while wet, and often has an unpleasant odor because of the volatility. An advantage of the topical drop application over the spray is that cats are often intolerant of sprays and would have to be physically restrained long enough, with use of the spray, to insure proper dose application. Clients and veterinary professionals should wear gloves when applying this product to prevent exposure to the drug.

INSECT GROWTH REGULATORS

Insect growth regulators are compounds that affect immature stages of insects and prevent maturation to adults. **Insect development inhibitors** and **juvenile hormone mimics** are types of insect growth regulators.

Methoprene (Precor found in products like Siphotrol and Ovitrol) and fenoxycarb are some of the first insect growth regulators incorporated into topical products and flea collars. While generally regarded as safe, the manufacturer of fenoxycarb voluntarily withdrew this product from the market in 1996 because of concerns over the results of government testing involving the use of high doses of fenoxycarb.

When incorporated into a flea collar, these compounds are distributed over the animal's skin. Female fleas absorb the drug and it is incorporated into the flea eggs. The drug-impregnated eggs hatch, but the larvae do not mature to adult fleas. Insect growth regulators are also effective if they come into contact with the immature stages of fleas; however, flea pupae in carpets are probably protected from methoprene because of the carpet fiber length and methoprene's propensity to adhere to fibers.

Lufenuron (Program) is an insect development inhibitor that is available as a tablet for dogs and cats, and an oral liquid for cats. Lufenuron interferes with development of the insect's chitin, which is essential for proper egg formation and development of the larval exoskeleton. The so-called "egg tooth" used by flea larvae to exit the egg is also made of chitin. Thus if flea larvae survive within the egg despite a defective shell, they will be unable to hatch. Because lufenuron is orally ingested and distributed throughout an animal's tissue fluids, a flea must bite the animal to be exposed to the drug. Lufenuron is distributed to fat and then leaches slowly back into the body fluids, providing a long duration of activity. Therefore the drug is given only once a month.

Methoprene, fenoxycarb, and lufenuron have no adulticidal activity (do not kill mature fleas). Therefore these products should be used as one component of a flea-control program along with environmental control of fleas and judicious application of an adulticide to kill mature fleas on an animal.

Pyriproxyfen (Nylar, found in products like Knockout) is a juvenile hormone mimic with a mechanism of action thought to be similar to, but

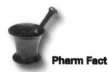

Pharm Fact

Insect growth regulators should be used as one component of a flea-control program.

perhaps more potent than, that of methoprene and fenoxycarb. Nylar is marketed for control of fleas in the environment but may also be formulated in a product for use on the animal. Early research suggests that pyriproxyfen may have some activity against adult fleas, but the effect is not immediate.

INSECT REPELLENTS

Insect repellents are used to repel insects and keep them off of animals. Repellent formulations include fly sprays, ear tags, and products applied to the tips of dogs' ears. Some of these products are insecticides as well as repellents. In horses and cattle, repellents prevent flies from laying eggs on the skin, reducing bot and warble infestations. In outdoor dogs, especially those with upright ears such as German Shepherds and Doberman Pinschers, flies sometimes continually bite the ear tips, producing oozing wounds and encrustations of black, scabby material (ear tip fly strike). Application of a repellent to the ears of these dogs reduces fly strike.

Some pyrethrins and pyrethroids have natural repellent properties. Butoxypolypropylene glycol (Butox PPG) is a repellent that has been incorporated into flea and tick spray products for use in dogs and cats. It is also used in equine fly repellents because it provides a shine that is of cosmetic value in show animals. Butoxypolypropylene glycol can cause dermal irritation if a harness or collar is applied over the area while the haircoat is still wet with spray.

Diethyltoluamide (DEET) is a common ingredient in repellent products formulated for use in people. It also was used with fenvalerate in the product Blockade (manufactured by Hartz), which was withdrawn from the market for several months because of reports that it caused death in several treated cats and dogs. Signs of toxicosis from this product include excitation, tremors, seizures, ataxia, and vomiting. People who use DEET in pure (100%) formulations have reported numbness of the lips or tingling associated with repeated use or application of large amounts.

OTHER EXTERNAL ANTIPARASITICS

Rotenone (Derris Powder) is a natural insecticide derived from derris root. It may be included with other insecticides in dips, pour-on liquids, and powders. Rotenone is toxic to fish and swine; therefore one must consider where runoff or rinsate from a dip or pour-on liquid will accumulate.

D-limonene, derived from citrus peels, purportedly has some slight insecticidal activity. When included in insecticidal products, it imparts a pleasant citrus smell to the haircoat.

Sulfur is sometimes included in tar and sulfur shampoos to help reduce skin scaling and to treat sarcoptic mange. These products are usually recognized by their strong sulfur odor.

Antiparasitic Drug Categories and Names

Internal antiparasitics

Antinematodals
  Piperazine
  Benzimidazoles
    Fenbendazole (Panacur)
    Mebendazole (Telmin, Telmintic)
    Thiabendazole (Equizole, Tresadermotic)
    Oxibendazole (Anthelcide EQ, Filaribits-Plus)
    Albendazole
    Oxfendazole
    Cambendazole
  Organophosphates
    Dichlorvos
    Trichlorfon
    Coumaphos
  Ivermectin (Ivomec, Eqvalan, Heartgard-30)
  Pyrantel
    Pyrantel pamoate (Strongid, Nemex)
    Pyrantel tartrate
  Morantel tartrate (Nematel)
  Febantel
    Levamisole
    Phenothiazine (Dyrex TF)
Anticestodals
  Praziquantel (Droncit)
  Epsiprantel (Cestex)
  Bunamidine (Scolaban)
Antiparasitics Used in Heartworm Treatment
  Thiacetarsamide sodium (Caparsolate)
  Melarsomine dihydrochloride (Immiticide)
  Milbemycin oxime (Interceptor)
  Diethylcarbamazine (Caricide, Nemacide, Filaribits)

Invermectin (Heartgard-30)
Antiprotozoals
  Sulfadimethoxine (Albon, Bactrovet)
  Metronidazole
  Amprolium (Corid)

External antiparasitics

Chlorinated Hydrocarbons
  Lindane
Organophosphates and Carbamates
  Chlorpyrifos (Dursban)
  Carbaryl (Sevin)
  Propoxur (Baygon)
Pyrethrins and Pyrethroids
  Resmethrin
  Allethrin
  Permethrin
  Tetramethrin
  Bioallethrin
  Fenvalerate
Amitraz
Imidacloprid (Advantage)
Fipronil (Frontline)
Insect Growth Regulators
  Methoprene (Siphotrol, Ovitrol)
  Fenoxycarb (Basus, Ectogard)
  Lufenuron (Program)
  Pyriproxyfen (Nylar)
Repellents
  Butoxypolypropylene glycol
  Diethyltoluamide
Other External Antiparasitics
  Rotenone (Derris powder)
  D-limonene
  Sulfur

Recommended Reading
Heartworm Infection

Allen TLC, et al: *Heartworm disease: practice tips for the veterinarian,* Proceedings of the North American Veterinary Conference in Orlando, Fla, Jan 1995.

Blagburn BL: Microfilaricidal therapy: review and update, *Vet Med* 89(7):630, 1994.

Dzimianski MT: Developing a heartworm prevention program, *Vet Med* 89(6):545, 1994.

Dzimianski MT et al: *Assessment of filaricidal activity of a new filaricide (RM 340) against immature and adult heartworms,* Proceedings of the American Heartworm Society Symposium, Charleston, SC, March 1989.

Hoskins JD: Canine heartworm disease, *Compend Cont Educ Vet* 18(3):348, 1996.

Immiticide package insert, Rhone Merieux, 1996.

Knight DH: *Seasonality of heartworm transmission and timing of prophylaxis,* Proceedings of the North American Veterinary Conference, Orlando, Fla, Jan 1995.

Knight DH: Heartworms in dogs and cats: reconsidering your treatment options, *Vet Med* 89(7):618, 1994.

Knight DH: Should every heartworm-infected dog be treated with an adulticide? *Vet Med* 89(7):620, 1994.

Tanner PA, Keister DM, Dunavent BB: *Clinical pathology changes in dogs with severe heartworm disease following treatment with immiticide,* Proceedings of the American Association of Veterinary Parasitologists, Abstract 75, Auburn, AL, March 1995.

Tanner PA, Winograd H, Keister DM: *Clinical field trials for treatment of mature and immature dirofilaria immitis infestation in dogs with severe heartworm disease,* Proceedings of the American Association of Veterinary Parasitologists, Abstract 82, Auburn, AL, March 1995.

Internal Parasites

Hendrix CM: Helminthic infections of the feline small and large intestines; diagnosis and treatment, *Vet Med* 90(35):456, 1995.

Herd RP: A 10-point plan for equine worm control, *Vet Med* 90(35):481, 1995.

Lindsay DS, Blagburn BL: Practical treatment and control of infections caused by canine gastrointestinal parasites, *Vet Med* 90(35):441, 1995.

External Parasites

Arthur R: Imidacloprid for flea control on dogs and cats, Tech Bulletin, Shawnee Mission, KS, 1996, Bayer Corporation.

Dubey JP, Blagburn BL: Advances in veterinary parasitology, *Compend Cont Educ Vet* 17(4):469, 1995.

Greek JS: Environmental flea control: general guidelines and recent advances, *Vet Med* 89(8)763, 1994.

Hepler DI: *Lufenuron: flea treatment for the '90s,* Proceedings of the North American Veterinary Conference in Orlando, Fla, Jan 1995.

Miller WH et al: Clinical efficacy of increased dosages of milbemycin oxime for treatment of generalized demodicosis in adult dogs, *JAVMA* 207(12):1581, 1995.

Mundell A: Demodicosis. In Birchard S and Sherding R, editors: *Manual of small animal practice,* Philadelphia, 1994, WB Saunders.

Smith CA: Searching for safe methods of flea control, *JAVMA* 206(8):1137, 1995.

Review Questions

1. The veterinary clinic where you work receives an advertisement touting a new flea product with "selective toxicity." Does this mean the product kills only certain parasites? To what does *selective toxicity* refer?

2. A client telephones and says the veterinarian told her a particular flea spray is safe to use on cats. She wants to know if she can use the spray on 4-day-old kittens that are covered with fleas. What is an appropriate response?

3. A client reports seeing "little white worm pieces" resembling grains of rice crawling around his dog's anal area. The client is upset because he believes that the medication dispensed last month by the doctor to eliminate hookworms was not effective. What is an appropriate explanation?

4. Promotional material for a new anthelmintic says that the drug is anticestodal, antinematodal, and antitrematodal. Against what types of parasites is this product likely to be effective?

5. The puppy dewormer commonly used in your clinic is described as a vermifuge. When dispensing this medication, what information or advice should you give to the client?

6. Owners of new puppies commonly say, "We don't need to have a stool sample checked. I give my puppy a once-a-month puppy dewormer." Which drug most likely has this client used? Which intestinal parasites are likely to be eliminated by this drug? Which will not be eliminated?

7. A new anthelmintic is classified as a benzimidazole. Is this drug likely to be antinematodal, anticestodal, or both?

8. How does ivermectin exert its antiparasitic effect?

9. Why do horses sometimes develop itchy skin after treatment with ivermectin?

10. Pyrantel pamoate (Strongid, Nemex) is considered very safe; however, some veterinary parasitologists say it should not be used with organophosphate flea products. What is the basis for this recommendation?

11. A client heard that some species of *Echinococcus* tapeworms have been implicated in certain malignant diseases of humans and now wants medication to rid his dog of this "dreaded parasite." Should you dispense praziquantel or epsiprantel?

12. A pet owner claims that the tapeworm medication you dispensed for her dog was not effective because she did not see any worms come out in the stool. What is an appropriate explanation?

13. A client telephones and says her dog was in a fight with a dog infected with heartworms. The client wants to know if her dog could contract heartworms from the bite wounds; she has not given heartworm preventive (ivermectin) to her dog in the past 2 months. What is an appropriate response?

14. An owner is concerned because he heard that the only way to eliminate heartworm infection is to inject the animal with strychnine, arsenic, or some other poison. What is an appropriate explanation for this client?

15. Why is melarsomine often preferred over thiacetarsamide as the treatment for adult heartworms?

16. In dogs being treated for heartworm infection, why is the most dangerous period (time when complications are most likely) a couple of weeks after the adult heartworms have been killed? What can be done to minimize problems during this time?

17. After adult heartworms are killed, what drugs can be used to eliminate microfilariae from the systemic circulation?

18. While assessing a dog with heartworm infection, the doctor comments that she cannot immediately start adulticide treatment with melarsomine or thiacetarsamide because the dog has too many heartworms. What is the significance of this comment?

19. What is the nature of Collies' increased risk of toxicosis from ivermectin?

20. A horse owner is concerned because he thinks his dog may have eaten some discarded ivermectin paste dewormer that he used on his horses. It happened about 4 hours previously. What signs of toxicosis should the owner look for? Is there an antidote for ivermectin toxicosis?

21. The doctor mentions that the biggest problem with ivermectin toxicosis in dogs is "keeping them alive long enough for them to recover." What is the significance of this comment?

22. If Collies are more likely to have toxicosis from ivermectin, why do they not have toxic effects from Heartgard-30 heartworm preventive?

23. What is the pharmacologic difference between ivermectin and milbemycin?

24. The doctor asks you to dispense an antibacterial to treat intestinal coccidia. What type of antibacterial should you dispense?

25. Why are insecticide sprays that are formulated for dogs and cats not normally used on cattle to prevent fly bites?

26. What precautions should be observed with use of lindane products?

27. A puppy becomes ill after being sprayed with a product containing chlorpyrifos. What signs would the puppy most likely show? What drug could help alleviate these signs?

28. What signs would a muscarinic acetylcholine receptor agonist cause? Would these signs be similar or opposite to the signs of organophosphate toxicity?

29. The veterinarian remarks that atropine does not "cure" organophosphate toxicity; it only obscures the signs. What is the significance of that comment?

30. A client telephones and says his 4-month-old cat is heavily infested with fleas. He has a spray product containing allethrin, and wants to know if he can safely use it on the cat. What is an appropriate response?

31. Why should aquarium fish be specially protected or removed from premises before use of pyrethrin foggers?

32. A dog's health record indicates that some years ago it was treated topically with amitraz. You are puzzled because you thought amitraz was only found in tick collars. For what condition was amitraz applied topically on this dog?

33. A client telephones and says his Cocker Spaniel just chewed up and swallowed most of a tick collar. The container says the active ingredient in the collar is amitraz. The owner asks if he should bring the dog to the clinic for examination. What is an appropriate response for this client?

34. What are the advantages and disadvantages of insect growth regulators and insect development inhibitors for flea control?

Key Terms

Addison's disease
adrenocorticotropic
    hormone (ACTH)
alcohol solutions
alcohol suspensions
anabolic effects
aqueous solution
arachidonic acid
biologic activity
catabolic effects
corticotropin-releasing
    factor (CRF)
Cushing's syndrome
eicosanoids
glucocorticoids
glucuronyl transferase
hyperadrenocorticism
hypoadrenocorticism
iatrogenic
leukotrienes
mast-cell tumor
mineralocorticoid
nonsteroidal
    antiinflammatory drugs
    (NSAIDs)
prostaglandins
renal papillary necrosis
steroidal
    antiinflammatory drugs
suspension
thromboxane

Antiinflammatories

12 Chapter

The Inflammation Pathway
Corticosteroids
Glucocorticoids
    Types of glucocorticoids
    Formulations of glucocorticoids
    Effects of glucocorticoids
Disease Caused by Glucocorticoid
    Excess
    Safe use of glucocorticoids
Nonsteroidal Antiinflammatory Drugs
    Phenylbutazone
    Aspirin
    Ibuprofen, ketoprofen, and
        naproxen

Flunixin meglumine
Meclofenamic acid
Dimethyl sulfoxide
Orgotein
Carprofen
Other Drugs Used to Fight
    Inflammation
Acetaminophen
Gold salts
Dipyrone
Piroxicam

Learning Objectives

*After studying this chapter,
you should know the following:*

The way inflammation is mediated and the antiinflammatory effects of
    glucocorticoids

The ways antiinflammatories are used

The way to select an appropriate antiinflammatory

Types of antiinflammatories and their clinical applications

Precautions in using antiinflammatories

Drugs that relieve pain or discomfort by blocking or reducing the inflammatory process are called *antiinflammatories*. Inflammation is a protective mechanism that increases the blood supply to a traumatized or infected area, increases migration of leukocytes (white blood cells) into the area, and increases the activity of phagocytes (cells that engulf and destroy foreign material and microorganisms). If this protective mechanism is activated inappropriately, such as with arthritis, severe allergic reactions, or autoimmune disease, antiinflammatory drugs are necessary to prevent excessive tissue damage.

There are two general classes of antiinflammatories: **steroidal antiinflammatory drugs** (corticosteroids) and **nonsteroidal antiinflammatory drugs (NSAIDs).** Most of these drugs relieve pain indirectly by decreasing inflammation; however, some also have direct analgesic (pain-relieving) activity. (A box listing antiinflammatories can be found at the end of this chapter.)

THE INFLAMMATION PATHWAY

After insult such as trauma, burns, and infection, tissues respond by producing substances that initiate the healing process. These substances also stimulate pain receptors, resulting in the perception of pain. If production of these inflammatory substances could be reduced or inhibited, stimulation of pain receptors could also be reduced. This is the general reason for antiinflammatory drug use.

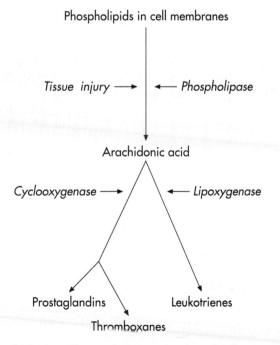

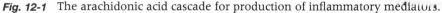

Fig. 12-1 The arachidonic acid cascade for production of inflammatory mediators.

When tissue is damaged by trauma, burns, or other insults, the enzyme phospholipase breaks down phospholipids in cell membranes, releasing **arachidonic acid** (Fig. 12-1). Arachidonic acid, in turn, is acted on by either the enzyme cyclooxygenase to produce **prostaglandins** and **thromboxanes,** or the enzyme lipoxygenase, which produces **leukotrienes,** another group of inflammation mediators. The prostaglandins, thromboxanes, and leukotrienes, referred to collectively as **eicosanoids,** diffuse out of the cell to initiate a very wide variety of physiologic reactions.

Corticosteroids, especially the glucocorticoids, reduce inflammation by blocking the action of phospholipase and hence stabilizing the cell's phospholipid membranes. This blocks the early portion of the pathway shown in Fig. 12-1, preventing production of most inflammatory mediators. NSAIDs have no effect on phospholipase but inhibit cyclooxygenase and, to varying degrees, lipoxygenase, reducing production of prostaglandins, thromboxane, and leukotrienes.

In addition to the eicosanoids, several other compounds, including histamine, kinins, substance P, and superoxide radicals, also contribute to the redness, swelling, heat, and pain associated with inflammation.

CORTICOSTEROIDS

The term *corticosteroids* refers to a group of hormones produced by the cortex (outer layer) of the adrenal gland. There are two groups of corticosteroids: **mineralocorticoids** and **glucocorticoids.** Although both groups of hormones are produced by the same gland, they have very different effects on the body.

Mineralocorticoids, as the name implies, affect the minerals in the body, such as sodium, potassium, and other electrolytes. Mineralocorticoids are involved with water and electrolyte balance in the body but have little or no antiinflammatory effect.

In contrast, glucocorticoids produce an antiinflammatory effect by inhibiting phospholipase and stabilizing cellular membranes; they also enhance deposition of glycogen in the liver. Glucocorticoids also affect glucose metabolism and generally cause an increase in blood glucose levels.

Every corticosteroid drug of either type produces both mineralocorticoid (sodium retention) and glucocorticoid (antiinflammatory, glycogen deposition) effects. These drugs may be classified as a glucocorticoid or a mineralocorticoid, depending on which effect predominates. Because we are focusing on antiinflammatory effects in this chapter, the remaining sections discuss glucocorticoids.

GLUCOCORTICOIDS

When veterinarians use the terms *cortisone* or *corticosteroids,* they are usually referring to glucocorticoids. Glucocorticoids are normally produced in the body in response to release of **adrenocorticotropic hormone (ACTH)** by

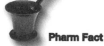

Pharm Fact

Every corticosteroid drug produces both mineralo-corticoid and glucocorti-coid effects.

the anterior pituitary gland. Release of ACTH from the anterior pituitary is in turn controlled by the hypothalamus through release of **corticotropin-releasing factor (CRF).** Production of hydrocortisone (cortisol) and cortisone by the adrenal gland provides the necessary negative feedback to curtail release of CRF and ACTH. Thus the CRF-ACTH-cortisol negative feedback loop (Fig. 12-2) is similar to that regulating production of other hormones, as described in Chapter 7.

Exogenous corticosteroids (glucocorticoids, such as prednisone) used in treatment have the same negative-feedback effect on the hypothalamus and pituitary gland as endogenous (internally produced) cortisol. As explained later, this negative feedback can result in potentially severe side effects if corticosteroids are used inappropriately.

Types of Glucocorticoids

Glucocorticoids are classified according to their duration of biologic activity. A glucocorticoid that exerts an antiinflammatory effect (biologic activity) for less than 12 hours is considered a short-acting glucocorticoid. Hydrocortisone is a short-acting glucocorticoid and a common ingredient in topical medications. Cortisone is another common short-acting glucocorticoid, but it is not used in veterinary medicine to any appreciable extent. Cortisone must be converted by the liver to hydrocortisone before it becomes active.

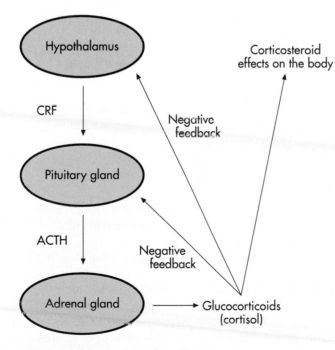

Fig. 12-2 Regulation of glucocorticoid production.

Many of the glucocorticoids used in veterinary medicine are classified as intermediate-acting glucocorticoids, exerting biologic activity for 12 to 36 hours. This includes such commonly used drugs as prednisone, prednisolone, triamcinolone (Vetalog), methylprednisolone, and isoflupredone. Prednisone must be converted by the liver to prednisolone to exert its maximal effect.

Long-acting glucocorticoids such as dexamethasone, betamethasone, and flumethasone exert their biologic activity for more than 48 hours.

Formulations of Glucocorticoids

Looking at the drugs stocked in the veterinary pharmacy or paging through a veterinary pharmacology text, you will notice that glucocorticoids are available in different formulations. For example, dexamethasone is available as dexamethasone and dexamethasone sodium phosphate. Why this difference?

Glucocorticoids are generally available in three liquid forms: **aqueous solutions, alcohol solutions,** and **suspensions.** The type of formulation determines its route of administration and use.

Glucocorticoids in aqueous (water) solution are usually combined with a salt to make them soluble in water. These salts include sodium phosphate or sodium succinate. Therefore dexamethasone sodium phosphate (Azium) and prednisolone sodium succinate (Solu-Delta-Cortef) are aqueous solutions of glucocorticoids. The advantage of aqueous forms is that they can be given in large doses intravenously with less risk than alcohol solutions and suspensions. (Suspensions should never be given intravenously.) The aqueous forms are often used in emergency situations such as with shock and CNS trauma because they can be delivered intravenously in large amounts and have a fairly rapid onset of activity.

Alcohol solutions of glucocorticoids usually do not contain a salt. Thus if the label of a vial of dexamethasone specifies the active ingredient as dexamethasone, without mention of sodium phosphate, it is likely an alcohol solution.

Suspensions of glucocorticoids contain the drug particles suspended in the liquid vehicle. Suspensions are characterized by their opaque appearance (after shaking), the need for shaking the vial before use, and the terms *acetate, diacetate, pivalate, acetonide,* or *valerate* appended to the glucocorticoid name. When in suspension, glucocorticoids are in a large, crystalline form that must be dissolved before the drug can be absorbed from the injection site. When injected into the body, the crystals dissolve over several days, releasing small amounts of glucocorticoid each day and providing prolonged action. Topical preparations of glucocorticoid suspensions using the acetate ester are very lipid soluble and are used in topical ophthalmic medications.

Suspensions of glucocorticoids must be stored within a certain temperature range. Extremely hot or cold temperatures cause development of larger crystals, delaying release of drug from the injection site because there is less surface area for dissolving and increasing irritation at the injection site. (Larger crystals cause an inflammatory response.)

Effects of Glucocorticoids

Because glucocorticoids affect many different types of cells in the body, they produce a wide variety of effects and side effects. Glucocorticoids decrease inflammation by blocking formation of prostaglandins and other autocoids. Glucocorticoids prevent release of lytic enzymes that would destroy cells and attract other inflammatory cells to the site of tissue damage. Glucocorticoids reduce capillary permeability (leaking), which decreases swelling in an injured area and loss of fluid from the systemic circulation. In addition to decreasing inflammation, glucocorticoids also inhibit fibroblasts that normally produce scar tissue. Although this can prevent damage caused by contraction of scar tissue, it also delays healing of wounds.

Although glucocorticoids can combat allergic reactions or inflammatory processes, they can also have detrimental effects. Glucocorticoids suppress T-lymphocytes and decrease the effectiveness of cell-mediated immune responses. Because glucocorticoids also decrease release of substances that attract macrophages, neutrophils, and monocytes, there is greater opportunity for infection or cellular damage. Generally, antibody formation is not adversely affected by glucocorticoids.

Glucocorticoids should not be used in animals with systemic fungal infections because of the potential for further spread of the mycotic agent. Vaccines containing modified-live (attenuated) viruses should be avoided in animals receiving glucocorticoids because glucocorticoids may allow replication of the virus in the animal.

Use of glucocorticoids dramatically alters the hemogram (blood count), and recent use of glucocorticoids should be considered when hematologic results are interpreted. Glucocorticoids cause lymphocytes, eosinophils, and monocytes to become sequestered (taken up, or stored) within the lungs, spleen, and other organs, thereby decreasing the number observed in systemic circulation. In contrast, glucocorticoids increase the number of platelets and neutrophils in circulation, giving rise to neutrophilia. The combination of neutrophilia, lymphopenia, and monocytopenia is characteristic of glucocorticoid administration or stress, which causes release of endogenous cortisol from the adrenal glands.

In the gastrointestinal (GI) tract, glucocorticoids increase gastric acid secretion and decrease mucus production, predisposing the patient to ulceration. Glucocorticoids should not be used with other drugs, such as NSAIDs, that also increase the risk of GI ulceration.

Corticosteroids are said to be catabolic because they enhance catabolism (breakdown) of protein. **Catabolic effects** are manifested as muscle wasting (atrophy), thinning of the skin, loss of hair (alopecia), and decreased bone density. The pot-bellied appearance of dogs that have been treated with glucocorticoids for a long period is primarily associated with weakening of abdominal muscles.

Many ophthalmic drops and ointments contain glucocorticoids for relieving inflammation. These preparations must not be used if corneal ulceration is present. The catabolic effect of corticosteroids can further damage the cornea, resulting in a deepening ulcer and possible corneal perforation. Many manufacturers of ophthalmic preparations market products that may

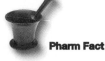

Pharm Fact

The antiinflammatory effects of glucocorticoids can delay healing and predispose the patient to infection.

or may not contain glucocorticoids. When dispensing ophthalmic drops or ointments, the veterinary technician should be certain that the packaged preparation is exactly what has been prescribed.

As discussed in Chapter 7, exogenous glucocorticoids can induce premature parturition or abortion in cattle and mares. After 20 days of gestation, bitches abort 2 to 5 days after receiving large doses of glucocorticoids.

Glucocorticoids increase blood glucose levels by stimulating gluconeogenesis (conversion of protein amino acids to glucose) and glycogenolysis (breakdown of glycogen stores to glucose). Elevated blood glucose levels can cause problems in animals with diabetes mellitus or require a change in the dose of insulin. Generally, if a glucocorticoid is to be used for only a short period, little change is made in the insulin dose; however, blood glucose levels should be monitored in animals receiving large glucocorticoid doses or long-term treatment with glucocorticoids.

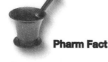

Pharm Fact

Overuse of a glucocorticoid drug may produce iatrogenic hyperadrenocorticism.

DISEASE CAUSED BY GLUCOCORTICOID EXCESS

Overproduction of glucocorticoids by the adrenal cortex, because of tumors or other pathologic conditions, results in a condition called **hyperadrenocorticism,** or **Cushing's syndrome.** Underproduction of glucocorticoids by the adrenal cortex, because of immune-mediated disease or other pathologic states, results in a condition called **hypoadrenocorticism,** or **Addison's disease.**

A state of hyperadrenocorticism can be produced by overuse of exogenous glucocorticoids, such as with long-term administration of large doses to control a pruritic skin problem. This type of treatment-induced disease is termed **iatrogenic.**

The signs of Cushing's syndrome are related to the effects of glucocorticoids and include alopecia, atrophy, pot-bellied appearance, slow healing of wounds, polyuria, polydipsia, and polyphagia. Alopecia and atrophy do not become apparent until the animal has been treated for weeks. However, increased water consumption, urination, and appetite become apparent soon after the animal begins receiving glucocorticoids.

If an animal begins to show signs of iatrogenic hyperadrenocorticism after being treated with glucocorticoids for several weeks, the veterinary professional should not immediately stop use of the drug. This would be inappropriate because the animal could suddenly go from a state of hyperadrenocorticism to a state of hypoadrenocorticism. This is related to the feedback mechanism that regulates cortisol production. Normally when the level of endogenous cortisol becomes elevated, release of CRF from the hypothalamus and ACTH from the pituitary is inhibited, which in turn removes the stimulus for cortisol production and prevents excessively high levels of cortisol. When exogenous glucocorticoids are administered for inflammation, pruritus, or other conditions, they exert the same type of negative feedback on the hypothalamus and pituitary. Stimulation of the adrenal cortex is shut down as long as the exogenous glucocorticoids are administered.

If the animal is receiving glucocorticoids daily, lack of stimulation of the adrenal cortex can cause the adrenal gland to shrink or atrophy. If glucocorticoid administration is suddenly stopped after weeks of daily use, the atrophied adrenal cortex may be unable to resume production of endogenous cortisol immediately. The resultant low blood cortisol levels may cause weakness, lethargy, vomiting, and/or diarrhea.

Safe Use of Glucocorticoids

Glucocorticoids can produce a wide variety of undesirable side effects. Following are guidelines for safe use of these potent drugs:

- If another drug such as an NSAID can accomplish the same result, use it rather than a glucocorticoid.
- Use the smallest dose that provides a clinical response, and reduce the dose as the clinical condition improves.
- Avoid continuous use of glucocorticoids because this suppresses the adrenal cortex and promotes atrophy. Consider alternate day use of an intermediate-acting glucocorticoid such as prednisolone.
- Do not use glucocorticoids with long biologic activity (for example, dexamethasone) or repository forms of glucocorticoids on a frequent basis because they may cause iatrogenic Cushing's syndrome.

If an animal has been receiving glucocorticoids for an extended period, the dose should be gradually reduced to allow the adrenal cortex to regain its ability to function normally.

Most of these precautions pertain to dogs. Cats seem to be more resistant to development of Cushing's syndrome and are relatively tolerant of long-term use of glucocorticoids.

NONSTEROIDAL ANTIINFLAMMATORY DRUGS

The advantage of NSAIDs versus corticosteroids centers around the many side effects of glucocorticoids as compared with the few adverse effects of NSAIDs. This is an especially important area of drug development in human medicine because of the frequency of glucocorticoid side effects in people.

Most NSAIDs work by blocking the activity of cyclooxygenase and subsequent production of prostaglandins. Although most NSAIDs do not block formation of leukotrienes, some (such as ketoprofen and ibuprofen) inhibit lipoxygenase and prevent production of leukotrienes. NSAIDs reduce discomfort and pain associated with inflammation, but they are not very effective analgesics and do not relieve severe visceral pain (for example, organ pain as experienced with colic) or severe somatic pain (such as with broken bones and trauma).

NSAIDs are tightly bound to plasma proteins, and hypoalbuminemia (low blood albumin level) may allow higher levels of NSAIDs to reach tissues, thereby enhancing their beneficial effects but also increasing the possibility of detrimental side effects. The major side effects of NSAIDs occur in the GI

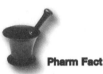

Pharm Fact

Because of the adrenal atrophy in animals treated for long periods with glucocorticoids, the dose should be gradually reduced before administration is halted.

tract. PgE and PgI_2 normally decrease the volume, acidity, and pepsin content of gastric secretions released during normal digestion. These "good" prostaglandins also stimulate secretion of sodium bicarbonate to neutralize the acidic stomach contents entering the intestine. They also increase perfusion of the gastric mucosa, stimulate gastric and enteric mucus production, and stimulate turnover and repair of the GI epithelial cells. Most NSAIDs block production of all prostaglandins, including good prostaglandins. The net effect is similar to that caused by glucocorticoids.

Animals experiencing adverse reactions to NSAIDs often have diarrhea, anorexia manifested as digested blood in the stool, and ulceration of the GI tract. Sucralfate and H2 blockers (for example, cimetidine or ranitidine) are often used to treat NSAID-induced GI ulcerations (see Chapter 4). Another fairly new drug, misoprostol, is similar in composition and effect to PgE. It is sometimes used to counteract the antiprostaglandin effect of NSAIDs on the GI tract, but like the other drugs, will not prevent ulcer formation in animals receiving high doses of NSAIDs.

Most NSAIDs also block beneficial prostaglandins in the renal blood supply. PgE_2 is released during conditions such as shock, dehydration, and blood loss, which decrease blood flow to the kidney. This prostaglandin normally causes dilation of the renal vasculature, allowing continued perfusion of kidney cells despite the decreased blood pressure and reduced overall renal perfusion. If these hypotensive conditions occur while an animal is being treated with NSAIDs, the kidney is unable to compensate for the overall decrease in renal perfusion and parts of the kidney may die from ischemia (low oxygen availability). This condition, called **renal papillary necrosis,** can result in significant kidney damage.

As a general rule, horses are very tolerant of NSAIDs. Dogs are generally less tolerant than horses, but there is some variability from drug to drug. Cats generally tolerate most NSAIDs poorly, except for a few of the "safer" ones such as aspirin, but even these relatively safe drugs must be used cautiously, at significantly reduced dosages, in cats.

Recently, research has shown that cyclooxygenase, the enzyme blocked by NSAIDs, exists in two forms. Cyclooxygenase-1 (COX-1) is thought to be the form that is involved in normal regulatory functions in the body. Thus COX-1 would be the enzyme that produces prostaglandins that normally increase protective mucus in the stomach and maintain renal perfusion. Cyclooxygenase-2 (COX-2) is thought to be an enzyme that is associated with the prostaglandin production during inflammation. Because two forms of cyclooxygenase have been identified, an NSAID that inhibits primarily COX-2 without significantly inhibiting COX-1 would theoretically be able to decrease inflammation without decreasing production of the normal "helpful" prostaglandins in the kidneys and stomach.

Phenylbutazone

Phenylbutazone is one of the most commonly used NSAIDs in equine medicine. It has been used for years in horses for relief of musculoskeletal inflammation. It is used to a lesser degree in dogs and cattle. Phenylbutazone decreases inflammation primarily by inhibiting cyclooxygenase and subsequent prostaglandin formation. NSAIDs do not break down existing prostaglandins, but simply prevent further production of new prostaglandins. Therefore inflammatory processes that have already been initiated by existing prostaglandins are less affected by the NSAIDs.

As with most other NSAIDs, phenylbutazone is metabolized by the liver. The primary metabolite of phenylbutazone is oxyphenbutazone, which is also an active antiinflammatory agent. Phenylbutazone is highly protein bound (greater than 99% in horses), and the relative amount of free drug available for distribution to tissues varies considerably if the animal has low blood albumin levels (hypoalbuminemia) or the NSAID is displaced from the protein by other protein-bound drugs (that is, other NSAIDs, sulfonamides, or phenytoin).

Before using phenylbutazone or any other NSAID in an animal already receiving other medications, check the package insert for information on drug interactions. For example, phenylbutazone induces increased hepatic metabolism of itself and other drugs metabolized with the same enzyme system (for example, phenytoin, digitoxin). Similarly, other drugs such as barbiturates and corticosteroids that use the same hepatic microsomal enzymes for metabolism increase phenylbutazone metabolism, resulting in a shorter half-life and overall decreased concentrations attained in the body. Thus the effectiveness of phenylbutazone or other drugs may be altered by concurrent administration of several medications.

The adverse effects of phenylbutazone are similar to those of other NSAIDs: risk of GI ulceration; renal papillary necrosis if renal perfusion is decreased; and retention of water and sodium from decreased renal function, which is more common in dogs than horses. Retention of water and sodium is particularly dangerous in animals with congestive heart failure because it increases the workload on the heart.

Two other adverse effects of phenylbutazone are bone marrow suppression resulting in neutropenia, thrombocytopenia, and anemia and tissue necrosis if the drug is injected intramuscularly or subcutaneously. Bone marrow suppression is more common in people and dogs than horses. Blood dyscrasias (abnormal blood cells) have been reported in dogs.

In horses, phenylbutazone should be given intravenously or by mouth. Accidental perivascular injection (outside the vein) can cause severe inflammation and tissue necrosis. Accidental injection of phenylbutazone into the carotid artery can cause marked central nervous system (CNS) stimulation (that is, seizures and collapse). For these reasons, the veterinary professional must be careful to ensure that this drug is administered properly.

Phenylbutazone should not be used in cats because of their low tolerance of the drug and the availability of safer NSAIDs such as aspirin.

Aspirin

Aspirin (acetylsalicylic acid) is a fairly safe NSAID to use in most animal species. Owners commonly give aspirin to their pets without advice from the veterinarian. Aspirin belongs to a larger group of compounds known as the *salicylates,* which include bismuth subsalicylate, found in antidiarrheal preparations such as Pepto-Bismol.

Aspirin fights inflammation by blocking the cyclooxygenase pathway. By blocking production of prostaglandins and thromboxanes, inflammation is reduced. Because thromboxane normally promotes platelet aggregation, thromboxane inhibition by aspirin is used to decrease platelet clumping. Because only the megakaryocyte precursors of platelets (but not the platelets themselves) are capable of regenerating thromboxane, the aggregating activity of platelets is significantly diminished with aspirin use. Daily aspirin doses are often given to reduce the likelihood of clot formation and subsequent blockage of coronary blood vessels in people at risk for heart attack.

Dogs with heartworm infection often have narrowed pulmonary vessels caused by proliferation of the endothelial lining of the vessel, an effect stimulated by thromboxanes. By using aspirin to inhibit thromboxanes and reduce platelet clumping, the degree of proliferation can be stopped and even reversed to some extent, thereby enhancing blood flow through the pulmonary arteries.

Cats with hypertrophic cardiomyopathy, a condition in which the heart muscle thickens, resulting in stiff ventricular walls and reduced cardiac output, often have "turbulent" blood flow through the diseased heart. This turbulent flow causes platelets to clump and form clots. Because these clots usually form on the left side of the heart, they flow with the blood into the aorta and commonly lodge at the caudal bifurcation (forking) of the dorsal aorta, where it divides to pass into the hind legs. The resulting clot, often called a saddle thrombus, can markedly reduce blood flow to the hind legs, resulting in eventual loss of the use of the limbs. Aspirin is used in these cats to reduce clot formation associated with hypertrophic cardiomyopathy.

Because of its short half-life and GI side effects in horses, aspirin is not used very often for analgesia in horses. However, it has been part of the treatment protocol for uveitis (inflammation of the iris and ciliary body of the eye).

Like other NSAIDs, aspirin is metabolized by the liver. Aspirin is conjugated with (joined to) glycine and glucuronic acid by the liver enzyme glucuronyl transferase. Because cats have little of this enzyme, aspirin is metabolized much more slowly in cats than in other species. Aspirin has a half-life of 1.5 hours in people, approximately 8 hours in dogs, and 30 hours in cats. Thus as with many other drugs, the aspirin dosage for cats is lower than dosages in other species and usually consists of one "baby aspirin" tablet (81 mg) every 2 or 3 days. If used prudently, aspirin is one of the safest and most effective NSAIDs for cats.

Pharm Fact

Aspirin should be used cautiously in cats because of their limited ability to metabolize salicylates.

Ibuprofen, Ketoprofen, and Naproxen

Ibuprofen, ketoprofen, and naproxen are derivatives of propionic acid and share common modes of action and side effects. Like other NSAIDs, these drugs work by blocking cyclooxygenase and subsequent prostaglandin formation. These NSAIDs also block leukotriene formation and thus reduce inflammation associated with this other branch of the arachidonic cascade. Naproxen is marketed as the veterinary product Naprosyn. A ketoprofen product, Ketofen, is approved for use in horses. All three drugs are available as over-the-counter (OTC) human medications. (Ibuprofen is marketed as Advil, naproxen is marketed as Aleve, and ketoprofen is marketed as Orudis.) Practicing veterinary technicians should recognize the brand names and understand the potential dangers when well-meaning owners indiscriminately give these drugs to their animals.

Few adverse reactions with these drugs have been reported in horses, although gastric mucosal damage and renal papillary necrosis are possible. In contrast, after 2 to 6 days of treatment, dogs consistently experience vomiting. GI toxicity is more frequent in dogs than other species and reflects their sensitivity to the GI effects. Because of the fairly high incidence of side effects and the availability of safer NSAIDs, these propionate derivatives are not usually recommended for use in dogs.

Flunixin Meglumine

Flunixin meglumine (Banamine, Meflosyl, generic versions) is used primarily in equine medicine for treatment of colic. Flunixin is a cyclooxygenase inhibitor, so it has an antiinflammatory effect, and also has an analgesic component that is more potent than that of other NSAIDs such as phenylbutazone and of some narcotic agents such as pentazocine (Talwin), meperidine (Demerol), and codeine. In addition to analgesic and antiinflammatory effects, flunixin also blocks the effects of endotoxins (poisons produced within the body) associated with colic in horses.

In dogs, flunixin meglumine provides analgesia superior to that of aspirin or phenylbutazone. It has been used as an analgesic in dogs with hip dysplasia, arthritis, intervertebral disk disease, and anterior uveitis. However, dogs are very sensitive to the GI side effects of flunixin. Some clinicians recommend using flunixin for no longer than 3 days because of the risk of vomiting, hemorrhagic gastroenteritis, and pyloric ulceration. In contrast, horses are relatively resistant to side effects and can receive up to 5 times the recommended dose without major side effects.

Although flunixin has also been used in an extra-label manner in cattle, swine, and other species, the doses are based on anecdotal evidence rather than controlled clinical trials.

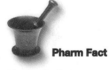

Pharm Fact

Horses tolerate treatment with flunixin and meclofenamic acid quite well, but dogs usually experience GI side effects.

Meclofenamic Acid

Meclofenamic acid (Arquel) has been available for use in equine medicine for over 20 years. It is most commonly administered as granules that are mixed in the feed, and accumulates in appreciable quantities in the joint fluid after oral administration. This drug has antiinflammatory and analgesic actions and is used in horses to treat lameness associated with joint inflammation. It has also been used to treat chronic joint degenerative diseases in dogs, such as hip dysplasia or chronic arthritis.

Like flunixin, meclofenamic acid is well tolerated in horses (up to 4 times the recommended dose) but can produce GI signs in dogs with long-term use. When dogs are being treated with meclofenamic acid, the owner should be advised to watch for anorexia, diarrhea, or changes in stool color (melena) that might indicate GI side effects. In pregnant rats, meclofenamic acid has produced minor skeletal abnormalities in the fetus. Although this effect has not been documented in pregnant mares, use of meclofenamic acid in pregnant mares should be avoided.

Dimethyl Sulfoxide

Dimethyl sulfoxide (DMSO) is an NSAID that works by a different mechanism than the drugs discussed previously. The primary antiinflammatory mechanism of DMSO involves inactivation of the destructive process caused by superoxide radicals produced by inflammation. These superoxide radicals produce hydroxyl radicals and hydrogen peroxide, which damage cells. DMSO traps the hydroxyl radicals while the metabolite of DMSO traps oxygen radicals. The combined activity reduces the cellular damage produced by the inflammatory process.

DMSO is used topically and parenterally, primarily in horses. DMSO is also a component of some otic (ear) preparations used in dogs and cats. DMSO is widely used in extra-label ways to treat a variety of conditions, including CNS trauma, mastitis, mammary swelling associated with nursing, postoperative pain, burns, and other superficial trauma. However, the only approved uses are for acute injury associated with trauma or as an antiinflammatory in otic preparations.

DMSO is known for its ability to penetrate intact skin and has been used as a vehicle to carry dissolved drug into the body when applied topically. DMSO can also carry toxins or harmful substances when it enters an animal or penetrates the skin of the person applying it. The skin in the area of application should be thoroughly cleansed to avoid absorption of bacterial toxins or other chemicals such as oil, grease, and insecticides. DMSO is also available as an industrial-grade solvent. Although considerably less expensive than the medical-grade form, the industrial-grade should never be used on veterinary patients because of toxic impurities such as benzene that are found in many of these products. People applying DMSO should protect themselves by wearing high-quality rubber gloves during topical application.

The smell of DMSO resembles garlic or raw oysters. This odor is evident during topical application, and the drug can sometimes be tasted after it is absorbed by the body.

After DMSO is applied topically, erythema (redness), edema, and pruritus may develop at the application site. These reactions reflect release of histamine and other vasoactive amines from mast cells in the skin. Although the cutaneous reaction is usually mild, a more severe reaction may occur if the animal has **mast-cell tumors.** DMSO causes these large aggregates of mast cells to release large amounts of histamine.

If given intravenously to horses, DMSO can cause hemolysis and passage of hemoglobin in the urine (hemoglobinuria). Severe hemolysis and release of hemoglobin can adversely affect the kidneys; therefore hemolysis should be minimized by using DMSO solutions with a concentration below 20% for IV administration.

In large doses, DMSO has produced defects in the offspring of hamsters and avian species. Although these effects have not been demonstrated in other

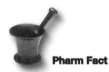

Pharm Fact

The person applying DMSO should wear high-quality rubber gloves for protection against inadvertent absorption of toxins.

species, the use of DMSO in pregnant animals should be weighed against any benefits the drug may provide. A conservative approach would include use of another NSAID that has been documented as safe for use in pregnant animals.

Orgotein

Like DMSO, orgotein (superoxide dismutase) exerts its antiinflammatory effect by inactivating superoxide radicals. This drug is marketed only as a veterinary product and is used to prevent or reduce joint damage. Superoxide radicals associated with inflammation degrade hyaluronic acid, the main component in joint fluid that is responsible for joint fluid viscosity and lubrication of the joint. Orgotein works as an enzyme, superoxide dismutase, to convert superoxide radicals into oxygen and hydrogen peroxide, which is then converted to water and oxygen, thus preserving the integrity of hyaluronic acid. Orgotein is most commonly used to treat horses with joint and vertebral disease.

Carprofen

Carprofen (Rimadyl) is a new NSAID labeled for relief of pain and inflammation in dogs. Unlike other NSAIDs commonly used in veterinary medicine, carprofen more selectively targets inhibition of COX-2, the enzyme thought to primarily produce prostaglandins associated with inflammation. By having less inhibition of COX-1, the prostaglandins associated with the protection of the GI tract and renal blood flow, carprofen should have less side effects than other NSAIDs. Clinical trials in dogs have shown that some degree of intestinal irritation still occurs, but the incidence is very low and overall side effects occur significantly less when compared with other NSAIDs such as aspirin. Even exaggerated doses produced minimal changes in the histologic appearance of the GI tract. Renal blood flow studies in rats indicated carprofen did not have any deleterious effects on urinary volume production or electrolyte excretion.

OTHER DRUGS USED TO FIGHT INFLAMMATION

Acetaminophen

Acetaminophen is not an antiinflammatory drug. However, because of its analgesic and antipyretic (fever reducing) properties, it is often grouped with NSAIDs. Unlike NSAIDs, acetaminophen (Tylenol) does not block prostaglandin formation associated with inflammation, but reduces the perception of pain by a mechanism not clearly defined and decreases the effect of endogenous pyrogens (substances that increase fever).

Acetaminophen does not cause the GI upset, ulcers, or interference with platelet clumping associated with NSAIDs. However, the metabolites of acetaminophen can have other severe side effects, especially in cats. Acetaminophen is normally conjugated with glucuronic acid and sulfate for metabolism and elimination. A small portion of acetaminophen

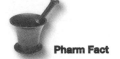

is also metabolized to a toxic metabolite. In most species this toxic metabolite is quickly conjugated with glutathione to form a nontoxic metabolite. Because of the relatively less effective glucuronide and sulfate conjugation in cats, more of the toxic metabolite tends to be produced. Unfortunately, the supply of glutathione needed by the liver to biotransform this toxic metabolite to a nontoxic metabolite is limited in the cat. Therefore the toxic metabolite accumulates in the liver and other tissues, producing cellular destruction. In addition to liver damage, the red blood cells are also severely affected. The hemoglobin in red blood cells (RBCs) is converted to methemoglobin, which is much less capable of efficient oxygen transport. Increased RBC hemolysis and Heinz bodies are evident on blood smears. Cats with methemoglobinemia have chocolate-colored mucous membranes and dark urine caused by methemoglobin in the blood and urine.

An acetaminophen dose of 50 mg/kg to 60 mg/kg can poison a cat. A single "extra-strength" acetaminophen tablet (500 mg) can kill an average-size cat. In dogs, a higher dose (above 150 mg/kg) is required before signs of hepatic necrosis, weight loss, and icterus (jaundice) become evident.

Phenacetin is a compound found in many "cold" preparations. This drug is metabolized to acetaminophen and thus can produce acetaminophen toxicity in susceptible species and individual animals.

Treatment of acetaminophen toxicity focuses on providing the sulfhydryl groups of glutathione to convert the toxic metabolite to its nontoxic form. The drug most commonly used to treat acet-aminophen toxicity is acetylcysteine (Mucomyst), a mucolytic agent used in treatment of respiratory infections.

Gold Salts

Gold salts, such as aurothioglucose, are used in human medicine for treatment of rheumatoid arthritis. These compounds are apparently taken up by macrophages and possibly prevent release of lysosomal enzymes. Gold salts also decrease histamine release from mast cells and inhibit prostaglandin formation. In veterinary medicine, gold salts have been used to treat severe immune-mediated skin problems such as the various forms of pemphigus.

Dipyrone

Dipyrone inhibits prostaglandin formation by blocking cyclooxygenase. Its antiinflammatory capacity is weak compared with its analgesic properties and its ability to decrease fever. Dipyrone has been used to relieve smooth muscle spasm and pain in horses, dogs, and cats, but other, more potent analgesics are more commonly used.

Piroxicam

Piroxicam (Feldene), an NSAID formulated for use in people, is sometimes used in small animal medicine. It is also being used as an antineoplastic agent for certain types of tumors.

Antiinflammatory Drug Categories and Names

Corticosteroids

Mineralocorticoids
Glucocorticoids
  Hydrocortisone
  Cortisone
  Prednisone
  Prednisolone
  Triamcinolone (Vetalog)
  Methylprednisolone
  Isoflupredone
  Dexamethasone
  Betamethasone
  Flumethasone

Nonsteroidal Antiinflammatory Drugs

Phenylbutazone
Aspirin

Ibuprofen, ketoprofen (Ketofen), naproxen
  (Naprosyn)
Flunixin meglumine (Banamine)
Meclofenamic acid (Arquel)
Dimethyl sulfoxide
Orgotein
Carprofen (Rimadyl)

Other Drugs Used to Combat Inflammation

Acetaminophen
Gold salts
  Aurothioglucose
Dipyrone
Piroxicam (Feldene)

Recommended Reading

Booth DM: Drug therapy in cats: a review article, *JAVMA* 196(10):1660, 1990.

Brayton CF, Schwark W: Use and misuse of DMSO. In Bonagura JD, editor: *Kirk's current veterinary therapy XII,* Philadelphia, 1996, WB Saunders.

Breider MA: Endothelium and inflammation, *JAVMA* 203(2).300, 1993.

DeGraves FJ, Anderson KL: Ibuprofen treatment of endotoxin-induced mastitis in cows, *Am J Vet Res* 54(7):1128, July 1993.

Godshalk CP et al: Gastric perforation associated with administration of ibuprofen in a dog, *JAVMA* 201(11):1734, 1992.

Hansen BD: Analgesics in severely ill dogs and cats. Proceedings of the North American Veterinary Conference, Orlando, Fla, Jan 1996.

Hansen BD: Prescription and use of analgesics in dogs and cats in a veterinary teaching hospital—258 cases, *JAVMA* 202(9):1485, 1993.

Holland M, Chastain CB: Use and misuses of aspirin. In Bonagura JD, editor: *Kirk's current veterinary therapy XII,* Philadelphia, 1996, WB Saunders.

MacAllister CG: Nonsteroidal anti-inflammatory drugs: their mechanism of action and clinical uses in horses, *Vet Med* 237, March 1994.MacAllister CG, Taylor-MacAllister C: Treating and preventing the adverse effects of nonsteroidal anti-inflammatory drugs in horses, *Vet Med* 241, March 1994.

MacAllister CG et al: Comparison of adverse effects of phenylbutazone, flunixin meglumine, and ketoprofen in horses, *JAVMA* 202(1):71, 1993.

May SA: Anti-inflammatory agents. In Robinson NE, editor: *Current veterinary therapy in equine medicine 3,* Philadelphia, 1992, WB Saunders.

Vonderhaar MA, Salisbury SK: Gastroduodenal ulceration associated with flunixin meglumine administration in three dogs, *JAVMA* 23(1):92, 1993.

Review Questions

1. What types of disease would an eicosanoid antagonist drug treat?
2. A pharmaceutical catalog advertises a reduced price for a corticosteroid drug listed as a mineralocorticoid. As your clinic's veterinary technician, should you consider purchasing the mineralocorticoid rather than the prednisone you usually order?
3. What effect does long-term administration of glucocorticoids have on the adrenal glands?
4. One topical cream contains cortisone and another contains betamethasone. Both are well-absorbed and well-applied to the skin. With long-term use, which is more likely to produce adrenal gland suppression?
5. Which glucocorticoid is more appropriate for IV use in emergency treatment of shock: dexamethasone or dexamethasone sodium phosphate?
6. Can prednisolone diacetate be safely given intravenously for treatment of shock?
7. What effect would overnight storage in subfreezing temperatures likely have on a vial of dexamethasone valerate?
8. Why are large doses of glucocorticoids generally not used in animals recovering from surgery?
9. Considering that glucocorticoids suppress the immune system, should vaccination of animals receiving prednisone for seasonal allergies be postponed until the animal is no longer receiving the medication?
10. Why are glucocorticoids and nonsteroidal antiinflammatory drugs said to be "ulcerogenic"?
11. On a complete blood count, how would numbers of neutrophils, lymphocytes, and monocytes be altered in an animal receiving glucocorticoids?
12. How do glucocorticoids differ from anabolic steroids in their effect on muscles?
13. By what mechanism does long-term glucocorticoid use cause a sagging, pendulous abdomen?
14. Why is it important to clearly label, and perhaps separately store, ophthalmic products containing glucocorticoids and those not containing glucocorticoids?
15. A client telephones and says that her mare has just aborted a near-term fetus. The doctor asks the client if she has recently given the mare any glucocorticoids, such as for relief of lameness. What is the reason for this question?
16. What is the difference between Addison's disease and Cushing's syndrome?
17. In animals with iatrogenic Cushing's syndrome caused by overzealous administration of glucocorticoids, why is glucocorticoid administration tapered off gradually rather than immediately stopped?
18. In an animal with low plasma albumin levels (hypoalbuminemia), should the normal dose of NSAIDs be increased or decreased? Why?

19. What two organ systems are most likely to be adversely affected by nonsteroidal antiinflammatory drugs?
20. Are NSAIDs nephrotoxic, like gentamicin or methoxyflurane?
21. Phenylbutazone is commonly used for pain relief in horses. Why is this drug not commonly used in dogs?
22. Why is the doctor particularly careful when injecting phenylbutazone into the jugular vein of horses?
23. Which NSAID can be used with relative safety in cats? Why are cats so intolerant of NSAIDs in general?
24. What is the logic in using aspirin in cats with dilative cardiomyopathy?
25. A client telephones and asks if it is safe to give Advil (ibuprofen), Orudis-KT (ketoprofen), or Aleve (naproxen) to his dog to relieve pain from chronic arthritis. What is an appropriate response?
26. Flunixin meglumine was used as a pain reliever in dogs for a while but seems to be used less now. It provides good analgesia in dogs, so why is it not used more often?
27. What precautions should you take when applying dimethyl sulfoxide to an animal's skin?
28. Why is dimethyl sulfoxide contraindicated for use in animals with mast-cell tumors?
29. You see an advertisement featuring industrial-grade dimethyl sulfoxide at a much lower price than you have paid for veterinary dimethyl sulfoxide. Is it advisable to purchase industrial-grade dimethyl sulfoxide for topical use on veterinary patients?
30. Considering that acetaminophen is less likely to produce GI upset than aspirin, why is acetaminophen not used to reduce inflammation?
31. What is the mechanism of acetaminophen intolerance in cats? What are signs of acetaminophen toxicosis in cats?
32. A client telephones and asks if it is safe to give an OTC human cold preparation containing phenacetin to his cat to relieve respiratory signs. What is an appropriate response?
33. How is carprofen different from other NSAIDs such as aspirin or phenylbutazone?

Chapter 1 Answers

1. *Proprietary* means "property" of a particular company. Therefore the proprietary, or trade, name has TM or ® appended to it. The proprietary name is also capitalized because it is a proper noun, like a person's name.
2. To find a generic equivalent for a given proprietary drug (for example, Lasix), consult a drug information reference to determine the nonproprietary name (that is, furosemide), then look in the index under that nonproprietary name. You should find several other trade names listed, as well as generic furosemide.
3. Generic drug manufacturers do not have to recoup the costs of research and development entailed in licensing of the original drug and therefore can sell the drug for less. Although most generic drugs perform adequately in veterinary patients, subtle differences in manufacturing occasionally cause alterations in drug absorption and bioavailability.
4. Tablets and caplets are both compressed powdered drug. A tablet is circular and a caplet is oblong (caplet shaped).
5. Enteric coating on a tablet prevents it from being exposed to the acidic environment of the stomach.
6. Per rectum. The drug is inserted through the anus and placed within the terminal end of the colon, where it dissolves and is absorbed across the colonic mucosa.
7. Sustained-release tablets dissolve slowly, releasing the drug over an extended period.
8. Drugs given intravenously *must* be solutions; drug particles in suspensions can obstruct narrow capillaries.
9. Syrups contain no alcohol, whereas elixirs have a relatively high alcohol content. Syrups are solutions of sugar (usually 85% sucrose) and water, along with a medication; elixirs are solutions of alcohol, water, a sweetener, and the medication.
10. Topical administration means applied to the surface of the body.
11. Lotions are applied without rubbing to the surface of the skin; liniments contain oils and are rubbed into the skin.
12. Medication applied into the ear canal should dissolve at body temperature; therefore an ointment is more appropriate.
13. A repository drug is designed to deliver an injectable drug over an extended period, much like the sustained-release oral formulations. If the standard formulation is given every 12 hours, the repository form is more likely to be given every 96 hours.
14. Extracts can be manufactured fairly inexpensively because they are made from ground-up animal or plant parts and are not chemically synthesized. A potential problem with extracts is the variability of drug concentration found in the animal or plant part used to make the extract.

15. "C" drugs are controlled substances. Of drugs that can be legally prescribed, C-II drugs have the most potential to be abused. (C-I drugs have "no medicinal value" and thus cannot be legally prescribed.) C-V drugs have the lowest potential for physical or psychologic addiction.

16. An indication is a condition for which a drug can be used; a contraindication is a condition for which the drug should *not* be used.

17. Not necessarily. Usually the veterinarian is left to use clinical judgement whether to use a drug under the conditions listed as *Precautions*. If pregnancy is mentioned as a precautionary condition, it usually means that data are lacking on safety of the drug for use in pregnant animals, but no serious complications have been reported. (Serious complications would be listed under *Warnings* or *Contraindications*.)

18. Any condition that would lead to death upon use of that drug is an absolute contraindication.

1. No. A valid relationship between the client, patient, and veterinarian does not exist in this case. The doctor has never examined the animal, does not know what type of medication was previously given for motion sickness, and does not know if there is any contraindication to dispensing the drug the owner wants.

2. This prescription does not list the veterinarian's telephone number, the date of the prescription, the client's complete address, the species of the animal, the Rx symbol, the strength of amoxicillin tablets to be given, which is very important, and how often the medication is to be given.

3.

2 g	= 2,000 mg
5 mg	= 0.005 g
14 lb	= 6.36 kg
23 kg	= 50.6 lb
83 kg	= 83,000,000 mg
65 kg	= 143 lb
0.4 kg	= 400 g
0.003 lb	= 1,363.6 mg
15 lb	= 6818.2 g
0.00043 kg	= 430 mg
25,488 mg	= 0.056 lb
0.0092 lb	= 4181.8 mg
25 ml	= 0.025 L
43 cc	= 43 ml
1.5 L	= 1500 ml
800 cc	= 0.8 L
0.055 L	= 55 ml
0.25 ml	= 0.00025 L

4. 15 lb = 6.82 kg = 102 mg of drug = 1 ml of drug solution.

5. 55 lb = 25 kg = 2 mg of drug = 2 of the 1-mg tablets. If this dose (2 mg) is given 4 times a day (q6h = every 6 hours), then 8 of the 1-mg tablets are given daily for 5 days, for a total of 40 tablets, at a cost of $14.

6. 16 lb = 7.27 kg. The dosage is 3 to 5 mg/kg, or a dose of 21.8 to 36.4 mg for this dog; this is approximately half of a 50-mg tablet given once daily. Half a tablet daily is 90 tablets for 180 days, at $2.70. 27 lb = 12.3 kg = dose of 36.8 to 61.4 mg; use 1 whole 50-mg tablet daily. One tablet daily for 180 days is 180

tablets, at $5.40. 66 lb = 30 kg = dose of 90 to 150 mg; use one 100-mg tablet, 1½ of the 100-mg tablets, or half of a 200-mg tablet; their respective costs would be $9.00, $13.50, and $6.30.

7. The dog is given 3.2 units per dose. The vial contains 100 units/ml × 10 ml = 1000 units. For this dog, the vial contains 312 doses. (Actually, it is 312.5 doses, but half of a dose is left unused.)

8. 10% solution = 10 g/100 ml = 0.1 g/ml = 100 mg/ml. 43% = 430 mg/ml.

9. 7.5% = 75 mg/ml = 9,750 mg in 130 ml.

10. The normal dose for this dog would be 0.22 mg/m² × 0.8 m² = 0.176 mg; 60% of that is 0.1056 mg. The elixir contains 0.15 mg/ml, so administer 0.704 or 0.7 ml.

11. 950 lb = 431.8 kg = 10,795 mg needed in 2 hours. 1.5% = 1.5 g/100 ml = 15 mg/ml. The mare requires 719.7 ml dripped in over 2 hours (120 minutes) = 5.99 ml/minute (60 seconds) = 0.1 ml/second = 1 drop/second.

12. 8 lb = 3.636 kg = 29.1 mg. The tablets are 15 mg, so the dog needs 2 tablets per dose. Each tablet costs $0.13 and the dog gets 2 tablets per day, so the daily cost is $0.26. Enough drug for 38 days can be dispensed for $10 (actually, 38.4 days).

13. 45 drops/30 seconds = 1.5 drop/second = 0.15 ml/second. 220-lb foal = 100 kg = 1,800 ml infused at 0.15 ml/second = 12,000 seconds = 200 minutes = 3.333 hours = 3 hours and 20 minutes. (20 minutes is one-third of an hour, not 33 minutes.)

14. Cool means 46° to 59° F. Room temperature is usually warmer than that (at least 68° F).

15. The veterinary technician cannot order such drugs. Only a veterinarian with a DEA certification number can order controlled substances.

16. A C-III drug has more potential for abuse than a C-V drug.

17. "Caution: Federal law prohibits the transfer of this drug to any person other than the (client and) patient for whom it was prescribed."

18. 2 years.

19. Surgical masks are porous enough to allow aerosolized drug to pass through. A single pair of latex surgical gloves does not provide complete protection.

20. If he is selling the drug to other practices, this constitutes illegal manufacture of a "new" drug, according to FDA regulations. His proposed label does not make it legal.

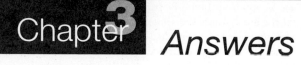
1. PO means per os, or given by mouth. IV means intravenous, or injected into a vein. SC means subcutaneous, or injected just deep to, or beneath, the skin. IM, or intramuscular, injections are administered into a muscle. The drug given intravenously will reach its peak in the plasma (blood) first because all the drug, if given as a bolus, is placed immediately into the blood. (There is no absorption phase.) If an IM injection is made into muscle that is well perfused and usually moving, absorption is also rapid. Drug absorption after SC and PO administration is slower and more variable because of the various factors that influence drug absorption.

2. If the lowest concentration of the therapeutic range is 50 μg/ml, concentrations of this drug will be in the subtherapeutic range after 2 hours. If the toxic range starts at 30 μg/ml, at 2 hours this animal will be very sick. Knowing this single concentration without knowing the therapeutic range is worthless.

3. The loading dose is the larger dose. It is given initially to establish concentrations within the therapeutic range. Once therapeutic drug concentrations in the body are established, smaller maintenance doses keep drug concentrations in the therapeutic range. The advantage of using the loading dose is that therapeutic concentrations are established quickly. If a maintenance dose is used initially, it may take hours or even days for the drug to gradually accumulate to its steady state within the therapeutic range.

4. Changing the dosage interval means adjusting the time between doses (q6h, or every 6 hours). In this case, the doctor is increasing the time between doses.

5. | 240 mg q12h | 160 mg q8h | 80 mg q4h |
    | 160 mg TID | 480 mg q24h | 120 mg QID |

   Divide the total daily dose (480 mg) by the number of times you want to give the drug in the new dosage regimen. For example, for use TID (3 times daily), 480 mg/3 = 160 mg. From a practical standpoint, the less frequently a client has to give medication, the greater the chance for client compliance with the directions. Therefore q24h or q12h use increases the likelihood of client compliance.

6. With an IV bolus the entire dose is injected within a few seconds. With an IV infusion the drug is "dripped" into the animal over minutes to hours. The bolus almost immediately produces very high concentrations in the blood (plasma) until it is distributed throughout the body. During this time, high concentrations can result in toxic signs if they exceed the therapeutic range. The IV infusion produces no prominent peak concentration but gradually increases concentrations in the body over time until steady state is achieved.

7. No. Blood in arteries flows in the opposite direction (away from the heart) of blood in veins (toward the heart). Injection into an artery produces high con-

centrations to a particular area or organ of the body. Injecting the drug into a vein would dilute it considerably before it reaches that area or organ.

8. The statement means that the drug will cause complications if it leaks out or is injected outside of the vessel (vein or artery). Some drugs can be extremely irritating to tissues if deposited outside the vein. In some cases the tissue becomes necrotic and sloughs. If you are attempting to administer a drug intravenously and inject it extravascularly, the area surrounding the injection site distends as it fills with the injected drug. The animal may also show a painful response. Within 8 to 24 hours, the injection site becomes warm, sensitive, and swollen.

9. Drugs administered by aerosolization are given with a nebulizer and inhaled into the respiratory tract. The highest concentrations are within the lumina of the respiratory tract.

10. An intracarotid injection sends the concentrated drug directly to the brain. Several drugs used in horses produce a violent reaction if inadvertently given in the carotid artery instead of in the jugular vein.

11. Intradermal injections (within the skin) are most superficial. SC injections are just deep to, or beneath, the skin. With IM injections the needle must pass through the skin and subcutaneous layers to reach the underlying muscles.

12. IP refers to intraperitoneal injection, within the peritoneal cavity of the abdomen.

13. a. Passive diffusion; b. Pinocytosis or phagocytosis; c. Active transport; d. Facilitated diffusion.

14. Passive diffusion of a drug into a cell is based on the drug's characteristics more than on energy expenditure by the cell. Therefore an antidote drug could passively diffuse into the cell. Active transport and pinocytosis or phagocytosis would not work because they depend on energy expended by the cell.

15. Facilitated diffusion and active transport require special proteins within the cell membrane to move drugs across the membrane. Numbers of these protein molecules are limited. If all the available protein molecules are occupied with transporting drug molecules across the membrane, the transport process is operating at its maximum speed. Because passive diffusion does not require special proteins for drug passage across the membrane, the maximum rate does not depend on a carrier system.

16. Bioavailability is the percentage of the drug administered that reaches the systemic circulation. 100% bioavailability = 1. Therefore only 25% of drug A reaches the systemic circulation, versus 40% of drug B. For drug A, 0.25×100 mg = 25 mg of drug in the body. For drug B, 0.40×100 mg = 40 mg of drug in the body. Therefore a 100-mg dose of drug B will produce higher concentrations after absorption. How much more would the dose of drug A have to be increased to achieve the same concentrations in the body that 100 mg of drug B achieves? Here's a simple way to find out: 100 mg of drug B $\times 0.40$ = X mg of drug A $\times 0.25$. Solving for X, 100 mg $\times (0.40/0.25)$ = 160 mg of drug A. This algebraic calculation is used when converting from tablet to liquid formulations of the same medication because tablets and liquid formulations usually have different bioavailabilities.

17. IV bolus administration produces high concentrations in the plasma shortly after administration. These high concentrations may produce toxic signs until plasma concentrations decrease as a result of distribution of the drug into the tissues and metabolism and excretion of the drug. For a drug with a narrow therapeutic index, there is not much difference between plasma concentrations of drug that provide benefit and plasma concentrations that cause toxicity. Thus it would be safer to use a route of administration that produces small fluc-

tuations in concentrations, such as by mouth or subcutaneously. Digoxin is usually used by mouth in veterinary medicine.

18. Drugs given subcutaneously and intramuscularly are placed into extracellular water (fluid). Being hydrophilic, they readily dissolve and diffuse away from the site of administration and through the fenestrations of capillary walls. Cells lining the intestinal lumen are tightly packed together so that hydrophilic drugs cannot pass between cells and do not readily penetrate cells, and hence are poorly absorbed.

19. As explained in answer 18, the drug passes through the fenestrations (gaps) between capillary cells.

20. Acidic drugs exist more in nonionized (lipophilic) form in increasingly acidic conditions. Alkaline drugs exist more in ionized (hydrophilic) form in increasingly acidic conditions. Therefore at a pH of 3, which is acidic, the alkaline drug would exist predominantly in the hydrophilic form and thus would be less well absorbed than the acid drug.

21. Acidic drugs in the lipophilic form in the stomach pH of 2 to 3 readily pass through the cell membranes and enter a more alkaline environment (pH 7.4) when they move into the cells lining the stomach. This more alkaline pH causes more of the nonionized molecules to become ionized (hydrophilic) and unable to diffuse through membranes, thus trapping them within the cells.

22.

Acidic drug pKa = 3	Placed in pH 6	Ionized (1:1000)
Acidic drug pKa = 2	Placed in pH 9	Ionized (1:10,000,000)
Acidic drug pKa = 5	Placed in pH 2	Nonionized (1:1,000)
Acidic drug pKa = 7	Placed in pH 5	Nonionized (1:100)
Acidic drug pKa = 7	Placed in pH 7	Ionized and nonionized equal
Alkaline drug pKa = 6	Placed in pH 9	Nonionized (1:1,000)
Alkaline drug pKa = 9	Placed in pH 8	Ionized (1:10)
Alkaline drug pKa = 5	Placed in pH 2	Ionized (1:1,000)
Alkaline drug pKa = 5	Placed in pH 8	Nonionized (1:1,000)

The ratio depicts the ratio of the lesser form to the predominant form. With the first drug (an acidic drug with pKa of 3, placed in pH 6), there are 1000 ionized molecules for every 1 nonionized molecule. With the third drug, there are 1000 nonionized molecules for every 1 ionized molecule.

23.

Drug A	Acidic drug pKa 3.4
Drug B	Acidic drug pKa 5.4
Drug C	Alkaline drug pKa 6.4
Drug D	Alkaline drug pKa 8.4

Determine which drug will exist predominantly in the hydrophilic form. Drug A, drug B, and drug D exist more in the hydrophilic form than in the lipophilic form. Looking at the difference between the pH of 7.4 and the respective pKa for each of those drugs, you find the greatest difference between drug A's pKa of 3.4 and the pH of 7.4 ($7.4 - 3.4 = 4$). The ratio of ionized to nonionized molecules is 10,000:1 (10,000 is 10^4). The other two drugs that also exist primarily in the ionized form have ratios of 100:1 for drug B and 10:1 for drug D.

24. Reabsorption of drugs from the renal tubules is passive and requires movement of drug molecules through the cell membrane. Thus a lipophilic drug is well reabsorbed, but a hydrophilic drug remains in the tubules and is excreted with the urine. If we alkalinize the urine (that is, make the renal tubular environment more alkaline), this acidic drug becomes more ionized (hydrophilic) and less is reabsorbed.

25. The enteric coating protects the drug from the acidic environment of the stomach so it can pass to the duodenum and be absorbed.

26. Pylorospasm slows gastric emptying. If the drug was not inactivated in the stomach, the only difference would be a delayed onset of action (assuming not much of the drug is absorbed from the stomach because it is an alkaline drug). If the drug was degraded by the acidic stomach environment, the onset of action would be delayed and a reduced amount of intact drug is absorbed.

27. If the intestinal transit time was accelerated (ingesta moving through more quickly), a tablet might not dissolve and be absorbed before it moves through the small intestine and into the colon, which does not absorb drugs as readily as the small intestine.

28. Highly hydrophilic compounds are not absorbed into the body from the GI tract and thus have little or no systemic effect. Even if the compound is absorbed across the gut wall, it might be eliminated by the liver (first-pass effect) and not reach the systemic circulation in significant concentrations. If toxic compounds are injected or absorbed across mucous membranes or damaged skin, they enter the systemic circulation directly producing toxicity.

29. In cold conditions, constriction of blood vessels near the body surface limits heat loss. This vasoconstriction reduces perfusion of superficial tissues, so a drug injected subcutaneously must diffuse farther to find an open capillary and be absorbed.

30. Fat is poorly perfused. Drugs injected into a fat pad are poorly absorbed and have significantly reduced effect on the body.

31. To cross the blood:brain barrier, drugs must be in the lipophilic form.

32. Redistribution is the movement of drug from tissue A, to the blood, and then to tissue B. The thiopental will diffuse from the brain, back into the blood, and then into the fat. As concentrations drop in the brain, breathing resumes and the animal may begin to awaken.

33. The dose should be decreased. With fewer protein molecules in the blood, there are fewer sites to bind drug. With more of the drug in the "free" form, more is distributed to tissues. A "normal" dose could produce higher concentrations of drug in the tissues, potentially producing toxicity.

34. Drug B is more likely to penetrate more fluid compartments because it is dissolved in 3 L of fluid. Because drug A is diluted in only 1 L of fluid instead of 3 L, its concentration (mg of drug in each ml of body fluid) would be higher.

35. Volume of distribution is usually called the *apparent* volume of distribution because it is always an approximation based on the drug concentration in the plasma only. So much digoxin moves out of the plasma and into the skeletal and cardiac muscle that concentrations within the plasma are very low. Looking at plasma concentrations, it appears that digoxin is diluted in a large volume of fluid. In fact, the drug is bound to sites outside the plasma.

36. Lower. More fluid in the body dilutes the drug, thereby reducing the concentration.

37. An antagonist to the insecticide would probably be ineffective because the insecticide has combined with a receptor in such a way that an antagonist cannot readily replace it at the receptor site. This is in contrast to a competitive agonist/antagonist situation, in which the effect of the agonist can be reversed by giving more antagonist.

38. Pentazocine has intrinsic narcotic activity when it combines with narcotic (opioid) receptors, but its effect is much weaker than that of oxymorphone. Therefore if pentazocine replaces oxymorphone at the opioid receptors, the degree of narcosis and analgesia is decreased but not totally eliminated. Using a true antagonist such as naloxone, which has little or no intrinsic activity, the narcosis and analgesia are completely reversed.

39. A chelator does not require a cellular receptor. A direct chemical reaction between the chelator drug and ions such as Ca^{++}, Mg^{++}, and H^+ produces the effect.

40. Cats have limited ability to conjugate glucuronide with drugs; drugs that depend on this process for normal metabolism and excretion are eliminated more slowly. The immature liver of young animals cannot biotransform drugs as readily as the liver in older animals; therefore hepatically biotransformed drugs must be used with caution in very young animals. This concern does not necessarily apply to drugs excreted exclusively by the kidneys because renal function is not normally reduced in the young animal or cats.

41. Hepatic metabolism of phenobarbital becomes more efficient over time. Because the phenobarbital is broken down more quickly, drug concentrations decrease more rapidly and less drug accumulates between doses. Thus a larger drug dose is necessary to compensate for more rapid metabolism.

42. Decreased blood flow to the kidneys means less drug delivered to the kidneys and subsequently less drug excreted by the kidneys. Therefore drug would accumulate in the body with each dose.

43. Penicillin is actively secreted into the renal tubule lumen and can achieve concentrations in the urine that may be much higher than those in the plasma. Thus the bacteria are killed in the urine by the higher concentrations attained through active secretion.

44. In enterohepatic circulation, the poison is excreted by the liver, dumped into the intestine, and then resorbed back into the body, where it can continue to cause damage. The poison adheres to the activated charcoal, decreasing its absorption. The charcoal must be given as long as the poison is being excreted back into the intestinal tract. Otherwise the poison will be reabsorbed and have a continued effect on the body.

45. Clearance is a measure of how quickly drug is removed from the blood. If IV fluids are administered, renal perfusion will increase, resulting in increased renal elimination of drugs. Rapid clearance means rapid movement of drug out of the blood and presumably from the body.

46.

Hour 0	0 µg/ml
Hour 1	24 µg/ml
Hour 2	19 µg/ml
Hour 3	12 µg/ml
Hour 4	9.5 µg/ml

Half-life is the time it takes for the plasma drug concentration to drop by half. In this example, from hour 1 to hour 3 the concentration dropped from 24 to 12 (half). If it took 2 hours for the concentration to drop from 24 to 12 µg/ml, the half-life is 2 hours. Note that from hour 2 to hour 4, the concentration dropped from 19 to 9.5 µg/ml (drop by half in 2 hours). Thus starting at any time, 2 hours later the drug concentration in plasma will be decreased 50%. Because the bottom end of the therapeutic range is 7 µg/ml, another dose should be given before the concentrations dip below that level. At hour 3, the concentration is 12 µg/ml; therefore 2 hours later at hour 5, the concentration should be $12 \div 2 = 6$ µg/ml, which would be below the therapeutic range. This drug would have to be given every 4 hours. (Of course, the peak and trough concentrations will increase until the drug achieves steady state). You can project what the concentration will be at 7 hours because you know the concentration at 3 hours and the half-life. At hour 3 the concentration is 12 μg/ml; therefore at hour 5 the concentration will be 6 μg/ml, and at hour 7 the concentration will be 3 μg/ml.

47. This is related to the time needed to reach steady state (5 times the half-life). Until steady state is achieved, drug concentrations are climbing. A drug with a long half-life, such as phenobarbital, does not achieve steady-state concentrations for days, as opposed to penicillin, which has a half-life of about 2 hours and reaches a steady state by 10 hours after the first dose. Because phenobarbital levels slowly increase over days, it may be present in very low concentrations during the first few hours (or days) after treatment begins. Therefore a loading dose might be used to establish therapeutic concentrations faster.

48. Theoretically the withdrawal time should be shorter for drug A because its half-life is so short. (The drug leaves the blood quickly.) Several other factors may enter into the withdrawal time, such as how long it takes for the drug to leave tissues (not just the blood) and the concentrations of residues in meat or other food products (eggs and milk) that are legally acceptable for human consumption.

1. *Gastric* refers to the stomach and *enteric* refers to the intestines.
2. The sympathetic nervous system shunts blood away from the GI tract and generally inhibits its function. The parasympathetic nervous system stimulates secretions and motility of the GI tract.
3. Acetylcholine is primarily associated with parasympathetic nervous system responses, and thus it or any drugs that act similarly would stimulate the GI tract. Epinephrine, norepinephrine, and other catecholamine drugs mimic the sympathetic nervous system response and hence depress the GI tract.
4. Prostaglandins are normally associated with inflammation. However, in the intestinal tract, prostaglandins are associated with production of protective mucus, normal cell turnover, intestinal motility, fluid secretions of the intestinal tract, and repair of the intestinal tract after injury.
5. The parietal, or oxyntic, cells of the stomach produce hydrochloric acid in response to stimulation of acetylcholine receptors by the parasympathetic nervous system, by stimulation of the H_2 receptors by histamine, and by gastrin receptor stimulation from gastrin release.
6. When the intestinal tract becomes irritated, impulses from the intestinal tract travel via the vagus nerve to stimulate the vomiting, or emetic, center.
7. Although vomiting in all of these cases is moderated by the vomiting center, the stimulus in each case is different. With motion sickness the stimulation originates from excessive stimulation of the vestibular apparatus in the inner ear. The distressed cat is likely vomiting from stimulation of the CRTZ by sympathetic neurotransmitters that work through the α receptors in the CRTZ. Digoxin most likely causes vomiting by direct stimulation of the CRTZ.
8. The vestibular apparatus normally uses histamine as a transmitter of excessive motion to the vomiting center and the CRTZ. Antihistamines block these impulses. They work better in dogs than cats because a dog's CRTZ has more histamine receptors and thus is more sensitive to histamine than a cat's CRTZ. This also means that antihistamines can quiet the dog's CRTZ better than a cat's.
9. Xylazine is an α_2 receptor stimulator. The CRTZ of cats has more α receptors than that of dogs, and hence is more sensitive to drugs that stimulate α receptors.
10. The CRTZ of cats has fewer dopamine receptors; therefore a vomiting cat is not helped much by an antidopaminergic drug. (However, dogs can benefit.) In addition, vomiting related to hairballs is usually associated with gastric stasis, so an antidopaminergic would probably not help even if the cat's CRTZ did have dopamine receptors.
11. You need something that acts quickly. Apomorphine produces emesis within seconds or minutes when placed in the conjunctival sac or injected intra-

venously or intramuscularly. Syrup of ipecac must pass into the intestinal tract before it can induce emesis and that takes time. The onset of action and efficacy of hydrogen peroxide are quite variable. In this situation, apomorphine seems to be the best choice.

12. In each case, vomiting should not be stimulated or should be stimulated only after further investigation. Cases a and b both involve corrosive substances that likely have burned or irritated esophageal tissues when swallowed. Inducing vomiting would bring them back up the esophagus and cause further damage. In case c, horses do not vomit. In case d, the dog has already vomited up the material; there is no need to induce further vomiting. In case e, vomiting should not be induced in patients with seizures; use gastric lavage after seizures are controlled. It has been 3 hours, so much of the poison is likely already absorbed. In case f, no acetaminophen remains in the GI tract to be removed by vomiting.

13. Xylazine is an effective emetic in cats.

14. Syrup of ipecac works by stimulating the GI tract, primarily the duodenum. It also exerts an emetic effect after it has been absorbed. Both of these take 10 to 30 minutes to occur. Therefore the ipecac may not have arrived in the duodenum at this point. Wait another 5 minutes.

15. No. The extract is much stronger than syrup. If the extract were given at syrup dosages, it would likely result in cardiotoxicity and death.

16. Simultaneous administration of syrup of ipecac and activated charcoal is not recommended because the charcoal adsorbs the ipecac, inactivating it. In addition, the ipecac coats the charcoal, preventing it from binding with any toxin.

17. Phenothiazine tranquilizers such as acepromazine block dopamine receptors in the CRTZ and decrease the histamine-mediated vomiting stimulated by the vestibular apparatus through their antihistamine effect.

18. Because phenothiazines are also alpha receptor blockers, they can block the vasoconstrictive effect of α_1 receptors on peripheral blood vessels, resulting in reflex vasodilation and a drop in blood pressure. If an animal is hypovolemic (low blood volume) from dehydration or any other cause, the blood pressure is low. The vasodilation from acepromazine or any other phenothiazine tranquilizer would further reduce the blood pressure.

19. Diphenhydramine (Benadryl) and dimenhydrinate (Dramamine) are antihistamines that block histamine transmission of impulses from the vestibular apparatus to the vomiting center and/or CRTZ.

20. An anticholinergic drug produces an effect opposite to that of acetylcholine, the neurotransmitter associated with parasympathetic nervous system responses. A parasympatholytic drug blocks or antagonizes an effect of the parasympathetic nervous system. Thus the terms *anticholinergic* and *parasympatholytic* are sometimes used interchangeably. Because these drugs block the parasympathetic nervous system, they have a general depressant effect on the GI tract.

21. Metoclopramide acts centrally by blocking dopamine receptors in the CRTZ. It acts locally by increasing tone of the distal esophagus, relaxing the pyloric exit of the stomach, and increasing gastric motility in the normal distal direction.

22. Acepromazine should generally not be used simultaneously with metoclopramide. Both drugs are antidopaminergic and affect other dopamine receptors in the CNS, producing sedation, tranquilization, and CNS depression. In addition, anticholinergic drugs such as atropine would block the acetylcholine activity by which metoclopramide stimulates gastric motility.

23. Cisapride (Propulsid) has been advocated for this use. Like metoclopramide, it increases gastric motility and tone, which in turn prevents the gastric atony that usually precedes hairball vomiting.

24. It depends on the cause of the diarrhea, such as maldigestion of food, hypersecretion, increased gut permeability, or increased gut motility.

25. See answer 24.

26. Segmental (circular) contractions of the gut create barriers to intestinal content flow. Therefore a drug that increases these is required. In addition, it would be preferrable for peristaltic waves, which normally push intestinal contents along, to be reduced. If the bowel becomes atonic (without tone) as a result of loss of segmental waves, even a slight peristaltic contraction will result in intestinal contents flowing readily along the GI tract.

27. Hypomotility is decreased intestinal movement, including segmental contractions. The intestinal tract essentially becomes a tube through which ingesta can easily slide. Diarrhea can be caused by small intestinal motility, but it usually results from acute irritation and lasts only a short time. Hypermotility associated with colonic irritation causes straining to pass feces even when no feces are present. This straining is called tenesmus.

28. See answer 27.

29. Opioid analgesics increase segmental contraction and decrease GI secretions in the small intestine. Anticholinergics simply cause intestinal atony (ileus).

30. Opioids can prolong the contact of an irritant or toxic substance with the intestinal tract wall, thereby facilitating absorption of the offending substance. This can prolong the stay of pathogens (bacterial or otherwise) within the intestinal tract.

31. Generally these drugs are anticholinergic and decrease intestinal contractions. These drugs are effective in treating spastic colon because they decrease acetylcholine-mediated tenesmus associated with colonic irritation.

32. Hypersecretory diarrheas can rapidly dehydrate an animal, especially young animals.

33. The bismuth subsalicylate in Pepto-Bismol is an aspirin-like compound that decreases prostaglandin formation and inflammation in the bowel. The protective coating is only of minor clinical significance.

34. Although intestinal disease could cause small bowel hemorrhage, the change in stool color is most likely related to bismuth administration, which turns the stool a dark color.

35. Bismuth subsalicylate (in Pepto-Bismol) must be used cautiously in cats because they do not metabolize salicylates (aspirin-like drugs) well.

36. If the diarrhea is caused by irritating substances or enterotoxins (toxins in the intestines), the offending substance can be adsorbed by these medications. This effect in animals is often questioned.

37. In some cases the kaolin-pectin combination can decrease absorption of orally administered drugs by adsorbing the drugs. Therefore any other oral drugs should be given 2 hours before the kaolin-pectin compound.

38. These irritant laxatives can cause explosive defecation and straining, and should not be used in animals with suspected intestinal impaction or in animals straining from the effects of colonic or anal surgery.

39. Phosphate enemas in cats (even phosphate soap enemas) can result in absorption of phosphate sufficient to produce severe and sometimes fatal blood electrolyte imbalances.

40. Use of oil-based laxatives for chronic constipation, hairballs, and other similar conditions can decrease absorption of vitamins A, D, E, and K, which are fat-soluble.

41. DSS (Colace) is used primarily as a stool softener. It works by breaking down the surface tension of water in much the same way a detergent does. This allows more water to enter the stool and soften it. In animals with a pelvic frac-

ture, a softened stool eases passage through the injured and/or narrowed pelvic canal. In bloated cattle, reduced surface tension reduces the bubbles of frothy bloat, facilitating eructation ("burping" of gas).

42. NSAIDs block formation of prostaglandins, which stimulate mucus production, normal perfusion, and healing of the stomach.

43. Local antacids simply neutralize stomach acid after it has been produced and can cause acid rebound. Systemic antacids inhibit or decrease acid production and thus are more effective at decreasing gastric hyperacidity.

44. No. Antihistamines primarily affect H_1 receptors but do not block H_2 receptors in the stomach.

45. A common misconception is that H_2 blockers are effective for common acute gastritis. They are used to decrease acidity in hyperacidity syndromes from diet or other causes. Vomiting has many causes; blocking acid production by using Pepcid-CD (famotidine) may do little if anything to correct the vomiting.

46. H_2 blockers decrease the stimulus for acid production. Omeprazole, the so-called *acid blocker*, prevents or decreases the amount of acid secreted into the lumen of the stomach by inhibiting the "proton pump" that moves hydrogen ions for hydrochloric acid into the stomach.

47. Sucralfate (Carafate). Antacids are often used with it, but generally it is a good idea to wait a couple of hours after sucralfate is given before giving the antacid. Sucralfate needs an acidic environment to facilitate its adhesion to the ulcer site.

48. Misoprostol (Cytotec) is a prostaglandin analog that is similar to the protective prostaglandins found in the GI tract. The side effects most commonly associated with misoprostol are related to overstimulation of the GI tract (for example, cramping, colic, and abdominal discomfort).

49. They are both used as ruminatorics to stimulate an atonic rumen.

50. Detergents such as poloxalene and DSS break down the water surface tension and viscosity, causing the bubbles of frothy bloat to break.

51. Sulfasalazine (Azulfidine) is broken down in the colon to an aspirin-like compound (aminosalicylate) that decreases inflammation. Because this occurs primarily in the colon, its major antiinflammatory effect is in the large intestine, not in the small intestine.

52. Tylosin causes severe diarrhea in horses.

53. Metronidazole (Flagyl). It can produce CNS signs even at "normal" doses. Signs include head tilt, staggering, disorientation, and even seizures.

54. Livestock producers often use oral electrolyte supplements because it is impractical to infuse IV fluids in calves or other young livestock that have scours (diarrhea). In small animals, significant dehydration should be corrected with IV fluids. Oral electrolyte solutions can be given after the animal's condition has improved.

55. The lipase in oral pancreatic supplements is very difficult to maintain in active form and is easily broken down in the acidic environment of the stomach. It is only active at a specific pH and at the proper temperature. Despite supplementation, fats still are not very well digested, resulting in greasy stools and poor weight gain.

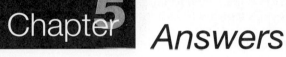

Chapter 5 *Answers*

1. Blood flows from the vena cava to the right atrium and then through the tricuspid valve into the right ventricle. It flows out the pulmonary valve to the pulmonary artery, to the lungs, and back to the heart through the pulmonary vein and into the left atrium. From the left atrium, the blood passes through the mitral valve into the left ventricle and then out through the aortic valve to the aorta.

2. The left ventricle is larger. It pumps blood to the entire body (except the lungs), whereas the right ventricle pumps blood only to the lungs.

3. The mitral valve is the left atrioventricular (AV) valve.

4. The sinoatrial (SA) node is the heart's pacemaker. The sympathetic nervous system increases the heart rate via the SA node; the parasympathetic nervous system decreases the heart rate.

5. SA node, atria, AV node, bundle branches, Purkinje fibers, apex of the ventricles.

6. The P wave represents atrial depolarization. The QRS complex represents ventricular depolarization. The interval between the P wave and the QRS complex is the time when impulses are passing through the AV node.

7. Depolarization occurs when sodium ions move into the cell. Repolarization occurs when potassium ions move out of the cell.

8. The refractory period is the time during which a cell cannot be depolarized again. A wave of depolarization that encounters a set of cells in the refractory period is halted because these cells cannot be depolarized, or can only be depolarized with a strong stimulus if in the relative refractory stage. This is similar to a forest fire progressing to an area that has been previously burned; the fire can go no further.

9. The rate of automaticity (inherent ability of cells to depolarize on their own without a stimulus) is determined by leakage of sodium ions into the cell. When this trickle of positively charged sodium ions causes the charge within the cell to rise to a particular threshold, the cell depolarizes (opens the fast sodium channels). The SA node "leaks" sodium faster than the AV node and thus fires more often.

10. When stimulated by an agonist, β_1 receptors increase the rate and force of cardiac contraction. β_2 Receptors are found on smooth muscles in the bronchioles (among other places), where they cause bronchodilation. Blocking β_2 receptors allows the bronchioles to constrict (bronchoconstriction) when stimulated by the parasympathetic nervous system. Stimulation of α_1 receptors causes vasoconstriction in the peripheral blood vessels. An α_1 agonist causes peripheral vasoconstriction; this is why epinephrine is included with lidocaine to retard lidocaine's absorption as a local anesthetic. A parasympathetic agonist slows the

rate (SA node effect) and force of cardiac contraction, slows conduction through the heart (AV node), and stimulates bronchoconstriction and GI tract motility and secretions.

11. A β_1 agonist would increase cardiac output by stimulating heart rate and contractility, and increase blood pressure. A β_2 agonist probably has little effect. An α_1 agonist causes peripheral vasoconstriction at the precapillary sphincters, "backing up" of blood in the arteries, and increasing arterial blood pressure. A parasympathetic agonist would reduce blood pressure by slowing the heart and reducing cardiac output.

12. a. Supraventricular (above the ventricles) tachycardia (increased rate); b. Supraventricular bradycardia; and c. Ventricular tachycardia.

13. Lidocaine is the drug of choice for emergency intervention of ventricular arrhythmias such as that which might be caused by a ventricular ectopic focus. It is given intravenously. It can be used in cats but the dose must be decreased.

14. If given by mouth, any lidocaine absorbed is removed by the first-pass effect, and it also causes GI irritation, thus lidocaine should not be given by mouth. Tocainide can be given by mouth but it is not used much in veterinary medicine. Instead, procainamide and quinidine (with the former used more often) are antiarrhythmic drugs that can be given by mouth.

15. Epinephrine is included with lidocaine in local anesthetic formulations to delay absorption of lidocaine from the site because it causes vasoconstriction. If injected intravenously with the lidocaine, epinephrine stimulates the heart and could worsen the arrhythmia. The veterinary technician should clearly mark the different forms of lidocaine so that in an emergency situation, the wrong vial is not accidentally grabbed in haste.

16. Quinidine is somewhat effective against ventricular ectopic foci; however, it tends to displace digoxin from its binding sites, increasing digoxin concentrations in plasma and increasing the possibility of digoxin toxicosis. When quinidine and digoxin are used together, the digoxin dose should be halved to prevent digoxin toxicosis.

17. Sustained-release medications are often formulated so the tablet dissolves very predictably from the outside inward at a controlled rate. If you break the tablet, this exposes the more readily dissolved drug inside of the tablet, negating the sustained-release effect.

18. The high sympathetic tone may be essential for the weakened heart to maintain adequate cardiac output. Reducing sympathetic tone by blocking the β_1 receptors in the heart may reduce contractility and kill the animal.

19. Most of the drugs that block arrhythmias also decrease the rate or force of cardiac contraction, the latter effect being a negative inotropic effect. In a heart that is marginally keeping up with the demands of the body, this can result in cardiovascular collapse.

20. Propranolol blocks β_1 receptors in the heart and is used to combat arrhythmias. However, it may also block the bronchodilating effect of the β_2 receptors in the airways, resulting in bronchoconstriction.

21. β-blocker drugs cause target tissues to develop more receptors, causing them to become more sensitive to the catecholamine drugs that β-blockers are intended to block. This is called *upregulation*.

22. β-blockers decrease sympathetic tone, which normally increases heart rate, thereby causing the heart rate to slow. Atropine blocks parasympathetic receptors that slow the heart rate, causing a slight increase in the heart rate. Epinephrine normally speeds the heart rate by stimulating β_1 receptors. However,

if those β_1 receptors are occupied by β-blockers, the epinephrine cannot stimulate the β_1 receptors and the heart rate does not increase.

23. When β-blockers are used for a long time, the body adapts by increasing the number of receptors on the cell surface (see answer 21). This increased number of receptors increases the cells' sensitivity to sympathetic stimulation from epinephrine, norepinephrine, dobutamine, or catecholamines. Because many of those receptors are still blocked by the β-blocker, the response (change in heart rate) to these β-stimulating compounds is not marked. However, when use of β-blockers is abruptly stopped, all of the receptors are open to the β-stimulating effect of the sympathetic nervous system. Thus a heart that had developed more β receptors while under the influence of β-blockers would now be very sensitive to even "normal" amounts of sympathetic nervous system stimulation and would develop tachycardia. In an animal with a diseased heart, this could result in heart failure or severe arrhythmias.

24. Diltiazem reduces the physical size of the heart in cats with hypertrophic cardiomyopathy, a disease in which the ventricular walls of the heart thicken so much that the heart cannot adequately pump blood.

25. All of the catecholamines must be delivered by injection, which makes it impractical for long-term use. The half-life of these catecholamines is very short so their effect lasts only minutes. Cells with sympathetic nervous system receptors *down regulate* after repeated exposure to catecholamines. (Receptors on the cell surface disappear, causing the cells to become less sensitive to catecholamines.) For these reasons, catecholamines are used only for a short time to improve contractility.

26. Digoxin is the usual choice.

27. Digoxin has a narrow therapeutic index, which means that beneficial concentrations are also very close to concentrations that produce toxicity. There is not much room for error in dosing or in the way the body metabolizes the drug (for example, if clearance were reduced from renal insufficiency).

28. In atrial fibrillation, the atria might be contracting at 200 beats/minute. Digoxin has a parasympathetic effect, slowing the conduction of impulses through the AV node. Therefore digoxin does not increase the atrial fibrillation itself, but decreases the number of impulses passing through the AV node and thus slows the ventricular contractions to a more efficient rate.

29. Owners should be instructed to look for anorexia, vomiting, and diarrhea.

30. Digoxin slows conduction through the SA node, so you would see bradycardia. AV node depression would increase the distance between the P wave (atrial depolarization) and the QRS complex (ventricular depolarization) in the phenomenon of first-degree AV block. Second-degree AV block occurs when occasionally there is a P wave without a corresponding QRS wave, indicating that the depolarization wave died out in the AV node.

31. Atropine blocks the parasympathetic effect of digoxin to some degree and would slightly increase conduction through the AV node and slightly increase the heart rate.

32. Hypokalemia (low blood potassium level) predisposes an animal to digoxin toxicosis at much lower concentrations than in animals with normal potassium levels. Furosemide is a diuretic that increases urinary excretion of potassium. Hypokalemia from furosemide use might increase the risk of digoxin toxicosis if the potassium level is not monitored.

33. Digoxin is primarily excreted by the kidneys. Renal disease would decrease clearance of digoxin from the body, allowing accumulation of digoxin and producing toxicosis.

34. Set up an algebraic equation: dose in tablet × 0.6 = dose in elixir × 0.75. 0.2 mg × 0.6 = X × 0.75 = 0.16 mg of elixir. To convert the other way, use the same equation and plug in the given dose of elixir and calculate X for the tablet: dose in tablet × 0.6 = 0.5 mg × 0.75 = 0.625 mg.

35. Capillary refill time reflects blood pressure and resistance to blood flow (that is, vasoconstriction). A high dose of vasodilator would dilate enough vessels to decrease the blood pressure and stimulate the sympathetic nervous system in an attempt to correct for the hypotension (this would be successful depending on the type of vasodilator that was used). The drop in blood pressure and reflex vasoconstriction would both impede return of blood to the capillaries; thus capillary refill time would be prolonged.

36. Renin is released from the kidney when blood pressure drops and renal perfusion decreases. Renin quickly converts inactive angiotensinogen to angiotensin I. Angiotensin I is, in turn, converted by angiotensin-converting enzyme (ACE) to angiotensin II. Angiotensin II is a potent vasoconstrictor. Angiotensin II also stimulates release of aldosterone, which increases sodium resorption from the kidneys, with water following the sodium back into the body. Although both these actions return blood pressure toward normal, they also increase the work load of the heart.

37. Hydralazine is an arterial vasodilator used to help control the effects of mitral valve insufficiency. Nitroglycerin is a venous vasodilator used to help reduce ascites (fluid accumulation within the abdomen) associated with right ventricular failure and pulmonary edema associated with left ventricular failure. Enalapril is an ACE inhibitor that prevents conversion of angiotensin I to the potent vasoconstrictor angiotensin II. It works on both the arterial and venous (veins) side of the circulatory system.

38. The vessels in dogs with heartworm disease are often damaged or altered sufficiently that they do not respond well to hydralazine.

39. Hypotension from the vasodilator is manifested as lethargy or staggering after rising.

40. The nitroglycerin patch can be cut into smaller pieces to reduce the dose.

41. Always wear latex gloves when applying nitroglycerin because topical formulations of the drug are easily absorbed through the skin.

42. Enalapril blocks formation of angiotensin II, a potent vasoconstrictor normally produced in response to falling blood pressure associated with congestive heart failure. In normal animals, little of this compound is produced and so enalapril has little effect.

43. ACE inhibitors such as enalapril block secretion of aldosterone, causing loss of sodium and retention of potassium. Hyponatremia (low blood sodium) or hyperkalemia (high blood potassium) can be worsened by the action of enalapril.

44. Loop diuretics work best in most veterinary patients when the goal is to reduce volume overload on the heart. Furosemide prevents reabsorption of sodium from the renal tubules; sodium remains in the urine and more water remains in the urine, producing diuresis. Furosemide does not cause a loss of sodium because in the distal convoluted tubule, much of the sodium in the urine is exchanged for potassium so that the body ends up conserving sodium but excreting increased amounts of potassium. In this way, furosemide can produce hypokalemia in some patients.

45. Digoxin is more likely to produce toxicity in hypokalemic patients. Hypokalemia can occur with use of furosemide. Therefore blood potassium concentrations should be monitored periodically in animals receiving both furosemide and digoxin.

46. Thiazide diuretics block resorption of sodium like loop diuretics, but they do it in the proximal portion of the distal convoluted tubules, where there is significantly less sodium reabsorption to be blocked. Hence they are much weaker diuretics than loop diuretics. Because sodium is exchanged for potassium in more distal parts of the nephron, there is a net loss of potassium with thiazide diuretics. Spironolactone is a competitive antagonist of aldosterone. Therefore it prevents reabsorption of sodium allowing sodium excretion and conserves potassium. This is the opposite effect of loop or thiazide diuretics.

47. Mannitol is an osmotic diuretic that does not alter sodium or potassium excretion. Mannitol's diuretic effect is from the mannitol molecules themselves.

48. Aspirin decreases clumping of platelets and thus reduces the risk of clots. In cats with hypertrophic cardiomyopathy, the heart wall thickens and clots can form thrombi in vessels, especially those in the rear legs. Aspirin use reduces that risk, but the dose used in cats is smaller and the dosage interval is longer than in dogs because cats do not metabolize aspirin well.

Answers

1. Once the animal is rehydrated, the cough may become productive. In addition, after the animal is rehydrated, the mucociliary apparatus may work better and the cough may "loosen up."
2. There are no cough receptors in the terminal bronchioles or alveoli.
3. Locally acting antitussives produce a soothing effect on the respiratory mucosa. They are usually in the form of cough drops, and veterinary patients do not keep them in their mouth long enough to derive any effect.
4. Butorphanol is the only antitussive with an approved form for use in veterinary patients. It is available only from veterinarians. Dextromethorphan is an OTC formulation found in cold and flu medications used by people. Codeine and hydrocodone are potent prescription antitussives that are controlled substances.
5. Migration of inflammatory cells into the respiratory tree causes the mucus in the mucociliary apparatus to become more sticky, impairing mucus movement out of the respiratory tree. Acetylcysteine breaks the disulfide bonds that contribute to this stickiness, making it easier for the mucociliary apparatus to move the mucus.
6. Animals often struggle when the nebulizer mask is placed over the face, which is undesirable in a hypoxic animal. If the nebulized drug is irritating, it can produce bronchoconstriction. Human patients can be instructed to breathe deeply to deliver drug deep into the respiratory tree, but veterinary patients usually do not breathe deeply during nebulization therapy.
7. Expectorants add fluid to, or dilute, the mucus in the airways, making it easier to be moved by the mucociliary apparatus. Mucolytics make the mucus less sticky and easier to move (see answer 5).
8. Guaifenesin (glycerol guaiacolate) is given intravenously as a muscle relaxant in equine surgery. For the respiratory effect (expectorant), guaifenesin is given orally. In the stomach it produces a mild irritation that stimulates the parasympathetic nervous system, resulting in increased respiratory secretions.
9. If the cat ingested a decongestant, you can expect to see signs associated with overstimulation of the sympathetic nervous system: tachycardia, apprehensive or nervous behavior, pacing, panting, and pupillary dilation. Decongestants generally act by stimulating α_1 receptors in the blood vessels of mucous membranes, causing vasoconstriction and reducing blood flow to the congested mucosa. This reduces the swelling and provides a "clearing" effect in the nasal passages. However, decongestants also stimulate other sympathetic receptors (in the heart and bronchioles), producing mild side effects at normal doses and marked sympathetic signs in larger doses.
10. The expectorant increases the fluidity of respiratory secretions, and the cough mechanism is needed to remove the extra fluid. Blocking the cough reflex with a strong antitussive impairs removal of respiratory secretions.

11. Parasympathetic nervous system stimulation normally causes increased bronchial secretions and bronchoconstriction. Therefore anything that blocks the parasympathetic nervous system allows the sympathetic nervous system to dominate, producing dry mucous membranes and bronchodilation. Because of the drying effect and reduced effectiveness of the mucociliary apparatus, atropine is rarely used as a bronchodilator, except in some toxicities in which the parasympathetic nervous system is overstimulated (for example, organophosphate insecticide poisoning).

12. Epinephrine also stimulates the heart (β_1 effect) and causes vasoconstriction of peripheral blood vessels (α_1 effect), two effects best avoided in the hypoxic animal because they increase the work load of the heart. Terbutaline and albuterol selectively stimulate β_2 receptors, although they also have some β_1 effects. Epinephrine use is usually confined to short-term, emergency use as a bronchodilator, or more commonly for reversing hypotension in some shock syndromes.

13. β-Blocker antiarrhythmics work by blocking β_1 receptors in the heart. However, some of them also block β_2 receptors in bronchiolar smooth muscle. If the β_2 sympathetic nervous system bronchodilating effect is blocked, the bronchoconstricting effect of the parasympathetic nervous system predominates.

14. β_2 Receptor stimulation normally produces cyclic AMP in the smooth muscle cells, which in turn produces the relaxation of the bronchiolar smooth muscles. Cyclic AMP is broken down by phosphodiesterase to terminate this effect. Methylxanthines inhibit this phosphodiesterase enzyme, and thus cyclic AMP persists for a longer period, prolonging smooth muscle relaxation.

15. The doctor wants to switch from "pure" theophylline to aminophylline, which contains about 80% theophylline and 20% salt and is often better tolerated in the GI tract than theophylline. The theophylline dose = 80% $\times$ aminophylline dose. Therefore, 200 mg theophylline = 0.80 $\times$ aminophylline dose = 250 mg aminophylline.

16. Antihistamines do not reverse cellular damage but only compete for histamine receptors (H_1) on cells, preventing further inflammation. The antihistamines given to a horse do nothing to reverse the inflammation caused by previous histamine release; however, because the horse will likely return to an environment containing allergenic dust and molds, the antihistamines can block further histamine effects. In the dog with an allergic reaction, histamine has already been released and combined with cellular receptors; therefore the antihistamine given after the fact does not block the effect. Only if the inflammatory reaction is continuing would the antihistamines be of any benefit.

17. If administration of the medication is stopped too soon, surviving resistant bacteria could multiply and produce a second infection that is much more difficult to control. The client should be advised to complete the medication as directed.

18. Diuretics often dehydrate the animal to some degree, which dries respiratory secretions and impairs function of the mucociliary apparatus.

19. Unless oxygen is humidified by bubbling it through water or some other mechanism, it is extremely dry and subsequently dries the respiratory membranes, decreasing the effectiveness of the mucociliary apparatus. High flows of oxygen to the nasal cavity can cause extreme drying of the nasal mucosa, producing significant irritation, or "oxygen burn".

1. *Exogenous* means it comes from outside the body (that is, is administered), whereas *endogenous* means it is a natural substance occurring in the body. Exogenous and endogenous hormones have the same effects on the body and on negative-feedback regulatory mechanisms. Exogenous hormone drugs are sometimes chemically modified to enhance their effect, but they generally have the same effects as endogenous hormones.

2. Hypothyroidism is characterized by reduced levels of the thyroid hormones T_3 and T_4. In primary hypothyroidism, the thyroid gland is unable to produce these hormones. However, the pituitary and hypothalamus are assumed to be normal. Because there is less T_3 and T_4 to provide negative feedback, the pituitary and hypothalamus glands keep producing TRH and TSH in an attempt to get the dysfunctional thyroid gland to produce T_3 and T_4; thus TRH and TSH levels would be normal to high.

3. T_3 is the biologically active hormone. T_4 often acts as a precursor that is converted by tissues to T_3. T_3 supplements are rarely used in veterinary medicine because they bypass the normal tissue T_4 to T_3 conversion, resulting in some tissues receiving more T_3 than they need while others receive less. T_4 (levothyroxine) is more commonly used as a thyroid hormone supplement.

4. Combination drugs containing T_3 and T_4 are formulated to provide the ideal T_3:T_4 ratio found in people, which is quite different from the ratio in dogs. These products are also much more expensive than the veterinary T_4 products. For these reasons, combination T_3 and T_4 products for people are rarely used in veterinary medicine.

5. In hyperthyroidism, metabolic processes are accelerated so the animal remains active or is more active than normal, loses weight, has a voracious appetite, and sometimes has diarrhea. Affected cats are often not brought to the veterinarian until they become very thin or the diarrhea becomes chronic.

6. Radioactive iodine and surgical removal of the thyroid tumor are effective in removing the cause of the hyperthyroidism; treatment with methimazole or propylthiouracil only control the overproduction of thyroid hormone. These drugs often have side effects that can range from mild anorexia to severe changes in blood cell production.

7. By blocking the β receptors in the heart (see Chapter 5), propranolol slows the heart rate and decreases arrhythmias. Hyperthyroid cats usually exhibit tachycardia that can make them a poor anesthetic risk for thyroid tumor removal. By using propranolol or another $β_1$ blocker, the veterinarian can slow the heart rate and stabilize electrical activity of the heart.

8. Diabetes mellitus is characterized by insufficient insulin production (or decreased sensitivity of insulin receptors to insulin's effect). Therefore diabetes

mellitus results in hyperglycemia (high blood glucose level), and animals with insulinoma often have hypoglycemia (very low blood glucose level), lethargy, trembling, and even hypoglycemic seizures.

9. The differences between the types of insulin relate to the routes of administration and the duration of activity. Regular (or crystalline) insulin is a short-acting insulin that is given intravenously to stabilize diabetic animals with very high blood glucose concentrations. Lente insulin is an intermediate-acting insulin most commonly used in diabetic canines. Ultralente insulin is a longer-acting insulin used to control the blood glucose levels in diabetic cats.

10. Adipose tissue is poorly perfused. Insulin injected into fat may remain at the site of injection and be very poorly absorbed, resulting in no insulin being delivered to the body.

11. The sulfonylurea hypoglycemic compounds are designed to "squeeze" more insulin out of the pancreatic β cells. This only works if there are enough functional pancreatic β cells. Most canine and feline diabetics have lost most or all of their β cells by the time they are brought to a veterinarian. Some diabetic cats have shown a moderate response to glipizide in the early stages of the disease.

12. The luteal phase derives its name from the corpus luteum, which forms at the site of a follicle that has ruptured and released its ovum. The corpus luteum produces progesterone that dominates this phase of the estrous cycle. The drug in question must somehow affect progesterone levels and therefore will only work during the luteal phase. An example would be prostaglandins, which decrease progesterone by lysing the corpus luteum. Estrus ("heat") generally occurs at the end of the follicular phase and at the beginning of the luteal phase of the estrous cycle.

13. GnRH drugs cause release of gonadotropins (that is, LH and FSH). Gonadotropin drugs (that is, HCG or eCG) have FSH and/or LH effects. GnRH drugs are seldom used in veterinary medicine because of their expense and because regular doses do not mimic the normal physiologic mechanism by which natural GnRH is released (in pulses).

14. Progesterone is produced by the corpus luteum. Progestins are drugs that resemble progesterone, but they may be modified to enhance their effect or to reduce side effects. Examples of progestins include altrenogest and norgestomet.

15. Large doses and prolonged use increase the risk of pyometra (uterine infection) and mammary hyperplasia (overdevelopment of mammary tissue), which may predispose the animal to mammary tumors.

16. Prostaglandins lyse the corpus luteum. This terminates progesterone production and mimics the end of diestrus. Prostaglandins can be used to induce proestrus and estrus by shortening the luteal phase, or to terminate the luteal phase should the corpus luteum persist longer than normal. Because progesterone is a key hormone in maintaining pregnancy and the corpus luteum is an important source of progesterone, prostaglandin use can terminate pregnancy by decreasing progesterone concentrations.

17. Prostaglandins are well absorbed through the skin and can lyse the human corpus luteum just as they do in animals. Therefore pregnant women should handle prostaglandin drugs cautiously or avoid them totally. Asthmatics are also at risk because prostaglandins can produce bronchoconstriction.

18. A progestin or a progesterone is used to mimic the luteal phase of the estrous cycle in transitional mares. Progestins are given for several days and then withdrawn to mimic lysis of the corpus luteum and stimulate return to proestrus.

19. Progestins suppress release of FSH and LH, and therefore delay follicular development during the follicular phase of the estrous cycle.

20. Because progesterone maintains pregnancy, it seems logical that giving pro-

gestins to a mare with a history of abortion would prolong the pregnancy and allow the mare to go full term. However, this only works when the cause of abortion is hypoluteoidism (decreased levels of progesterone from a poorly functioning corpus luteum). Abortion or premature birth is often unrelated to progesterone levels; in those cases, exogenous progestins would be of little use.

21. Megestrol is a progestin that suppresses the follicular phase of the estrous cycle by suppressing FSH and LH release. In so doing, this drug prevents proestrus from progressing to estrus and the corresponding release of an ovum or ova. Megestrol can produce all of the side effects of progesterone therapy: uterine changes that could lead to pyometra, changes in mammary tissue, and delayed parturition in pregnant animals.

22. Megestrol is a progestin. Progestins decrease the effectiveness of insulin, resulting in an increase of blood glucose. Megestrol use could destabilize insulin therapy in the controlled diabetic animal.

23. Megestrol acetate is a progestin; mibolerone is similar to testosterone. They both work by essentially the same mechanism (that is, inhibition of the follicular phase by suppressing LH and FSH release). Mibolerone suppresses more of the LH release than FSH release. Because the follicular phase is suppressed, no ova are released.

24. Most "mismating" injections are estrogen compounds, the most common being estradiol cypionate. Large doses cause the folds of the oviducts to enlarge to the point where they obstruct passage of the egg to the uterus. Many mismating injections fail because the injection must be given very soon after ovulation and before the ova reach the uterus.

25. Estrogen therapy can cause pyometra, aplastic anemia (bone marrow suppression), or persistent estrual behavior. Clients must be aware of possible side effects or adverse reactions to watch for signs but also to make an informed decision whether to proceed with the estrogen treatment.

26. Progesterones can cause changes in the uterus that result in pyometra. However, estrogens such as estradiol can enhance the progesterone effect and thus increase the risk of pyometra.

27. Prostaglandins are used most often to terminate early pregnancy in cattle and mares. $PgF_{2\alpha}$ lyses the corpus luteum, terminating production of progesterone, the hormone that helps maintain pregnancy. Unlike cattle and mares, the corpus luteum of dogs and cats is usually resistant to the effects of $PgF_{2\alpha}$ until late in pregnancy. Therefore exogenous prostaglandins are not likely to terminate early pregnancies in dogs or cats.

28. No. In cattle, the placenta also produces progesterone and therefore the drop in progesterone levels produced by the prostaglandin lysis of the corpus luteum would not be as great as in species in which the corpus luteum produces the majority of progesterone.

29. Corticosteroids can induce parturition and premature birth in mares and cows late in pregnancy by mimicking the elevated cortisol levels that occur before the onset of labor.

30. This dog may have uterine inertia, in which the uterus is exhausted. The veterinarian might try to stimulate labor by injecting oxytocin, which causes the uterus to contract. Prostaglandins would have no appreciable effect on the uterus because the corpus luteum has already regressed.

31. Megestrol acetate has been used to treat inappropriate elimination in male cats and excessive self-grooming in dogs and cats. The mechanism by which the drug alters behavior is unknown.

32. Perianal adenomas and adenocarcinomas occur in older male dogs and usually shrink with estrogen therapy.

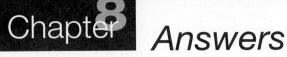

1. Although the animal appears to be comfortable while it lies undisturbed, it is likely to cry out and bite during positioning for radiography. Many sedatives do not have analgesic (pain killing) activity. This is a potentially dangerous situation because the animal appears to be without pain but can still respond to painful stimuli.

2. Barbiturates differ primarily in their duration of activity. Pentobarbital has an intermediate duration of action, whereas phenobarbital has a much longer duration of activity. Pentobarbital is given intravenously and is still used occasionally as an anesthetic; it is more often used to control seizures. Phenobarbital is used in tablet form for long-term seizure control.

3. Thiopental can produce severe inflammation or necrosis if injected perivascularly.

4. Infiltrate the site with 1 or 2 ml of procaine or lidocaine. Injection of saline or isotonic fluids around the site can also dilute the irritant effect of the barbiturate. Hot packs and massage can also be applied to the site.

5. Thiobarbiturates are slowly distributed to fatty tissue; therefore the majority of the initial dose of thiobarbiturate is distributed to well-perfused tissues such as the brain. If the dose for an obese animal is calculated by body weight, an excessive amount of the drug will go initially to the brain, resulting in an anesthetic overdose. As the drug is redistributed to the fat, the concentration in the brain decreases, resulting in an appropriate level of anesthesia. The initial dose of thiobarbiturate for obese animals should be calculated for the estimated lean body weight.

6. Bigeminy is a normal QRS wave followed by an abnormal QRS wave and indicates premature ventricular contraction caused by an ectopic focus. Bigeminy is common with many injectable anesthetic agents. Generally they spontaneously disappear within a few minutes without significant compromise of cardiac function. If ventricular arrhythmias become severe, the veterinarian can administer lidocaine intravenously.

7. Sighthounds, such as Greyhounds, Whippets, and Borzois, tend to be more sensitive to the effects of thiobarbiturates. Some veterinarians use methohexital for these breeds because it is metabolized faster than thiobarbiturates and is better tolerated.

8. Propofol can be used as a restraint for short diagnostic procedures. It has minimal analgesic activity and therefore is not a good choice for painful procedures such as manipulating fracture sites for radiographs. It is injected intravenously but does not cause tissue necrosis if injected perivascularly.

9. Telazol contains the dissociative anesthetic tiletamine as well as a benzodiazepine tranquilizer, zolazepam. Ketamine is a dissociative anesthetic similar to

tiletamine, and diazepam (Valium) is a benzodiazepine tranquilizer like zo-lazepam.

10. The eyes remain open and the corneas can dry out unless protected by a lubricant or other moisturizing agent.

11. Although it is not a controlled substance, ketamine has a high potential for abuse. Ketamine is often stolen during burglary of veterinary hospitals.

12. Dissociative anesthetics such as ketamine and tiletamine produce very poor muscle relaxation. They should not be used alone for procedures requiring retraction of muscle bodies or manipulation of joints. Although dissociative anesthetics reduce superficial pain, they do not provide sufficient control of visceral pain such as might be caused by manipulation of organs or bones.

13. Nitrous oxide produces a euphoric effect and reduces the effective dose required of more potent anesthetic gases to achieve surgical anesthesia.

14. Nitrous oxide should not be used in patients with gaseous distention of organs or cavities such as pneumothorax or even a normal rumen. The increased pressure within these areas could result in very serious complications. If nitrous oxide is used, 100% oxygen should be administered for a few minutes after cessation of nitrous oxide flow to prevent diffusion hypoxia.

15. Anesthetic induction and recovery are most rapid with isoflurane, somewhat slower with halothane, and relatively slow with methoxyflurane. An advantage of methoxyflurane is its excellent muscle-relaxing qualities.

16. Metabolism of methoxyflurane produces fluoride ions, which are nephrotoxic. Therefore methoxyflurane is contraindicated in animals receiving other nephrotoxic medications such as aminoglycoside antibiotics. It should also be used with caution in animals with impaired renal function.

17. Halothane sensitizes the heart to arrhythmias from epinephrine, which can be increased during periods of fear or stress.

18. Malignant hyperthermia is a syndrome characterized by a high body temperature. It has been associated with halothane anesthesia. Its cause is not well understood, and it is difficult to identify patients at risk. Halothane-induced malignant hyperthermia can be prevented by avoiding use of halothane.

19. Desflurane, sevoflurane, and enflurane are inhalant anesthetics with similar properties to, but are more costly than, isoflurane. They all share the qualities of a short induction and recovery period, as well as less epinephrine sensitization of the heart, as compared with halothane.

20. Acepromazine and other phenothiazine tranquilizers reduce anxiety and suppress the CRTZ that stimulates vomiting.

21. Acepromazine relaxes the penile retractor muscles in stallions, resulting in penile prolapse and possible penile injury. Penile prolapse is irreversible in some male horses.

22. Acepromazine causes the third eyelid (nictitating membrane) to extend across the eye, making an eye examination more difficult.

23. α_2 Receptors are found on neurons that release norepinephrine (an excitatory neurotransmitter). Stimulation of α_2 receptors by an α_2 agonist (stimulator) decreases norepinephrine release and therefore produces sedation. A drug that blocks the α_2 receptor site (an α_2 antagonist) would reverse the sedation caused by an α_2 agonist. Examples of α_2 agonists are xylazine, detomidine, and medetomidine. They are reversed by the α_2 antagonists yohimbine, tolazoline, and atipamezole.

24. Xylazine commonly produces vomiting in dogs and cats. Therefore xylazine should not be used with any condition in which an animal should not vomit, such as gastric torsion, bloat, or ingestion of a corrosive or caustic sub-

stance. Cattle are very sensitive to xylazine, so smaller doses are used in this species.

25. Xylazine causes vomiting in 50% of treated dogs. Corrosive substances should not be vomited up because they will further damage the esophagus.

26. Xylazine sometimes produces gastric distention from gas accumulation. This is especially true in deep-chested, large-breed dogs and can result in acute bloat and possibly gastric dilatation-volvulus, which is serious.

27. The sedative effects of xylazine and detomidine (α_2 agonists) persist long after the analgesic (pain-killing) effects have worn off. A horse that appears sedated can kick in response to painful stimuli after the analgesic effects have worn off.

28. Accidental injection into the carotid artery sends a concentrated bolus of drug directly to the brain, producing seizures or even sudden death.

29. The pulse may be somewhat stronger, reflecting vasoconstriction, followed by a drop in heart rate and a return of the pulse pressure to near normal. Within a few minutes the horse has bradycardia, but the pulse strength is near normal or slightly less than normal.

30. First-degree or second-degree AV block is not uncommon with larger doses of xylazine. This parasympathetic effect can be reversed by drugs that block the parasympathetic nervous system, such as atropine or glycopyrrolate (cholinergic receptor antagonists).

31. The doctor is most likely to use yohimbine (Yobine) to reverse the effects of xylazine. Ruminants are very sensitive to xylazine and should receive only small doses.

32. Oxymorphone is a much more potent analgesic than xylazine. For visceral pain (pain from organs, sensitive membranes lining organs, or bone pain), xylazine is much less effective than oxymorphone. A small dose of oxymorphone would probably be safe in a cat, but there is always the risk of "morphine mania" in cats receiving narcotics.

33. The statement comparing the analgesic activity of κ and σ agonism is true; however, most of the analgesia of opioids is produced by stimulation of μ receptors, and there is no mention about this in the brochure. Although this analgesic drug might be fairly weak because of the kappa receptor mechanism, it probably does not depress the respiratory system to any significant degree; the statement about fewer respiratory side effects is probably true. Analgesics with strong μ and κ receptor activity and minimal σ activity are preferred.

34. Many opioids make animals more sensitive to sounds or other stimuli. Therefore it is best to reduce auditory, visual, and tactile stimulation in these patients.

35. Butorphanol is used to control coughing (Torbutrol) and as an injectable analgesic (Torbugesic). Smaller doses are used for cough suppression; large doses produce a potent analgesic effect.

36. Butorphanol and nalorphine are partial narcotic agonists and antagonists because they reverse the effects (antagonistic activity) of potent narcotics (such as oxymorphone), but exert a narcotic effect of their own (partial agonist activity). These drugs are used for low-level analgesia or to partially reverse the sedative effects of oxymorphone while still maintaining some degree of pain relief.

37. Large doses of opioids can produce hallucinogenic effects in cats. If used in small doses, there are several narcotic drugs that seem to be fairly safe for use in cats, including meperidine (Demerol), oxymorphone, and buprenorphine (Buprenex).

38. A neuroleptanalgesic is a tranquilizer combined with a narcotic (opioid). Phenothiazine tranquilizers are often used with a potent narcotic because the tran-

quilizer's antiemetic effect controls the vomiting that opioids often produce. Innovar-Vet is an example of a neuroleptanalgesic.

39. The drug of choice for controlling status epilepticus is IV diazepam (Valium). IV pentobarbital or phenobarbital may also be used to control prolonged seizures. Diazepam given intravenously is metabolized very quickly and therefore has a short duration of effect. Because of diazepam's short duration, injectable barbiturates are sometimes used instead. Much of an oral dose of diazepam is removed by the first-pass effect, negating diazepam's use when given orally in dogs. For long-term control of seizures, oral phenobarbital is the drug of choice.

40. Phenobarbital induces hepatic enzyme formation, which speeds phenobarbital metabolism. As the body becomes more efficient at removing the drug, phenobarbital concentrations may decline below the therapeutic range, resulting in recurrence of seizures.

41. Primidone is metabolized to phenobarbital (and other compounds with weak anticonvulsant activity). Because the phenobarbital component of primidone exerts the majority of the anticonvulsant activity, it is more practical to use just phenobarbital. In addition, primidone may cause drug-induced hepatopathy, a fatal liver condition.

42. This dog is supposed to receive 60 mg 3 times a day (every 8 hours). Using the 0.5 grain tablets, 2 tablets = 2 × 0.5 grain = 1 grain = 60 mg. The label instructions are correct.

43. Animals treated with phenobarbital commonly have increased serum alkaline phosphatase activity, especially soon after therapy is initiated. As long as the other liver enzymes are not markedly elevated, it is unlikely that the increase of serum alkaline phosphatase alone indicates liver disease. In drug-induced hepatopathy, activity of all liver enzymes is markedly increased and there is often severe icterus (jaundice).

44. Phenytoin (Dilantin) was commonly used in human medicine but is relatively ineffective in dogs because the canine liver quickly removes the drug and it is difficult to keep drug concentrations within the normal therapeutic range.

45. Potassium bromide (KBr) is used in conjunction with phenobarbital in those animals that are refractory (continue to have seizures) to phenobarbital alone. Vomiting, diarrhea, and sedation are the primary side effects of KBr.

46. Inhibition of the CNS produces sedation. A disinhibitor "takes the brakes off" the CNS. This decreased suppression of excitatory responses allows increased CNS stimulation.

47. Theobromine is an ingredient of chocolate and is the toxic agent in chocolate toxicosis.

48. A single chocolate bar is unlikely to harm this large dog. Milk chocolate generally has a low concentration of theobromine. Ingesting large quantities of chocolate typically produces vomiting but little CNS stimulation. Baking chocolate, however, contains much more theobromine and poses a greater risk to dogs.

49. Doxapram (Dopram) is used to simulate breathing.

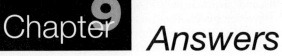

Chapter 9 Answers

1. The suffix *-cidal* indicates that the drug kills; *-static* indicates that the drug retards multiplication to keep the microbial population constant. A bacteriostatic drug requires a functional immune system to help eliminate bacteria; therefore a bactericidal drug is preferred in immunocompromised patients.

2. What is the MIC for each drug in different bacterial populations? In other words, what is the therapeutic range? Concentrations of 50 µg/ml are good if the therapeutic range is 20 to 60 µg/ml, but inadequate if the therapeutic range is 80 to 100 µg/ml. Because therapeutic ranges for antimicrobials vary among bacterial species, you cannot generalize about a drug's effectiveness without referring to specific types of bacteria.

3. The most susceptible bacteria die when exposed to low concentrations of the antibiotic. Therefore if low dosages are used or the drug is administered for only a few days, the susceptible bacteria die, leaving the most resistant bacteria to reproduce. With less competition for resources, these resistant bacteria multiply rapidly, and the previously effective antibiotic may be ineffective against these bacteria.

4. Most antibiotics are *not* broken down sufficiently by pasteurization of milk or by normal cooking of meat or egg products. Even low levels of antibiotics can produce allergic reactions or hypersensitivity reactions in people who are especially sensitive to certain antibiotics, such as penicillins. Exposure to low levels of antibiotics selects for more resistant bacteria, as explained in answer 3.

5. Penicillins are drugs that kill bacteria by interfering with cell wall formation. New wall formation only occurs when the bacteria divide. Therefore bacteria that are not actively dividing are not forming cell walls and hence these drugs cannot exert their effect.

6. Some antifungal agents (and antineoplastic drugs) do affect mammalian DNA or RNA as well as the bacterial DNA. However, more modern drugs, such as quinolones, act on specific enzymes found only in bacteria, sparing the DNA found in the cells of domestic animals.

7. Although penicillins are quite safe, they can produce a potentially severe allergic reaction in people or animals hypersensitive to these drugs. They can also alter the normal intestinal flora (bacteria) of some small mammals and exotic pets, resulting in severe and sometimes fatal diarrhea.

8. Tetracycline is often used at bacteriostatic concentrations. Penicillins require an actively dividing bacterial population to kill the bacteria by preventing bacterial cell wall formation. If tetracycline is used first, it halts bacterial multiplication, thus preventing the penicillins from exerting their effect.

9. It should be rephrased, "Bacteriostatic antibiotics should not be used with antibiotics that require actively dividing bacterial populations to exert their effect."

Thus penicillins, cephalosporins, and bacitracin should not be used in conjunction with bacteriostatic drugs. However, many other bactericidal drugs, such as aminoglycosides, kill bacteria, regardless of whether they are actively dividing. Therefore some bactericidal and bacteriostatic drugs *can* be used together.

10. If an animal reacts to one type of penicillin, it is likely to react to other penicillins. Reactions are less notable with oral penicillins. However, as a general rule, any adverse reaction to a penicillin should be considered an allergic reaction, and administration of any penicillin drug should be avoided thereafter to prevent anaphylaxis.

11. Staphylococcus bacteria and some other strains of bacteria secrete an enzyme (β-lactamase) that destroys the β-lactam ring of the penicillin molecule, rendering the antibiotic ineffective.

12. The *-oxacillins* (oxacillin, cloxacillin, dicloxacillin) are commonly used in food animals for treatment of conditions such as mastitis, where β-lactamase-producing bacteria are often found. A disadvantage is that oxacillins have a narrow spectrum of antibacterial activity, and they are ineffective against many bacteria that are susceptible to amoxicillin or penicillin G.

13. Clavulanate (clavulanic acid) and sulbactam are added to penicillins so that bacterial β-lactamase will attack the clavulanate molecule instead of the penicillin. These tablets are individually wrapped because these drugs absorb water from the environment and become somewhat soft.

14. Penicillin G is inactivated by gastric acid and thus would be useless if given by mouth. In this situation, you could use a penicillin formulated for oral use.

15. Hetacillin is metabolized to ampicillin.

16. The later the generation of cephalosporin, the more effective the drug is against gram-negative bacteria. First-generation cephalosporins are available in oral dosage forms; nearly all third-generation cephalosporins are injectables. Thus first-generation cephalosporins (oral forms) are usually dispensed to clients.

17. All three are enzymes produced by bacteria. β-Lactamase attacks the β-lactam ring of penicillins and cephalosporins. Penicillinase attacks penicillins, and cephalosporinase attacks cephalosporins.

18. Because bacitracin is used topically (on the skin), very little is absorbed and little reaches the kidneys to produce a toxic effect.

19. Puncture wounds are usually anaerobic. Aminoglycosides are taken up by bacteria in a process that is oxygen dependent. Therefore if oxygen is not present, aminoglycosides are not taken up by the bacteria.

20. Amikacin and the other aminoglycosides block protein production within the bacteria. This is not dependent on active division of the bacteria; therefore aminoglycosides are still effective if a bacteriostatic drug has been used first.

21. The kidneys (nephrotoxicity) and inner ear (ototoxicity).

22. Ulcerated or denuded skin, which is open to dermal or subcutaneous tissue, such as occurs with "road burn" abrasions or other open wounds, may absorb topically applied drugs much better than areas of intact skin. Systemic levels of the drug can become significant with frequent applications or application of concentrated solutions to areas of denuded skin.

23. Because older animals are more likely to have compromised renal function and because aminoglycosides are excreted exclusively by the kidneys, older animals need more time to eliminate a dose of aminoglycosides than a younger animal with normal renal function. The extended dosage interval maintains the same relative peak concentration of aminoglycoside while providing more time for drug concentrations to fall to a safe level (slower elimination because of decreased renal function). Animals with decreased liver (hepatic) function may

not need a reduced dose because the liver is not involved with elimination of aminoglycosides.

24. Ototoxicity is indicated by deafness or loss of balance (falling over, staggering, and nystagmus).

25. Aminoglycosides combine with nucleic acids as part of their normal bactericidal function. Pus and cellular debris contains many lysed cells with nucleic acids to which the aminoglycosides bind. If they bind to the cellular debris, the drug will not be taken up by the bacteria.

26. Perform a urinalysis to check for increased levels of protein and cellular casts in the sediment. These are found long before the blood urea nitrogen (BUN) or serum creatinine levels increase or the urine-specific gravity becomes "fixed."

27. Quinolone drugs attack the enzyme DNA gyrase, which is essential to DNA function. Because this enzyme is significantly different from mammalian DNA gyrase, quinolones have been formulated to attach only to the bacterial form, thus sparing the mammalian DNA function.

28. Most drugs cannot penetrate the prostate gland. Enrofloxacin (Baytril) is one of the few that can achieve therapeutic concentrations within the prostate.

29. Because large doses of quinolones produce degenerative lesions in joint cartilage of actively growing animals, enrofloxacin is contraindicated in small-breed and medium-breed dogs between 2 and 8 months of age. In large-breed and giant-breed dogs, this growth period can extend 1 year or longer.

30. The rapid cartilage and bone growth phase begins somewhere around 2 months of age. Thus quinolones may be used before that time in very young animals. However, for many infections, enrofloxacin should not be routinely used as the first drug of choice when there are many other more common antibiotics that will be equally as effective.

31. The more often a drug is used, the greater the risk for development of resistant bacterial strains. Because drugs like amoxicillin, tetracycline, or potentiated sulfonamides are still effective against common infections, they should be used instead of enrofloxacin. Enrofloxacin should be reserved for use in infections that do not respond to the more common antibacterials.

32. With approval of new fluoroquinolones like sarafloxacin, the regulatory agencies will increase their restriction on the extra-label use of other quinolones in food animals.

33. Any tetracycline is effective in treating these diseases. The aminopenicillins amoxicillin and ampicillin are also effective.

34. The human products (doxycycline, minocycline) cost more, but they penetrate body tissues more effectively than the older tetracyclines. Doxycycline and minocycline have greater spectra of antibacterial activity than oxytetracycline or tetracycline. They also produce less chelating of divalent ions in the gut when given by mouth.

35. Tetracycline and oxytetracycline chelate calcium and magnesium ions. Tetracycline that chelates with the calcium in milk is not absorbed.

36. Water-soluble tetracyclines (oxytetracycline, tetracycline) combine with bone or developing tooth enamel and stain them brownish yellow and decrease the strength of tooth enamel. Tooth discoloration would be a significant blemish in show animals. Large doses of these tetracyclines can impair bone growth to some degree.

37. Tetracyclines eliminate the normal bowel flora (nonpathogenic), allowing the more pathogenic bacteria to proliferate. This leads to enteritis and diarrhea.

38. If stored too long, tetracycline can break down to a compound with nephrotoxic effects, resulting in Fanconi syndrome.

39. By themselves and at normal dosages, sulfonamides are bacteriostatic. However, if used with trimethoprim or ormetoprim, they become bactericidal because they work at two different metabolic pathway sites in bacteria.

40. Enteric sulfas are formulated to work within the bowel lumen and are not absorbed to any large extent. Systemic sulfas are formulated to be absorbed into the systemic circulation.

41. Like the penicillins, many of the sulfas are actively secreted into the forming urine in the kidneys, producing high drug concentrations in the urine. These high drug concentrations in the urine can often eliminate cystitis, or bacterial infections in the bladder.

42. Because sulfa drugs attain high concentrations in the urine in the kidneys, dehydration may cause the drug to precipitate, forming crystals in the kidneys that can block urine flow. This problem is common with older sulfonamides.

43. Keratoconjunctivitis sicca ("dry eye") is caused by lack of tear production. Early signs include pawing at the eye, irritation, accumulation of matter around the eyes, or a loss of the normal glossy "shine" to the surface of the eye. Keratoconjunctivitis related to sulfonamide use can sometimes be reversed by stopping use of the drug. If normal tear function does not return, application of cyclosporine ophthalmic ointment can stimulate tear production.

44. Some cats with toxoplasmosis die after treatment with clindamycin. More study is needed to better define this problem.

45. Oral erythromycin causes severe and possibly fatal diarrhea if given orally to adult horses and ruminants. Oral tylosin is contraindicated in adult horses for the same reason. However, injectable erythromycin can be given to adult ruminants for treatment of respiratory infections.

46. Horses, swine, and nonhuman primates are sensitive to the cardiotoxic (heart toxicity) effects of tilmicosin. Because of the cardiac effects (tachycardia, arrhythmias) on nonhuman primates, the package insert recommends contacting a physician if accidental injection occurs. There have been several incidents of accidental injections, but none has produced any severe reactions.

47. Metronidazole (Flagyl) is effective in these cases.

48. Nitrofurans are rapidly excreted by the kidneys before they attain significant concentrations in tissues. They achieve high concentrations in the urine and thus can exert an antimicrobial effect on bacteria in the bladder.

49. In the past, chloramphenicol was commonly used because of its ability to penetrate tissues well. However, chloramphenicol use can cause fatal aplastic anemia. For this reason, chloramphenicol is banned in food-producing animals. Florfenicol, a recently introduced drug that is related to chloramphenicol, is approved for use in beef cattle to treat respiratory disease.

50. Rifampin is used with or without erythromycin to treat *Corynebacterium equi* infections in young foals. A side effect is discoloration of body secretions and urine to a reddish orange color that can resemble dilute blood.

51. Most dogs treated with amphotericin B sustain some renal damage. Although IV fluid therapy can reduce the renal insult, the results are not consistent and many animals still suffer from some degree of nephrotoxicosis.

52. Ketoconazole and itraconazole have fewer side effects than amphotericin B and nystatin, but their onset of action is usually delayed 5 to 10 days. Use of these drugs should be avoided in pregnant animals, if possible, but the ketoconazole and itraconazole are *not* contraindicated in pregnant animals.

53. Griseofulvin (Fulvicin) is a common treatment for dermatophytes (fungi) that cause ringworm. Cats are slow to metabolize this drug, and defects in fetuses have frequently been reported in cats treated with this drug while pregnant.

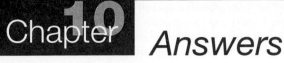

1. A compound that is strong enough to kill viruses on the floor of a dog run may be too strong to use on skin as a presurgical scrub. *Disinfectants* are formulated for use on inanimate objects, whereas *antiseptics* are for use on living tissue. You should ask about the spectrum of antimicrobial activity, including effectiveness against spores, protozoa, fungi, and the types of viruses.

2. By definition, a germicide kills "germs;" however, "germs" are undefined. Without more specific information, one cannot tell if this product is virucidal, bactericidal, or exactly what its properties consist of.

3. You should learn what effect this product has on living tissue. Hydrochloric acid is cheap and effective against almost all microorganisms, but it cannot be safely used as an antiseptic. The potential of an antiseptic to damage tissue must be considered along with its antimicrobial activity.

4. This would waste a lot of disinfectant. Many disinfectants are inactivated by fecal material or organic matter. A disinfectant cannot exert its antimicrobial effect until after this material has been removed. Therefore it would be more economical to remove the organic material first by hosing down the run and then applying the disinfectant.

5. Iodine is largely inactivated by organic material, including dirt, skin debris, and skin oils. The first and second scrubs remove the organic material, and the final scrub disinfects.

6. Viruses with a lipid envelope (enveloped viruses) are fairly easy to destroy with many disinfectants. However, naked or unenveloped viruses are more resistant to the effects of disinfectants and more difficult to inactivate. A particular virucidal compound may only kill certain types of viruses and leave the other viruses intact.

7. Disinfectants or antiseptics stored for extended periods are likely to lose some efficacy, although this can vary considerably among compounds. An additional concern is potential neurotoxic effects from repeated exposure to this particular antiseptic, hexachlorophene. Although used extensively in the past, hexachlorophene is now used less commonly than other antiseptics because of the risk of toxicity.

8. No, they are different compounds. Chlorhexidine is a guanidine found in many antiseptics such as Nolvasan. It does not have the neurotoxic potential of hexachlorophene (a phenol).

9. Although the alcohol is a good antiseptic, it denatures (alters the structure of) protein and may form a protective coagulum over the wound, preventing antiseptics from reaching the bacteria in underlying tissue. Another antiseptic such as povidone-iodine would be more effectively used.

10. No. Alcohol does not penetrate fecal material very well; microorganisms in the fecal material remaining on the thermometer are likely to be unaffected by the

alcohol. In addition, alcohol is not very effective against unenveloped viruses, and these viruses could survive immersion in alcohol.

11. Benzalkonium chloride is a quaternary ammonium compound. It has good antibacterial activity against gram-negative and gram-positive bacteria, but is largely ineffective against spores, fungi, and unenveloped viruses.

12. One of the first things to consider is inadequate rinsing of disinfectant cleaning solutions from the run surface. Strong disinfectants can irritate skin, causing contact dermatitis. Make sure the runs are thoroughly rinsed of disinfecting compounds.

13. Chlorines can corrode metal.

14. Chlorine vapors are very irritating to the mucous membranes and eyes. Personnel and animals in a poorly ventilated area that has been disinfected with chlorine may develop respiratory and ocular irritation.

15. Color-fast bleach typically is composed of concentrated hydrogen peroxide, which is generally a poor disinfectant.

16. Iodophor scrubs usually contain soap for removing dirt and debris from the skin. That soap can be irritating if placed within a wound. An iodophor solution is more appropriate for use in an open wound.

17. The free iodine in iodine solutions (often called "iodine-based" products) is quickly used up when placed at the antiseptic site. In an iodophor, the iodine is combined with a carrier that allows the free iodine to slowly leach into the application area over time.

18. Chlorhexidine is more inactivated by fecal material and organic debris than are chlorine and iodine, but chlorhexidine is more effective than these compounds after a thorough cleansing of the application area.

19. Chlorhexidine forms a precipitate when mixed with "hard" water containing mineral salts, such as saline (sodium chloride solution). This reduces the effectiveness of chlorhexidine. Distilled water contains no salts and is a more appropriate diluent.

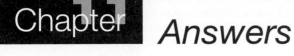
1. *Selective toxicity* usually refers to the drug's selective nature to kill the parasite, with minimal toxic effect on the host animal.

2. As a rule of thumb, all antiparasitic drugs should be used with caution in very young, old, debilitated, weakened, and pregnant animals. Neonates are very sensitive to even "safe" compounds because they have much less ability to metabolize compounds than mature animals. Although it is always a good idea to check with the doctor first, the client should be advised to avoid using insecticides on very young kittens.

3. The client has probably observed tapeworm segments, for which an anticestodal drug must be used. The hookworm medication previously dispensed would most likely not be effective against tapeworms. Many antinematodal drugs (drugs for "round" worms such as ascarids and hookworms) are not effective against cestodes (tapeworms). The hookworm infection has probably been eliminated, but the medication was not intended to work against the tapeworm infection.

4. Anticestodals are effective against some types of tapeworms. Antinematodals are effective against some types of roundworms. Antitrematodals are effective against some types of flukes. This general information does not specifically state against which parasites the drug is effective.

5. Vermifuges cause the animal to expel live worms. They are most frequently used with roundworm infections. The client should expect to see live worms in the animal's stool. In puppies with large numbers of roundworms, this can be quite upsetting to clients if they have not been forewarned.

6. One of the most common over-the-counter puppy dewormers is piperazine. It is very safe and fairly effective against ascarids and related roundworms, but it has no effect on hookworms, whipworms, tapeworms, or coccidia, some of which are usually found in young puppies. Therefore clients may have a false sense of security because they administered the piperazine (a vermifuge) and saw worms pass in the stool. However, the puppy could still be infected with other types of parasites.

7. Most benzimidazoles are very effective against nematodes. Although some benzimidazoles (mebendazole and fenbendazole) have activity against a limited range of cestodes, you would need to see the specifications on the new compound to see if it shares a similar anticestodal quality.

8. Ivermectin paralyzes the nervous system of parasites by enhancing the inhibiting effects of glutamate and GABA neurotransmitters. (It depresses the nervous system).

9. The ivermectin will kill many types of parasites, including *Onchocerca* organisms. The microfilariae of *Onchocerca* organisms migrate in the dermis and,

when killed by the ivermectin, can produce an inflammatory reaction. The signs subside fairly quickly with administration of corticosteroids.

10. The effect of pyrantel pamoate mimics that of acetylcholine, the neurotransmitter whose action is also enhanced by exposure to organophosphate or carbamate insecticides. Using pyrantel and organophosphates together can cause nicotinic CNS signs such as tremors and shaking, followed by paralysis.

11. Although both praziquantel (Droncit) and epsiprantel (Cestex) are effective against *Taenia* and *Dipylidium* tapeworms, only praziquantel is listed as effective against *Echinococcus* tapeworms.

12. Most modern anticestodals kill the tapeworms; the dead worms are digested and are not evident in the stool.

13. The microfilariae circulating in the blood of dogs infected with heartworm are not infective until after they have undergone the required molts within a mosquito. Thus even a transfusion of blood from a dog with circulating microfilaria is not likely to result in development of adult heartworms in the animal receiving the blood.

14. Both thiacetarsamide (Caparsolate) and melarsomine (Immiticide) are arsenical compounds. In fact, the antidote for an overdose of melarsomine is BAL, a common antidote for arsenic poisonings. The client has some cause for concern; however, you should assure the client that the doctor is aware of the side effects and that these drugs are generally safe when used at the dosages required for heartworm treatment.

15. Melarsomine can be given by deep IM injection, whereas thiacetarsamide must be given by IV injection and can cause tissue sloughing if injected perivascularly. In addition, melarsomine seems to have less of an adverse effect on the liver than thiacetarsamide. Melarsomine is given only twice, whereas 4 doses of thiacetarsamide are required.

16. As the adult heartworms die and decompose within the heart, parts of the dead worms (emboli) pass from the heart through the pulmonary artery to the lungs, where they can lodge in small capillaries and produce a significant inflammatory reaction. During this time, the animal must be kept calm to reduce "showering" of the lungs with emboli. Aspirin and glucocorticoids are sometimes given to decrease inflammation and reduce blood clot formation in the lungs.

17. Ivermectin, often in the liquid injectable form (Ivomec), is commonly used to eliminate microfilariae. Milbemycin (Interceptor) may also be used as a microfilaricidal agent.

18. Animals with caval syndrome, in which the heartworms are backed up all the way into the vena cavae, are often severely affected by degeneration of large numbers of dead heartworms. Dogs with severe heartworm disease usually require surgical removal of some of the adult worms.

19. The problem seems to be a breed-specific difference in permeability of the blood-brain barrier to ivermectin. In Collies, the blood-brain barrier is somewhat permeable to ivermectin, allowing the drug to pass to enter the brain to reach receptor sites in the brain.

20. Ivermectin inhibits the CNS, causing CNS depression: sedation leading to coma, ataxia progressing to full loss of motor control, and loss of vision and visual reflexes. Respiration is often depressed, and bradycardia may be present. There is no antidote and the only treatment is supportive care.

21. The effects of ivermectin toxicosis can persist for days or weeks. In that time, body functions must be maintained, which entails considerable nursing care.

22. The dose of Heartgard-30 used for heartworm prevention is only 0.006 mg/kg, compared with the microfilaricidal dosage of 0.05 mg/kg that is more likely to produce toxicosis in Collies. Even so, the manufacturer of Heartgard 30 recom-

mends observing Collies and Collie-crossbreeds for signs of adverse reaction after administration of Heartgard.

23. The drugs differ very little. In fact, their chemical structures share many similarities. Although the respective manufacturers say there are significant differences (perhaps for competitive reasons), from a clinical standpoint these drugs have virtually identical effects and uses.

24. Although coccidia are protozoa and not bacteria, sulfonamides are very effective against many coccidia.

25. Some insecticidal sprays formulated for dogs and cats may be safely used on livestock with regard to the animal's health; however, there is always the concern over contamination of the human food supply. In addition, use of insecticidal sprays for livestock would be prohibitively expensive because of the large volume of spray needed.

26. Lindane is a chlorinated hydrocarbon like DDT. It persists in the environment and can become a long-term environmental contaminant. Lindane is poorly metabolized by cats and therefore should never be used on them.

27. Chlorpyrifos is an organophosphate. Signs of intoxication include salivation, lacrimation, urination, defecation and diarrhea, dyspnea, and emesis (SLUDDE), with miosis (pinpoint pupils). Chlorpyrifos may also cause trembling, ataxia, and mydriasis (dilated pupils). Atropine is used to counteract the SLUDDE signs. Pralidoxime is also used to help regenerate the acetylcholinesterase that is inactivated by the organophosphate.

28. If a compound stimulates the muscarinic receptors (muscarinic agonist effect), the animal will show parasympathetic nervous system stimulation signs (SLUDDE). Organophosphates and carbamates enhance the parasympathetic nervous system effects on the body by blocking the enzyme that normally breaks down the neurotransmitter acetylcholine. In blocking the acetylcholinesterase enzyme, the acetylcholine acts longer, enhancing the effect of acetylcholine on its receptor.

29. Atropine does not reverse the bond between acetylcholinesterase and the organophosphate molecule; thus atropine does not really "fix" the problem. Atropine only blocks the muscarinic acetylcholine receptors so that acetylcholine cannot produce its effect. Atropine decreases parasympathetic stimulation, evident as a resolution of SLUDDE signs. Because the problem is not "fixed," however, clinical signs return when the atropine wears off. Pralidoxime *does* break apart the organophosphate from the acetylcholinesterase, liberating the enzyme so it can function again.

30. Pyrethrins and pyrethroids, including allethrin, are usually very safe. Advise the client to carefully follow label instructions and use only a small amount of spray.

31. Fish readily absorb pyrethrins from water. Unless precautions are taken to prevent the fogger mist from getting into the fish tanks, the fish are likely to die.

32. Amitraz was originally formulated as a dip for treating demodectic mange.

33. Amitraz is a very potent toxin when ingested. There are reports of severe toxicity resulting from accidental ingestion of amitraz flea collars. The owner should bring the animal to the clinic immediately so the doctor can induce vomiting and possibly use yohimbine as a reversal agent.

34. Insect growth regulators and insect development inhibitors interrupt the life cycle of the insect (for example, a flea). Because they emulate natural hormones or compounds found only in fleas and not in mammals, they are considered very safe to use in households. Although they interrupt the life cycle, they do not kill adult fleas. Therefore many of these compounds must be used in conjunction with traditional insecticides.

Answers

1. Eicosanoids are compounds involved with the inflammatory process. An eicosanoid antagonist would likely be used as an antiinflammatory agent.

2. Mineralocorticoids affect the balance of electrolytes such as sodium and potassium in the body. Glucocorticoids such as prednisone have antiinflammatory effects. Unless you need mineralocorticoids, you should not order these tablets instead of prednisone.

3. Exogenous glucocorticoids inhibit pituitary release of ACTH, which normally stimulates the adrenal cortex function. Lack of ACTH stimulation causes the adrenal cortex to atrophy (shrink) to some degree.

4. Betamethasone is a very potent, long-acting corticosteroid that has biologic activity for several days; cortisone is far less potent and has a much shorter effect (24 hours or less). After absorption through the skin, the potent, long-acting corticosteroids are more likely to exert a systemic effect than less-potent, shorter-acting corticosteroids.

5. Dexamethasone sodium phosphate is an aqueous (water) solution of dexamethasone that is given in large IV doses to fight shock. Dexamethasone is available as an alcohol or other nonaqueous solution and should not be injected intravenously.

6. Prednisolone diacetate is a suspension; suspensions should not be given intravenously.

7. Dexamethasone valerate is a suspension. The crystals in some suspensions may be altered when exposed to extremes in temperature or very rough handling. This change in crystal characteristics can result in irregular absorption of an injectable suspension or pain on injection.

8. Glucocorticoids usually inhibit fibroblasts, which are involved in wound healing. Fibroblasts are also involved with scar formation, so when excessive scar formation would be undesirable, glucocorticoids are sometimes used to minimize scarring.

9. Glucocorticoids tend to suppress the immune response but do not significantly affect antibody formation. Vaccination should still produce adequate immunity. However, some manufacturers of modified-live vaccines do not recommend vaccination of animals receiving glucocorticoids because of possible replication of the virus in the animal.

10. Both groups of drugs inhibit prostaglandin production in the stomach and other tissues. Prostaglandins help protect the stomach lining from the hydrochloric acid secreted by the stomach. Glucocorticoids and NSAIDs interfere with this normal defense mechanism against gastric acid, allowing an ulcer to form. Glucocorticoids also increase gastric acid production to some extent, making an ulcer more likely to form.

11. The CBC would likely show neutrophilia (increased), lymphopenia (decreased), and monocytopenia (decreased). This is the same pattern observed with a "stress leukogram" in which endogenous glucocorticoids are elevated.

12. Glucocorticoids are catabolic and favor the breakdown of tissues and protein. Anabolic steroids have the opposite effect and favor tissue (muscle) development, which is the reason they are sometimes used (illegally) by athletes.

13. The muscle wasting produced by corticosteroids causes the abdominal muscles to become weakened and thin. This loss of muscle tone makes the abdomen more pendulous.

14. Application of corticosteroids to an eye with a corneal ulcer can cause the ulcer to deepen and perhaps even perforate into the anterior chamber. Accidental dispensing of an ophthalmic product containing corticosteroids for a patient with a corneal ulcer would be grounds for a malpractice suit.

15. Corticosteroids can induce parturition, resulting in a premature birth or abortion in mares and females of some other domestic species.

16. Addison's disease is another name for hypoadrenocorticism. Cushing's syndrome is another name for hyperadrenocorticism. An easy way to remember this is that Addison begins with a vowel and *hypo* ends in a vowel; Cushing begins in a consonant and *hyper* ends in a consonant.

17. As explained in answer 3, prolonged administration of glucocorticoids causes adrenocortical atrophy. If glucocorticoid administration were to be stopped immediately, the atrophied adrenal cortex would not be able to produce adequate amounts of cortisol and the animal would slip into a state of hypoadrenocorticism, which can be fatal. By gradually reducing the dose of glucocorticoids, the adrenal glands are allowed time to return to their fully functioning state. This may take up to 6 months.

18. NSAIDs are highly bound to blood proteins such as albumin. If blood albumin levels are lower than normal, more of the drug dose will be nonprotein bound and free to enter tissues from the blood. Thus more drug reaches the target sites. This could produce toxicity. Therefore the dose should be decreased slightly to compensate for this effect.

19. The GI tract and kidneys are most likely to be adversely affected, with ulcers and renal papillary insufficiency.

20. No. NSAIDs do not damage the kidneys unless blood pressure or blood volume is decreased. In those situations, they block the protective mechanism by which the kidneys maintain adequate blood flow to the renal tissues. The decreased blood flow deprives the kidneys of adequate oxygen, resulting in cell death and a condition called *renal papillary necrosis.*

21. Horses seem to be resistant to the GI side effects of NSAIDs. However, dogs and cats are much more sensitive to the ulcerogenic (ulcer-causing) effects of these drugs.

22. If inadvertently injected into the carotid artery, phenylbutazone produces severe CNS stimulation, including seizures and collapse. If the drug is injected outside the vein, it can cause severe irritation of perivascular tissues and may even result in sloughing of those tissues.

23. Aspirin is probably the safest NSAID to use in cats. However, the drug should be given only every 2 to 3 days. Cats do not tolerate NSAIDs very well because they are less efficient than other species in conjugating them in the liver, which slows drug elimination.

24. One aspect of dilative cardiomyopathy is excessive clot formation. Aspirin usually retards clot formation.

25. All three of these drugs belong to the same class of NSAIDs that can cause severe gastric ulceration in dogs. Therefore aspirin is a better choice.

26. Flunixin meglumine, a potent NSAID, is well tolerated in horses but easily produces gastric and duodenal bleeding and ulceration in dogs.

27. Dimethyl sulfoxide is rapidly absorbed through the skin and can carry skin contaminants, including bacterial toxins, into the body. The veterinary technician should always wear latex gloves when applying the drug to patients.

28. Mast-cell tumors are aggregates of the cells that produce histamine and other mediators of inflammation. Dimethyl sulfoxide causes these cells to spontaneously release their inflammatory mediators, resulting in a severe adverse reaction.

29. Industrial-grade dimethyl sulfoxide may contain contaminants such as benzene or formalin. These compounds can be carried into the body as the dimethyl sulfoxide penetrates the skin. Only medical-grade dimethyl sulfoxide solution should be used on patients.

30. Acetaminophen is not an antiinflammatory drug, and therefore does not reduce inflammation. Acetaminophen decreases pain perception and reduces fever. It is less likely to produce stomach upset because it does not block prostaglandins as do NSAIDs.

31. Metabolism of acetaminophen yields a toxic intermediate metabolite that, in most mammals, is quickly metabolized to a nontoxic final metabolite. Cats have limited capacity to conjugate this toxic metabolite with glutathione, so the toxic metabolite accumulates and causes toxicity. Conversion of hemoglobin to methemoglobin discolors the blood to a dark "chocolate" color, causing the mucous membranes of affected cats to turn dark. Often the urine is darkened by the methemoglobinuria.

32. Tell the client not to give this medication to his cat. Phenacetin is metabolized to acetaminophen, which can cause toxicity in cats. Such "cold" preparations often contain several different ingredients (for cough, stuffy noses, sore throat, and other symptoms), any of which may be harmful to animals.

33. Carprofen is selective for inhibition of cyclooxygenase-2 enzyme while having less inhibition of cyclooxygenase-1. This decreases the inflammation while preserving the normal protective functions of the prostaglandins in the GI tract and kidneys.

Index

A

Abbreviations used in prescriptions, 13
Absolute refractory period, 106
Absorption
    distribution, metabolism, excretion (ADME), 39
    effect of route of administration on, 39-40
ACE; *see* Angiotensin-converting enzyme
ACE inhibitors; *see* Angiotensin-converting inhibitors
Acepromazine (PromAce), 79, 80, 81, 89, 110, 152, 177-178, 183, 184
Acetaminophen (Tylenol), 132, 285-286
Acetate, 276
Acetazolamide, 122
Acetic acid, 243
Acetonide, 276
Acetylcholine, 76, 108, 114, 134, 187, 252
Acetylcholinesterase, 91, 134, 252, 260
Acetylcysteine (Mucomyst), 132, 286
Acetylsalicylic acid, 42, 122, 281-282
Acid blockers, 90
Acidic drug versus alkaline drug, 42, 43
Acidosis, 170
ACTH; *see* Adrenocorticotropic hormone
Activated charcoal, 81, 86-87
Active transport, 36
Addison's disease, 278
Adenocarcinoma, perianal, 160, 164
Adenoma, perianal, 160, 164
Adenosine triphosphate (ATP), 103
ADME; *see* Absorption, distribution, metabolism, excretion
Administration of drugs, 32-35
Adrenaline, 107, 136

Adrenergic agonists, 107
Adrenergic antagonists, 107, 108
Adrenergic drugs, 113
Adrenergic receptors, 107
Adrenocorticotropic hormone (ACTH), 155, 274-275
Adsorbents, antidiarrheals and, 86-87
Adult animals, effect of drugs on, 63
Adulticide, 254
Advantage; *see* Imidacloprid
Adverse reactions, 7
Advil; *see* Ibuprofen
Aerobic bacteria, 211
Aerophagia, 123, 179
Aerosol administration of drugs, 34
AErrane; *see* Isoflurane
Age differences, biotransformation and, 62, 63
Agonists, 57-60
Albendazole, 249, 258
Albon; *see* Sulfadimethoxine
Albumin, 53
Albuterol, 136
Alcohol, 61-62, 236, 239-240
Alcohol solutions of glucocorticoids, 276
Aldosterone, 117, 119, 121
Aleve; *see* Naproxen
Alkaline drug versus acidic drug, 42, 43
Allergic reactions, 9, 201, 206
Allethrin, 263
Alpha receptors, 77
Alpha$_2$ agonists, 179, 180, 181
Alpha$_2$ antagonists, 190
Altrenogest (Regu-Mate), 157, 158, 161-162
American Animal Hospital Association, 22
American Heartworm Society, 253

American Veterinary Medical Association (AVMA), 21
Amikacin, 175, 198-199, 210, 211, 212, 215
Aminoglycosides, 36, 210, 211-215
Aminopenicillins, 203, 208
Aminopentamide (Centrine), 82, 85
Aminophylline, 122, 136-139, 189
Aminosalicylic acid, 92, 221, 222
Amitraz (Mitaban), 264
Ammonium chloride, 133
Amoxicillin (Amoxil; Amoxi-Tabs; Robamox-V; Utimox), 3, 67, 203, 204, 205, 208
Amoxil; *see* Amoxicillin
Amoxi-Tabs; *see* Amoxicillin
Amphetamines, 189
Amphojel, 89
Amphotericin, 228
Amphotericin B, 210, 227-228
Ampicillin, 203, 208
Amprolium (Corid), 258
Ampules, 5
Anabolic steroids, 156-157, 163-164
Anaerobic bacteria, 211
Analgesics, 169, 181-184
    narcotic, 84, 181-184
    neuroleptanalgesics, 184
    opioid, 84, 181-184
Anased; *see* Xylazine
Anemia, aplastic, 161
Anesthetic cocktails, 24
Anesthetics, 169-177
    barbiturates, 169-172
    dissociative, 173-174
    inhalant; *see* Inhalant anesthetics
    propofol, 172-173
    sedatives; *see* Tranquilizers and sedatives
Anestrus, drugs used in treatment of, 159
Angel dust, 174
Angina pectoris, 118
Angiotensin II, 116-117, 119
Angiotensin-converting enzyme (ACE), 116-117
Angiotensin-converting enzyme (ACE) inhibitors, 118-119
Angiotensinogen, 116-117
Antacids, 88-90, 218
Antagonists, 57-60

Anthelcide EQ; *see* Oxibendazole
Anthelmintics; *see* Antiparasitics
Antiarrhythmic drugs, 108-113, 136
    β-blocker, 111-112
    calcium channel blocker, 112-113
    inhibiting sodium influx, 109-111
Antibiotics; *see* Antimicrobials
Antibloat medications, 91
Anticestodals, 249, 253
Anticholinergics, 82, 85
Anticonvulsants, 90, 184-189, 226
    clonazepam, 188
    diazepam, 187-188
    phenobarbital, 185-186
    phenytoin, 187
    potassium bromide, 188-189
    primidone, 186-187
    valproic acid, 189
Antidiarrheals, 83-87, 218
    adsorbents, 86-87
    hypersecretion and, 85-86
    intestinal motility and, 84-85
    protectants, 86-87
Antidopaminergics, 78
Antiemetics, 81-83
Antifungals, 227-230
Antihistamines, 82, 139-140
Antiinflammatories, 272-289
    acetaminophen, 285-286
    acetylsalicylic acid, 281-282
    Addison's disease and, 278
    adrenocorticotropic hormone, 274-275
    aspirin, 281-282, 283
    carprofen, 285
    categories of, 287
    corticosteroids, 273, 274, 275, 281, 287
    Cushing's syndrome and, 278
    dimethyl sulfoxide, 284-286
    dipyrone, 286
    eicosanoids, 274
    flunixin meglumine, 283
    glucocorticoids, 274-278, 287
    gold salts, 286
    hyperadrenocorticism and, 278
    hypoadrenocorticism and, 278
    iatrogenic diseases and, 278
    ibuprofen, 282-283

Antiinflammatories—cont'd
  inflammation pathway and, 273-274
  ketoprofen, 282-283
  leukotrienes, 274, 279
  meclofenamic acid, 283-284
  mineralocorticoids, 274
  naproxen, 282-283
  nonsteroidal antiinflammatory drugs, 273,
      274, 277, 279-285, 287
  orgotein, 285
  phenylbutazone, 280-281, 283
  piroxicam, 286
  prostaglandins, 274, 279-280
Antimicrobials, 67, 91-92, 140-141, 196-233
  aminoglycosides, 36, 211-215
  antifungals, 227-230
  bacitracins, 210
  categories of, 229-230
  cephalosporins, 208-210
  classes of, 203-230
  concern over residues from, 200-201
  effects of, against cell membrane, 202
  effects of, against cell metabolism, 203
  effects of, against cell wall, 201-202
  effects of, against nucleic acids, 203
  effects of, at ribosomes, 202
  goals of therapy with, 198-199
  mechanisms of action of, 201-203
  penicillins, 203-208
  potentiated sulfonamides, 220-223
  quinolones, 215-217
  resistance of microorganisms to, 199-200
  sulfonamides, 186, 220-223
  tetracyclines, 217-220
  types of, 197
Antinematodals, 249-252
  benzimidazoles, 249-250
  febantel, 252
  ivermectin, 251
  organophosphates, 250-251
  piperazines, 249
  pyrantel, 251-252
Antineoplastic agents, handling of, 22-24
Antiogensin I, 116-117
Antiparasitics, 246-271
  amitraz, 264
  anticestodals, 253

Antiparasitics—cont'd
  antinematodals, 249-252
  antiprotozoals, 258-259
  carbamates, 260-263
  categories of, 268
  chlorinated hydrocarbons, 259
  external, 258-267, 268
  fipronil, 265-266
  in heartworm treatment, 253-258
  imidacloprid, 265
  insect growth regulators, 266-267
  insect repellents, 267
  internal, 248-258, 268
  organophosphates, 260-263
  principles of use of, 247-248
  pyrethrins, 263-264
  pyrethroids, 263-264
Antiprostaglandins, 86
Antiprotozoals, 249, 258
Antirobe; *see* Clindamycin
Antisedan; *see* Atipamezole
Antiseptics, disinfectants and; *see* Disinfectants
    and antiseptics
Antispasmodics, 85
Antithyroid drugs, 150
Antitrematodal compounds, 249
Antitussives, 129-131
  butorphanol, 130
  codeine, 131
  dextromethorphan, 131
  hydrocodone, 131
Antiulcer drugs, 42, 88-90
Aplastic anemia, 161
Apnea, 190
Apomorphine, 80, 183
Apramycin, 211
Aqueous solutions of glucocorticoids, 276
Arachidonic acid cascade, inflammatory
    mediators and, 273, 274
Arquel; *see* Meclofenamic acid
Arrhythmias, 108-113
Arsenic, 248
Artificial insemination, 158
Ascarids, 249
Ascites, 55, 118
*ASHP Technical Assistance Bulletin on Handling
    Cytotoxic and Hazardous Drugs*, 22

Aspiration pneumonia, 79

Aspirin, 42-43, 44-45, 88-89, 122, 169, 186, 222, 255, 281-282, 283, 285

Asthma, 139

Atenolol, 111

Atipamezole (Antisedan), 181, 190-191

ATP; *see* Adenosine triphosphate

Atrioventricular (AV) block, 112, 114, 180

Atrioventricular (AV) node, 102

Atropine, 82, 85, 112, 114, 181

Augmentin, 208

Aura, 184

Aurothioglucose, 286

Automaticity, 101, 106

Autonomic nervous system, cardiovascular function and, 106-108

AV block; *see* Atrioventricular block

AV node; *see* Atrioventricular node

Avermectins, 251

AVMA; *see* American Veterinary Medical Association

Azium; *see* Dexamethasone sodium phosphate

Azulfidine; *see* Sulfasalazine

B

Bacitracin A, 210

Bacitracins, 210

Bacterial cell membrane, 202

Bacterial cell wall, 201

Bacterial nucleic acids, effects of antimicrobials against, 203

Bacterial toxins, 77

Bactericidal chemicals, 197, 204, 235

Bacteriostatic chemicals, 197, 204

Bactrovet; *see* Sulfadimethoxine

BAL; *see* British Anti-Lewisite

Banamine; *see* Flunixin meglumine

Banminth; *see* Pyrantel

Barbiturates, 53, 61-62, 79, 90, 138, 169-173, 226, 227, 281

Baygon; *see* Propoxur

Baytril; *see* Enrofloxacin

Benadryl; *see* Diphenhydramine

Benzalkonium chloride, 240

Benzathines, 206, 207

Benzimidazoles, 249-250, 258

Benzodiazepine tranquilizers, 178, 187, 227

Beta blockers, 90, 111-112, 138, 151

Beta-adrenergic agonists, 136

Beta-lactam ring, 205

Beta-lactamases, 205

Betamethasone, 276

Bigeminy, 171, 172

Biguanides, 243

Biliary excretion, 65-66

Bioallethrin, 263

Bioavailability, 39, 45-49

Biotransformation, 61-63

Bismuth subsalicylate, 86, 218, 282

Bleach, 241, 242

Bloat, 91

Blockade, 267

Blood concentrations of drugs, 39, 40, 48, 66

Blood flow, dynamics of, 100-101

Blood-brain barrier, 50-51, 52, 204

Borreliosis, 218

Bovilene; *see* Fenprostalene

Bradycardia, 108-109

Bradypnea, 190

Brand name of drugs, 3, 6

Brevital; *see* Methohexital

British Anti-Lewisite (BAL), 255

Bromocriptine, 163

Bronchoconstriction, 134

Bronchodilators, 122, 134-139

   β-adrenergic agonists, 136

   methylxanthines, 136-139

Bucket analogy of drug dosages and dosage interval, 32

Bulk laxatives, 87

Buprenorphine (Buprenex), 181, 183, 184

Butorphanol (Torbugesic; Torbutrol), 59, 130, 181, 182, 183

Butoxypolypropylene glycol (Butox PPG), 267

Butyrophenones, 178, 184

C

C-1 drugs; *see* Schedule I drugs

Caffeine, 136-139, 189

Calcium antacids, 89

Calcium channel blockers, 90, 112-113

Calcium gluconate, 163

Cambendazole, 249

Canine distemper virus, 238

Caparsolate; *see* Thiacetarsamide sodium

Caplets, 4

Captopril, 118-119

Carafate; *see* Sucralfate

Carbamates, 260-263

Carbaryl (Sevin), 260

Carbenicillin, 203

Carbonic anhydrase inhibitors, 122

Cardiac anatomy, 100-101

Cardiac function, normal, 100-108

Cardiomyopathy, hypertrophic, 282

Cardiovascular system, drugs affecting, 99-127

    antiarrhythmic drugs, 108-113

    aspirin, 122

    autonomic nervous system and, 106-108

    bronchodilators, 122

    carbonic anhydrase inhibitors, 122

    cardiac anatomy and, 100-101

    categories of, 123

    depolarization, repolarization, and refractory
        periods and, 103-106

    diuretics, 119-122

    dynamics of blood flow and, 100-101

    electrical conduction through heart and,
        101-103

    normal cardiac function, 100-108

    positive inotropic agents, 113-115

    sedatives, 123

    tranquilizers, 123

    vasodilators, 115-119

Caricide, 257

Carmilax, 89

Carprofen (Rimadyl), 285

Castor oil, 87

Catabolic effects, 163, 277

Catalepsis, 173

Catecholamines, 113, 152, 181

Categories of controlled substances, 7

Cathartics, 87

Cefa-Dri, 209

Cefadroxil, 209

Cefa-Lak, 209

Cefa-Tabs, 209

Cefotaxime, 209

Cefoxitin, 209

Ceftiofur, 209

Cell membrane, effects of antimicrobials against,
    202

Cell metabolism, effects of antimicrobials
    against, 203

Cell wall, effects of antimicrobials against,
    201-202

Center for Veterinary Medicine, FDA, 217

Central nervous system (CNS) stimulants, 79,
    139-139, 189-191

    atipamezole, 190-191

    doxapram, 190

    methylxanthines, 189-190

    tolazoline, 190-191

    yohimbine, 190-191

Centrally acting antitussive, 130

Centrally acting emetics, 80

Centrine; *see* Aminopentamide

Cephalexin, 209

Cephaloridine, 210, 213-214

Cephalosporins, 205, 208-210, 213-214, 220

Cephalothin (Keflin), 209, 214

Cephapirin, 209

Cestex; *see* Epsiprantel

Cestodes, 249

Charcoal, activated, 81, 86-87

Chelation, 218

Chelators, 60

Chemical name of drugs, 2-3

Chemoreceptor trigger zone (CRTZ), 77-79

Chemotherapy spill kit, 23

Cheque Drops; *see* Mibolerone

Chewable heartworm preventive, 4

Chewable vitamins, 4

Chewing cud, 75

Chitin, effect of lufenuron on, 266

Chloramphenicol, 170, 185, 210, 225-226, 227

Chlorhexidine, 236, 239, 243

Chlorinated hydrocarbons, 259

Chlorine, 236

Chlorine compounds, 241-242

Chlorothiazide, 121

Chlorpromazine (Thorazine), 81, 86

Chlorpyrifos (Dursban), 260, 261, 262

Chocolate toxicity, 189

Cholinergic antagonists, 108

Cholinergic receptors, 108

Chromosomes, drug resistance and, 199-200

Chronic obstructive pulmonary disease, 140

Cilia, 132

Cimetidine (Tagamet), 42, 89-90, 93, 280

Ciprofloxacin, 215, 216

Cisapride (Propulsid), 83

CL; *see* Corpus luteum

Claforan, 209

Clavamox, 205, 208

Clavulanic acid, 205, 208

Clindamycin (Antirobe), 223, 226

Clonazepam (Klonopin), 178, 187, 188

Cloprostenol (Estrumate), 157

Clorox; *see* Sodium hypochlorite

Cloxacillin, 203, 205, 208

CNS stimulants; *see* Central nervous system
    stimulants

Coagulum, 240

Cocaine, 189

Coccidiostats, 249

Cocktails, anesthetic, 24

Cod liver oil, 88

Codeine, 131, 181, 182, 283

Colace; *see* Docusate sodium succinate

Colonic functions, 75

Color-fast bleaches, 242

Combot, 250

Compazine; *see* Prochlorperazine

Compendium of Veterinary Products, 6

Competitive antagonism, 59

Composition statement of drug in drug
    reference, 7

Compounding, drug, 24-25

Congestive heart failure, 119

Contraceptives, 160-161

Contradictions in drug reference, 9

Controlled substances, 7, 20-21, 131

Controlled Substances Act of 1970, 21

Conversion factor, ratio method of dosage
    calculation and, 15

Convulsions, 184

Cor pulmonale, 129

Corid; *see* Amprolium

Corpus luteum (CL), 154

Corrosives, vomiting and, 79

Corticosteroids, 89, 93, 139, 140, 152, 160, 162,
    163, 170, 171, 206, 227, 273, 274, 275,
    281

Corticotropin-releasing factor (CRF), 275

Cortisol, 228, 275

Cortisone, 274, 275

Cough, 129-130

Cough center, 129

Cough suppressants, 130

Cough syrups, 5

Cough tablets, 4

COX-1; *see* Cyclooxygenase-1

COX-2; *see* Cyclooxygenase-2

Creams, 5

CRF; *see* Corticotropin-releasing factor

CRF-ACTH-cortisol negative feedback loop, 275

Cross-resistance, 205

CRTZ; *see* Chemoreceptor trigger zone

Crystalluria, 216, 222

Cushing's syndrome, 278

Cyclic AMP (cAMP), 138

Cyclooxygenase, 274, 279, 280

Cyclooxygenase-1 (COX-1), 280, 285

Cyclooxygenase-2 (COX-2), 280, 285

Cyclosporine, 222

Cystorelin, 156

Cythioate (Proban), 262

Cytobin; *see* Liothyronine

Cytomel; *see* Liothyronine

Cytotec; *see* Misoprostol

Cytotoxic agents, 22

D

Darbazine; *see* Prochlorperazine

DDT, 259

DEA; *see* Drug Enforcement Administration

DEA certification number, 21

Deafness, 213

DEC; *see* Diethylcarbamazine

Decongestants, 131-134

DEET; *see* Diethyltoluamide

Dehydration, therapeutic, 141

Delayed neurotoxicity syndrome, 261

Delta receptors, 182

Demerol; *see* Meperidine

Depolarization, cardiac, 103-106

Derris Powder; *see* Rotenone

DES; *see* Diethylstilbestrol

Description of drug in drug reference, 7

Desflurane (Suprane), 176

Detomidine (Dormosedan), 177, 178-181, 183, 184

Dexamethasone, 152, 162, 227, 255, 276

Dexamethasone sodium phosphate (Azium), 276

Dextromethorphan, 131

Dextrose, 118

Diabetes mellitus, 151

Diacetate, 276

Diazepam (Valium), 45, 49, 90, 173, 178, 187-188, 227

Dichlorvos, 251, 262

Dicloxacillin, 203, 205, 208

Diethylcarbamazine (DEC), 250, 257

Diethylstilbestrol (DES), 156-157

Diethyltoluamide (DEET), 267

Diffusion, passive, 35-36

Diffusion hypoxia, 175

Digitoxin, 281

Digoxin, 40, 89, 110, 113-114, 121

Dihydrostreptomycin, 211

Dilantin; *see* Phenytoin

Diltiazem, 112-113

Dimenhydrinate (Dramamine), 82

Dimercaprol, 255

Dimethyl sulfoxide (DMSO), 255, 284-285

Dinoprost tromethamine (Lutalyse), 157, 162

Dioctyl sodium succinate (DSS), 91

Diphenhydramine (Benadryl), 82

Diphenoxylate (Lomotil), 84-85

Dipyrone, 286

Disinfectants and antiseptics, 197, 234-245
   alcohols, 239-240
   appropriate use of, 236-237
   biguanides, 243
   categories of, 244
   chlorine compounds, 241-242
   iodine compounds, 242
   iodophors, 242
   phenols, 238-239
   quarternary ammonium compounds, 240-241
   selection of, 237-238
   terminology for, 235-236
   types of, 238-244

Disinhibition, 189, 191

Dispensing medication, 12-14

Dissociative anesthetics, 173-174

Dissolution of drug, 46, 47

Distribution, drug, 50-56

Diuresis, 119-122

Diuretics, 119-122, 141
   loop, 120-121
   osmotic, 122
   potassium-sparing, 121
   thiazide, 121

DMSO; *see* Dimethyl sulfoxide

DNA, effects of antimicrobials against, 203

DNA gyrase, 215

Dobutamine, 113

Docusate sodium succinate (Colace), 88

Domitor; *see* Medetomidine

Dopamine, 163, 177

Dopaminergic antagonists, 78

Dopram; *see* Doxapram

Dormosedan; *see* Detomidine

Dosage calculations, 14-19
   factor label method, 15-17
   ratio method, 14-15, 16, 17
   stoichiometry, 15-17

Dosage forms, 4-6

Dosage interval, 33

Dosage regimen, 32-35

Down-regulation, 112, 113, 117

Doxapram (Dopram), 181, 190

Doxycycline, 170, 217, 218, 219-220

Dramamine; *see* Dimenhydrinate

Drip rate for IV infusion, calculation of, 19

Droncit; *see* Praziquantel

Drontal, 252

Drontal-Plus, 252

Droperidol, 80, 178, 183, 184

Drug absorption, 39-44

Drug clearance, half-life and, 66-67

Drug compounding, 24-25

Drug distribution, 50-56

Drug elimination, 64-68
   hepatic, 65-66
   renal, 64-65
   routes of, 64

Drug Enforcement Administration (DEA), 11, 21, 131

Drug handling, 19-24

Drug information, sources of, 6

Drug interactions, biotransformation and, 61-62

Glucocorticoids—cont'd
  safe use of, 279
  suspensions of, 276
  types of, 275-276
Gluconeogenesis, 149, 278
Glucosuria, 151
Glucuronic acid, 285
Glutamate, 251
Glutaraldehyde, 243
Glycerin, 88
Glycerol guaiacolate, 133
Glycogenolysis, 149, 278
GnRH; *see* Gonadotropin-releasing hormone
Goiter, 147-148
Gold salts, 286
Gonadotropin-releasing hormone (GnRH), 154, 156, 160
Gonadotropins, 156, 159
GOZE-2-SLEEP, 7
Grains, 186
Grand mal seizures, 185
Griseofulvin (Fulvicin), 229-230
Guaifenesin, 133

H

H_2 antagonists, 89-90
H_2 blockers, 93, 280
H_2 receptors, 76
Half-life
  clearance and, 66-67
  steady-state concentrations and, 67, 68
Halogens, 241, 242
Halothane (Fluothane), 64, 171, 173, 176
HCG; *see* Human chorionic gonadotropin
Heart
  autonomic nervous system and, 106-108
  electrical conduction through, 101-103
  normal function of, 100-108
Heart block, 112, 114, 180
Heart disease, vasoconstriction in, 115-117
Heartgard-30; *see* Ivermectin
Heartgard for Cats; *see* Ivermectin
Heartgard-30 Plus; *see* Ivermectin
Heartworm, 4, 118, 122, 251, 253-258
Heat, 154
  foal, drugs used in, 159

Heaves, 140
Hemoglobin, 286
Hepatic elimination of drugs, 65-66
Hepatotoxicity, 132
Hetacillin, 203, 208
Hexachlorophene, 239
Histamine, 76, 78, 82, 134, 136, 139, 140, 274
Hormonal control of estrous cycle, 153-156
Hormonal therapy, 145
Human chorionic gonadotropin (HCG), 156, 159
Humulin; *see* Recombinant human insulin
Hyaluronic acid, 285
Hycodan; *see* Hydrocodone
Hydralazine, 117-118
Hydrocarbons, chlorinated, 259
Hydrocodone (Hycodan), 131
Hydrocortisone, 275
Hydrogen peroxide, 81, 242, 243
Hydrophilic colloids, 87
Hydrophilic nature of drug, 38, 41, 42, 50, 51
Hyperadrenocorticism, 278
Hyperalgesia, 180
Hyperglycemia, 151
Hyperkalemia, 119
Hypermotility, 84
Hypersecretion, antidiarrheals and, 85-86
Hypersensitivity
  drug, 9, 201, 206
  flea-bite, 262
Hyperthermia, malignant, 176
Hyperthyroidism, 147, 149-151
Hypertonic salts, 87-88
Hypertrophic cardiomyopathy, 282
Hypoadrenocorticism, 160, 278
Hypoalbuminemia, 53, 64, 281
Hypoglycemic agents, 153
Hypokalemia, 114, 120-121
Hypomagnesemia, 114
Hypomotility, 84
Hypoproteinemia, 170
Hypotension, 64, 117, 120
Hypothermia, 176
Hypothyroidism, 146-149
Hypovolemia, 120
Hypoxic, 133-134

I

I-131; *see* Radioactive iodine

Iatrogenic diseases, 278

Ibuprofen (Advil), 279, 282-283

Ictus, 184

ID injection; *see* Intradermal injection

Idiopathic epilepsy, 184

Idiosyncratic reaction to phenobarbital, 186

Illegal manufacturing of drug, 24

IM administration of drugs; *see* Intramuscular administration of drugs

Imathal; *see* Pyrantel

Imidacloprid (Advantage), 265

Imidazole antifungals, 228

Immiticide; *see* Melarsomine dihydrochloride

Imodium; *see* Loperamide

Imodium A-D; *see* Loperamide

Implants, 5

Inderal; *see* Propranolol

Indomethacin (Indocin), 88-89

Induced biotransformation, 61-62

Inflammation pathway, antiinflammatories and, 273-274

Inhalant anesthetics, 174-177
  halothane, 176
  isoflurane, 176-177
  methoxyflurane, 175
  nitrous oxide, 174-175

Inhibin, 154

Inhibitory neurotransmitters, 251

Injectable drugs, 5

Innovar-Vet,184, 183

Inotropic agents, 111, 113-115

Insect development inhibitors, 266

Insect growth regulators, 266-267

Insect repellents, 267

Insecticides, 260-264

Inspissated mucus, 130

Insulin, 151-152

Insulin-dependent diabetes mellitus, 151

Insurmountable antagonism, 59

Interceptor; *see* Milbemycin oxime

Internal antiparasitics, 248-258, 268

Internal parasitics, terminology for, 248-249

Intestinal motility
  antidiarrheals and, 84-85
  drug absorption and, 47-49

Intraarterial injection, 34-35

Intradermal (ID) injection, 35

Intramuscular (IM) administration of drugs, 35, 39-40, 41, 49

Intraperitoneal (IP) injection, 35

Intravenous (IV) administration of drugs, 34, 40

Intravenous infusion, 34

Iodine, radioactive, 150-151

Iodine compounds, 242

Iodophors, 236, 242

Ion trapping, drug absorption and, 44-45, 46

Ionized drug molecules, 42, 44, 45

IP injection; *see* Intraperitoneal injection

Ipecac, syrup of, 80-81

Iron supplements, 218

Irreversible antagonism, 59

Irritant laxatives, 87

Isoflupredone, 276

Isoflurane (AErrane; Forane), 173, 176-177

Isopropamide, 82, 85

Isopropyl alcohol, 239

Isoproterenol, 136

Itraconazole, 228

IV administration of drugs; *see* Intravenous administration of drugs

IV bolus, 34

Ivermectin (Eqvalan; Heartgard for Cats; Heartgard-30; Heartgard-30 Plus; Ivomec), 248, 251, 252, 256-258

Ivomec; *see* Ivermectin

J

Juvenile hormone mimics, 266

K

Kanamycin, 211, 215

Kaolin and pectin (Kaopectate), 87, 218, 223

Kappa receptors, 182

KCS; *see* Keratoconjunctivitis sicca

Keflex, 209

Kennel cough, 130

Keratoconjunctivitis sicca (KCS), 222

Ketamine, 21, 173-174

Ketoconazole, 228

Ketoprofen (Ketofen; Orudis), 279, 282-283

Kinins, 274

Klonopin; *see* Clonazepam

Knockout, 266-267

L

LA-200, 218
Lactose, 118
Lasix; *see* Furosemide
Laughing gas, 174
Laxatives, 87-88
Let-down, 156
Leukotrienes, 136, 274, 279
Levamisole, 252
Levothyroxine (Soloxine; Synthroid), 148-149
LH; *see* Luteinizing hormone
Lidocaine (Xylocaine), 45, 50, 109-110, 171
    with epinephrine, 110
D-Limonene, 267
Lincomycin, 223, 226
Lincosamides, 223, 224
Lindane, 259
Liniments, 5
Liothyronine (Cytobin; Cytomel), 148, 149
Lipophilic nature of drug, 38, 41, 42, 50, 52
Lipoxygenase, 274
Liquid forms of drugs, 5
Liquid ketamine, 174
Loading dose, 33
Local anesthesia, 169
Locally acting antitussive, 130
Locally acting emetics, 80
Lomotil; *see* Diphenoxylate
Loop diuretics, 120-121
Loperamide (Imodium; Imodium A-D), 84-85
Lotions, 5
Lozenges, 4
Lubricants, 87-88
Lufenuron (Program), 266
Lutalyse; *see* Dinoprost tromethamine
Luteal phase of estrous cycle, 154, 155
Luteinizing hormone (LH), 154, 156, 159, 160
Lyme disease, 218
Lysol, 238

M

M-99; *see* Etorphine
Maalox, 89
Macrodantin, 225
Macrolides, 223-224
Maintenance dose, 33

Malabsorption, 92-93
Malathion, 262
Maldigestion, 92-93
Malignant hyperthermia, 176
Malpractice, 9
Mannitol, 60, 122, 228
Manufacturing, illegal, of drug, 24
Mast cell tumors, 76, 284
Material safety data sheet (MSDS), 23
Mebendazole (Telmin; Telmintic), 249, 250, 258
Meclofenamic acid (Arquel), 283-284
Medetomidine (Domitor), 177, 178-181
Medication dispensing, 12-14
Meflosyl; *see* Flunixin meglumine
Mefoxin, 209
Megestrol acetate (Ovaban), 160, 164
Melarsomine dihydrochloride (Immiticide),
    254-255
Melena, 86
Meningitis, 204
Meperidine (Demerol), 181, 183, 283
Mercury, 248
Metabolite, 61
Metamucil, 87
Methemoglobin, 286
Methemoglobinemia, 286
Methimazole (Tapazole), 150
Methohexital (Brevital), 170, 172
Methoprene, 266, 267
Methoxyflurane (Metofane; Penthrane), 64,
    171, 175, 176, 220
Methylcarbamate, 260, 262
Methylprednisolone, 139
Methylxanthines, 136-139, 189-190
Metoclopramide (Reglan), 83
Metofane; *see* Methoxyflurane
Metronidazole (Flagyl), 92, 224-225, 258
MFO system; *see* Mixed function oxidase system
Mibolerone (Cheque Drops), 160-161
MIC; *see* Minimum inhibitory concentration
Micotil; *see* Tilmicosin
Microbicidal disinfectants, 235-236
Microbiostatic disinfectants, 235-236
Microfilaremia, 256
Microfilariae, 254
Microfilaricides, 252, 254, 256
Midazolam (Versed), 178

Milbemycin oxime (Interceptor), 256-258
Milk of Magnesia, 87-88
Milk-discard times, 206
Mineral oil, 88, 91
Mineralocorticosteroids, 274
Minimum inhibitory concentration (MIC), 198
Minocycline, 217, 218
Miosis, 260
Misoprostol (Cytotec), 90, 280
Mitaban; *see* Amitraz
Mitral insufficiency, 117
Mixed function oxidase (MFO) system, 61-62
Mixed-function oxidase enzyme system, 185
Molded tablets, 4
Monogastric animal, 75
Morantel tartrate (Nematel), 252
Morphine mania, 85, 183
Morphine sulfate, 181, 183
Mosby's Veterinary Drug Reference, 6
MSDS; *see* Material safety data sheet
Mu receptors, 182
Mucociliary apparatus, 129
Mucolytics, 131-134
Mucomyst; *see* Acetylcysteine
Multidose vials, 5
Muscarinic receptors, 260
Mustard, powdered, and water, 81
Myelosuppression, 226

N

Nadolol, 111
Naked viruses, 238
Nalidixic acid, 215
Nalorphine, 183
Naloxone, 58-59, 80, 182-183
Naproxen (Aleve; Naprosyn), 282-283
Narcotic analgesics, 84, 85, 181-184
Natural penicillins, 203
Naxcel, 209
Nebulization, 132, 141
Negative feedback system, endocrine system
    and, 145-146
Negative inotropic drugs, 111
Nemacide, 257
Nematel; *see* Morantel tartrate
Nematodes, 249
Nemex; *see* Pyrantel

Neomycin, 47-49, 199, 210, 211, 213
Neostigmine (Stiglyn), 91
Nephrotoxicity, 211, 213
Nephrotoxicosis, 210
Nervous system, drugs affecting, 168-195
    analgesics; *see* Analgesics
    anesthetics, 169-177
    anticonvulsants; *see* Anticonvulsants
    categories of, 191
    central nervous system stimulants; *see* Central
        nervous system stimulants
    sedatives; *see* Tranquilizers and sedatives
    tranquilizers; *see* Tranquilizers and sedatives
Neurodermatitis, 164
Neuroleptanalgesics, 184
Newborn animals, effect of drugs on, 63
Nicotinic receptors, 260
Nifedipine, 112
Nitrofurans, 225
Nitrofurantoin (Furandantin), 225
Nitroglycerin, 118
Nitrous oxide, 174-175
Noncompetitive antagonism, 59, 60
Nonionized drug molecules, 42, 44, 45
Nonprescription Drugs and Ophthalmic Drugs, 6
Nonproductive cough, 130
Nonproprietary name of drugs, 3, 7
Nonreceptor-mediated reactions, 60
Nonsteroidal antiinflammatory drugs (NSAIDs),
    88-89, 171, 273, 274, 277, 279-285
    aspirin, 281-282
    carprofen, 285
    dimethyl sulfoxide, 284-285
    flunixin meglumine, 283
    ibuprofen, 282-283
    ketoprofen, 282-283
    meclofenamic acid, 283-284
    naproxen, 282-283
    orgotein, 285
    phenylbutazone, 280-281
Nonsystemic antacids, 89
Norepinephrine, 107, 112, 113, 177, 178-179,
    181, 187
Norfloxacin, 215
Norgestomet, 157
Nosocomial infections, 235
NSAIDs; *see* Nonsteroidal antiinflammatory
    drugs

Nucleic acids, effects of antimicrobials against, 203
Nuflor; *see* Florfenicol
Numorphan; *see* Oxymorphone
Nylar, 266-267
Nystagmus, 213
Nystatin, 227-228

O

Occupational Safety and Health Administration (OSHA), 22
Off-label drug use, 7, 8
Ointments, 5
Omeprazole, 90
Ophthalmic drops and ointments, 277-278
Opioid analgesics, 84, 181-184
Optimmune, 222
Oral administration of drugs, 45-49
Oral electrolyte replacements, 92
Organophosphates, 91, 250-251, 260-263
Orgotein, 285
Ormetoprim, 220, 221, 222
Orudis; *see* Ketoprofen
OSHA; *see* Occupational Safety and Health Administration
Osmotic diuretics, 122
Ototoxicity, 211, 213, 243
Ovaban; *see* Megestrol acetate
Ovitrol, 266
Oxacillin, 203, 205, 208
Oxfendazole, 249
Oxibendazole (Anthelcide EQ; Filaribits-Plus), 249, 250
Oxidants, 243
Oxybarbiturates, 170
Oxygen, 141
Oxymorphone (Numorphan), 58-59, 172, 181, 183, 184
Oxyntic cells, 76, 89
Oxyphenbutazone, 281
Oxytetracycline, 217, 218, 219, 220
Oxytocin, 156, 163

P

P wave, 101
Package inserts, 6
Package label, drug information on, 6

2-PAM; *see* Pralidoxime
Panacur; *see* Fenbendazole
Pancreatic enzyme powder, 6
Pancreatic enzyme supplements, 92-93
Pancrezyme, 93
Parasympatholytic drugs, 82
Paregoric, 84-85
Parenteral administration of drugs, 34, 49-50
Parietal cells, 76, 89
Partial agonists, 59-60, 181, 183
Partial antagonists, 59-60, 183
Parvovirus, 239, 241
Passive diffusion, 35-36, 37, 65
Pastes, 5
PCP; *see* Phencyclidine
PCV; *see* Premature ventricular contraction
PDR; *see* *Physicians' Desk Reference*
Peak drug concentration, 67
Pedialyte, 92
Penicillin, 65, 198, 203-208, 210, 215, 217, 220
    amoxicillin, 208
    ampicillin, 208
    bacterial resistance to, 205-206
    cloxacillin, 208
    dicloxacillin, 208
    natural, 203
    oxacillin, 208
    penicillinase-resistant, 203
Penicillin G, 203, 204, 206-207, 208
Penicillin V, 203, 207-208
Penicillinase-resistant penicillin, 203
Penicillinases, 205
Pentazocine (Talwin), 181, 183, 283
Penthrane; *see* Methoxyflurane
Pentobarbital, 7, 170, 188, 226, 227
Pentothal; *see* Thiopental
Pepcid; *see* Famotidine
Pepcid-CD, 90
Pepto-Bismol, 86, 218, 282
Per os (PO) administration of drugs, 34, 40
Percentage solution, 18
Perianal adenocarcinoma, 160, 164
Perianal adenoma, 160, 164
Peristaltic contractions, intestinal motility and, 84
Perivascular injection, 35
Permethrin, 263, 264

Peroxides, 243

Petit mal seizures, 185

PgE; *see* Prostaglandin E

pH of environment, effect of, on absorption, 41-44

Phagocytosis, 36-37

Pharmacokinetics, 29-73

  active transport, 37

  agonists, 57-60

  antagonists, 57-60

  biotransformation, 61-63

  clearance, 66-67

  dosage interval, 33

  dosage regimen, 32-35

  drug absorption, 39-44

  drug distribution, 50-56

  drug elimination, 64-68

  facilitated diffusion, 36, 37

  half-life, 66-67, 68

  hepatic elimination of drugs, 65-66

  hydrophilic nature of drug, 38, 41

  ion trapping, 44-45, 46

  lipophilic nature of drug, 38, 41

  movement of drug molecules in body, 35-38

  nonreceptor-mediated reactions, 60

  oral administration of, 45-49

  parenteral administration of, 49-50

  passive diffusion, 35-36

  ph of environment, 41-44

  physical transport, 36-37

  plasma protein binding, 53, 55

  renal elimination of drugs, 64-65

  routes of administration, 32-35, 39-40

  steady-state concentrations, 67, 68

  therapeutic range, 30-31, 32

  tissue perfusion, 51-53, 54

  volume of distribution, 54-56

  ways in which drugs exert effects, 56-60

  withdrawal times, 67-68

Pharmacy procedures, 11-28

Phenacetin, 286

Phencyclidine (PCP), 174

Phenobarbital, 21, 61-62, 67, 138, 170, 178, 185-187, 188, 189, 226, 227

Phenolic compounds, 238-239

Phenolphthalein, 87

Phenols, 236, 238-239

Phenothiazine dewormers, 252

Phenothiazine tranquilizers, 80, 81, 82, 152, 177, 178, 184

Phenylbutazone, 88-89, 280-281, 283

Phenylephrine, 133

Phenylethylmalonamide, 186

Phenylpropanolamine, 133

Phenytoin (Dilantin), 90, 138, 187, 226, 281

Phosphate salts, 87-88

Phosphodiesterase, 138

Physical transport, 36-37

Physicians' Desk Reference (PDR), 6

Physician's GenRx, 6

Physiologic pH, 43

Pine oil, 133, 238

Pinocytosis, 36-37

Piperacillin, 203

Piperazines, 249, 250

Piperonyl butoxide, 263

Piroxicam (Feldene), 286

Pivalate, 276

pKa, 43-44

Placenta, drugs crossing, 50-51

Plasma concentrations of drugs, 39, 40, 48, 66

Plasma protein binding, drug distribution and, 53, 55

Plasmids, drug resistance and, 199-200

PMSG; *see* Pregnant mare serum gonadotropin

Pneumonia, aspiration, 79

PO administration of drugs; *see* Per os administration of drugs

Poison Control Center, 79

Poison Prevention Packaging Act of 1970, 14

Poisons, drugs as, 2

Poloxalene, 91

Polymyxin B, 210

Polypeptide antibiotics, 210

Polyvinylpyrrolidone, 242

Positive inotropic agents, 113-115

Postictal phase of seizure, 185

Potassium bromide, 188-189

Potassium clavulanate, 205

Potassium iodide, 133

Potassium-sparing diuretics, 121

Potentiated sulfonamides, 220-223

Pour-on, 262-263

Povidone-iodine, 239, 242

Powdered mustard and water, 81

P-QRS interval, 102

P-R interval, 102

Pralidoxime (2-PAM), 261

Praziquantel (Droncit), 252, 253

Prazosin, 119

Precautions in drug reference, 7

Precor, 266

Prednisolone, 61, 276

Prednisolone sodium succinate (Solu-Delta-
Cortef), 276

Prednisone, 61, 139, 152, 160, 227, 275, 276

Pregnancy
drugs crossing placenta in, 50-51
drugs used to prevent, maintain, and
terminate, 160-163
progesterone and, 155

Pregnant mare serum gonadotropin (PMSG),
156

Preictal phase of seizure, 184

Premature ventricular contraction (PVC), 108

Prescriptions, 12-14
abbreviations used in, 13
components of, 12-13
outlines for writing, 12

Preventic, 264

Primidone, 138, 186-187, 226

Primor, 220

Priscoline; *see* Tolazoline

Proban; *see* Cythioate

Procainamide, 109, 110

Procaine, 171, 206, 207

Procaine penicillin G, 206-207

Procan-SR, 110-111

Prochlorperazine (Compazine; Darbazine), 81,
82

Prodrugs, 61

Productive cough, 130

Progesterone, 152, 155, 157, 158, 159, 161-162,
163

Progestins, 157, 158-159, 161-162, 164

Proglottids, 253

Program; *see* Lufenuron

Pro-Kill, 262

Prolactin, 163

PromAce; *see* Acepromazine

Prophylactic use of antihistamines, 140

Pro-Powder, 262

Propoxur (Baygon), 260

Propranolol (Inderal), 111, 136, 138, 151, 170,
227

Proprietary name of drugs, 3, 6

Propulsid; *see* Cisapride

Propylene glycol, 118

Propylthiouracil, 150

Pro-Spot; *see* Fenthion

Prostaglandin E (PgE), 75-76, 85, 121

Prostaglandins, 75-76, 136, 155-156, 157-159,
162, 163, 221, 274, 279

Protamine zinc insulin (PZI), 152

Protectants, antidiarrheals and, 86-87

Protein-bound fraction, 53

Protozoacidal chemicals, 235

Psyllium, 87

Purgatives, 87

Pyogenic infections, 214-215

Pyrantel (Banminth; Imathal; Nemex; Strongid),
251-252, 257

Pyrantel pamoate, 252

Pyrethrins, 262, 263-264, 267

Pyrethroids, 263-264, 267

Pyriproxyfen, 266-267

PZI; *see* Protamine zinc insulin

Q

QRS complex, 103, 109, 171, 172

Quaternary ammonium compounds, 236,
240-241

Quinidine, 90, 109, 110, 170, 227

Quinolones, 203, 215-217, 227

R

Radioactive iodine (I-131), 150-151

Ranitidine (Zantac), 89-90, 280

Ratio method of calculating drug dosages,
14-15, 16, 17

Receptor, 56-57, 58, 60

Recombinant human insulin (Humulin), 152

Reconstituted drugs, 20

Redistribution of drug, 52-53, 54

Refractory period, cardiac, 103-106

Reglan; *see* Metoclopramide

Regu-Mate; *see* Altrenogest

Relative refractory period, 106

Renal elimination of drugs, 64-65
Renal papillary necrosis, 280
Renin-angiotensin system, 115-117, 119
Repolarization, cardiac, 103-106
Repository forms of injectable drugs, 5
Reproduction, drugs affecting, 153-165
  anestrus and, 159
  contraceptives, 160-161
  corticosteroids, 162
  drugs used to control estrous cycling, 158-159
  ergot alkaloids, 163
  estrogen, 156-157
  foal heat and, 159
  gonadotropin-releasing hormone, 156 158
  gonadotropins, 156, 159
  hormonal control of estrous cycle, 153-156
  pregnancy and, 160-163
  progesterone, 161-162
  progestins, 157, 158-159, 161-162
  prostaglandins, 157-158, 162
Residues, 200-201
Resistance, drug, 199-201, 247
Resmethrin, 263, 264
Resorb, 92
Respiratory system, drugs affecting, 128-143
  antihistamines, 139-140
  antimicrobials, 140-141
  antitussives, 129-131
  bronchodilators; *see* Bronchodilators
  categories of, 142
  corticosteroids, 139
  decongestants, 131-134
  diuretics, 141
  expectorants, 131-134
  mucolytics, 131-134
  oxygen, 141
Rest and restore system, 75, 107-108
Resting state, 103
Reversible antagonism, 59
Ribosomes, effects of antimicrobials at, 202
Ricinoleic acid, 87
Rifampin, 203, 226-227
Rimadyl; *see* Carprofen
Ringworm, 229
Riopan, 89
RNA, effects of antimicrobials against, 203
Robamox-V; *see* Amoxicillin

Rolaids, 89
Rompun; *see* Xylazine
Rotenone (Derris Powder), 262, 267
Roundworms, 249
Routes of administration of drugs, 32-35
RU486, 163
Ruminal tympany, 91
Ruminants, 75
Ruminatorics, 91

S

SA node; *see* Sinoatrial node
Saddle thrombus, 282
Salicylates, 186, 221, 222, 282
Sanitizers, 235
Sarafloxacin (Saraflox), 215, 216, 217
SC injection; *see* Subcutaneous injection
Schedule I (C-I) drugs, 21
Schedules of controlled substances, 7
Seasonal anestrus, 159
Second-gas effect, 175
Sedatives, tranquilizers and; *see* Tranquilizers
  and sedatives
Segmental contractions, intestinal motility and,
  84
Seizures, 184-185
  ketamine anesthesia and, 173
  phenothiazines and, 82
  quinolones and, 217
  vomiting and, 79
Semisolid dosage forms, 5
Septra, 220
Serum concentrations of drugs, 39, 40, 48, 66
Sevin; *see* Carbamyl
Sevoflurane (Ultane), 176
Side effects, 7
Sig, prescriptions and, 13
Sigma receptors, 182
Silica packets, 20
Single-dose vials, 5
Sinoatrial (SA) node, 101
Siphotrol, 266
SLUDDE signs, 260-261
Sodium citrate, 133
Sodium hypochlorite (Clorox), 241
Sodium influx, antiarrhythmic drugs inhibiting,
  109-111

Sodium phosphate, 276

Sodium succinate, 276

Sodium valproate, 189

Sodium-potassium-ATPase pump, 103

Soloxine; *see* Levothyroxine

Solu-Delta-Cortef; *see* Prednisolone sodium
     succinate

Solutions, 5, 46
  percentage, 18

Somatostatin, 151

Special K, 174

Species differences, biotransformation and, 62,
    63

Spironolactone, 121

Spore form of bacteria, 236

Sporicidal chemicals, 235

Spot-on, 262-263

SQ injection; *see* Subcutaneous injection

SR formulations; *see* Sustained-release
    formulations

Status epilepticus, 184

Steady-state concentrations, half-life and, 67, 68

Sterilizers, 235

Steroidal antiinflammatory drugs, 273

Steroids, anabolic, 156-157

Stiglyn; *see* Neostigmine

Stoichiometry, dosage calculations and, 15-17

Stool softeners, 87-88

Streptomycin, 211

Strongid; *see* Pyrantel

Strychnine, 79, 82, 188, 189, 248

Subcutaneous (SC; SQ) injection, 35, 40, 41, 49

Substance P, 274

Sucralfate (Carafate), 90, 280

Sulbactam, 205

Sulfa drugs, 220-223

Sulfachlorpyridazine, 220

Sulfadiazine, 220, 222

Sulfadimethoxine (Albon; Bactrovet), 42-43,
    220, 258

Sulfamethoxazole, 220

Sulfapyridine, 221, 222

Sulfasalazine (Azulfidine), 91-92, 220, 221, 222

Sulfonamides, 186, 217, 220-223, 249, 258

Sulfonylurea compounds, 153

Sulfur, 267

Supercoiling, 215

Superinfection, 206

Superovulation, 156

Superoxide dismutase, 285

Superoxide radicals, 274

Supona, 260

Suppositories, 4

Suprainfection, 206

Suprane; *see* Desflurane

Supraventricular arrhythmia, 109

Surgical scrubs, 242

Surital; *see* Thiamylal

Surmountable antagonism, 59

Suspensions, 5, 276

Sustained-release (SR) formulations, 4, 46-47,
    138

Sympathomimetics, 113

Synergistic effect, 138

Synthroid; *see* Levothyroxine

Syrup of ipecac, 80-81

Syrups, 5

Systemic antacids, 89-90

Systemic sulfas, 220

T

T wave, 103

T_3; *see* Triiodothyronine

T_4; *see* Thyroxine

Tablets, 4

Tachycardia, 108-109

Tachypnea, 129, 176

Taeniacides, 253

Tagamet; *see* Cimetidine

Tagamet-HB, 90

Taktic, 264

Talwin; *see* Pentazocine

Tapazole; *see* Methimazole

Target tissues, 39

Task, 250

Telazol, 173, 174, 178, 227

Telmin; *see* Mebendazole

Telmintic; *see* Mebendazole

Tenesmus, 84

Tennis match cats, 173

Terbutaline, 136

Terminology
    for disinfectants and antiseptics, 235-236
    for internal parasitics, 248-249
    for therapeutic agents, 2-6

Terpin hydrate, 133
Testosterone, 160, 163, 164, 228
Tetracycline, 19, 89, 175, 217-220
Tetramethrin, 263
Theobromine, 136-139, 189-190
Theophylline, 90, 122, 136-139, 189
Therapeutic dehydration, 141
Therapeutic range, 30-31, 32
Therapeutic window, 30
Thiabendazole (Equizole; Tresaderm Otic), 249,
    250
Thiacetarsamide sodium (Caparsolate), 254-255
Thiamin, 258
Thiamylal (Surital), 170, 173
Thiazide diuretics, 121, 152
Thiobarbiturates, 170-172
Thiopental (Pentothal), 52-53, 170
Thorazine; *see* Chlorpromazine
Thromboxanes, 274, 282
Thyroid disease, 146-151
    hyperthyroidism, 149-151
    hypothyroidism, 146-149
Thyroid extract, 148
Thyroid hormones, 146-147
Thyroid storms, 149
Thyroid supplements, 5-6
Thyroidectomy, 150
Thyroid-releasing hormone (TRH), 147, 148
Thyroid-stimulating hormone (TSH), 146-147,
    148
Thyrotoxicosis, 149
Thyroxine (T_4), 147, 148
Ticarcillin, 203
Tight junctions, 50
Tiguvon, 262-263
Tiletamine, 173, 174, 178
Tilmicosin (Micotil), 224
Timolol, 111
Tincture, 5, 242
    of iodine, 242
    of opium, 84-85
Tissue perfusion, 49, 51-53, 54
T-max, 37
Tobramycin, 211, 215
Tocainide, 109
Tolazoline (Priscoline), 181, 190-191

Topical administration of drugs, 5, 34
Torbugesic; *see* Butorphanol
Torbutrol; *see* Butorphanol
Total daily dose, 33
Toxic synergism, 138
Trade name of drugs, 3, 6
Tranquilizers
    benzodiazepine, 178, 187, 227
    phenothiazine, 80, 81, 82, 152, 177, 178,
        184
    and sedatives, 123, 169, 176, 177-181
        acepromazine, 177-178
        clonazepam, 178
        detomidine, 178-181
        diazepam, 178
        droperidol, 178
        medetomidine, 178-181
        midazolam, 178
        xylazine, 178-181
        zolazepam, 178
Transduction, 200
Transitional estrus, 159
Trematodes, 249
Tresaderm Otic; *see* Thiabendazole
TRH; *see* Thyroid-releasing hormone
Triamcinolone (Vetalog), 276
Tribrissen, 220
Trichlorfon, 251
Triiodothyronine (T_3), 146-147, 148
Trimethoprim, 220, 221-222
Troches, 4
Trough drug concentration, 67
TSH; *see* Thyroid-stimulating hormone
Tums, 89
Tylan; *see* Tylosin
Tylenol; *see* Acetaminophen
Tylosin (Tylan), 92, 223-224, 226
Tympany, 180

U

Ultane; *see* Sevoflurane
Unenveloped viruses, 238
Universal antidote, 81
Up-regulation of β-adrenergic receptors, 112
U.S. Department of Agriculture (USDA), 11
Utimox; *see* Amoxicillin

V

Vagal stimulation, 82
Valerate, 276
Valium; *see* Diazepam
Valproic acid, 189
Vapona, 260
Vasoconstriction, 49-50, 115-117
Vasodilators, 50, 115-119
  angiotensin-converting enzyme inhibitors,
    118-119
  hydralazine, 117-118
  nitroglycerin, 118
  prazosin, 119
  vasoconstriction in heart disease, 115-117
Vd; *see* Volume of distribution
Vegetative form of bacteria, 236
Ventricular arrhythmia, 109
Ventricular fibrillation, 108
Verapamil, 112
Vercom, 252
Vermicides, 248-249
Vermifuges, 249, 253
Versed; *see* Midazolam
Vetalog; *see* Triamcinolone
Veterinary Drug Handbook, 6
Veterinary Pharmaceuticals and Biologicals, 6
Vials, 5
Viokase, 93

Virucidal chemicals, 235
Vitamins, chewable, 4
Volatile liquids, vomiting and, 79
Volatile oils, 133
Volume of distribution (Vd), 54-56
Vomiting, induction of, emetics and, 79-80
Vomiting reflex, emetics and, 77-79

W

Warnings in drug reference, 8-9
Wheal and flare reaction, 82
White petrolatum, 88
Withdrawal time, 67-68, 201, 206

X

Xenobiotics, 49
Xylazine (Anased; Rompun), 78, 80, 171, 172,
    173, 177, 178-181, 183, 184, 190
Xylocaine; *see* Lidocaine

Y

Yohimbine (Yobine), 80, 181, 190-191, 264
Young animals, effect of drugs on, 63

Z

Zantac; *see* Ranitidine
Zolazepam, 174, 178, 227

V

Vagal stimulation, 82
Valerate, 276
Valium; *see* Diazepam
Valproic acid, 189
Vapona, 260
Vasoconstriction, 49-50, 115-117
Vasodilators, 50, 115-119
    angiotensin-converting enzyme inhibitors,
       118-119
    hydralazine, 117-118
    nitroglycerin, 118
    prazosin, 119
    vasoconstriction in heart disease, 115-117
Vd; *see* Volume of distribution
Vegetative form of bacteria, 236
Ventricular arrhythmia, 109
Ventricular fibrillation, 108
Verapamil, 112
Vercom, 252
Vermicides, 248-249
Vermifuges, 249, 253
Versed; *see* Midazolam
Vetalog; *see* Triamcinolone
Veterinary Drug Handbook, 6
Veterinary Pharmaceuticals and Biologicals, 6
Vials, 5
Viokase, 93

Virucidal chemicals, 235
Vitamins, chewable, 4
Volatile liquids, vomiting and, 79
Volatile oils, 133
Volume of distribution (Vd), 54-56
Vomiting, induction of, emetics and, 79-80
Vomiting reflex, emetics and, 77-79

W

Warnings in drug reference, 8-9
Wheal and flare reaction, 82
White petrolatum, 88
Withdrawal time, 67-68, 201, 206

X

Xenobiotics, 49
Xylazine (Anased; Rompun), 78, 80, 171, 172,
      173, 177, 178-181, 183, 184, 190
Xylocaine; *see* Lidocaine

Y

Yohimbine (Yobine), 80, 181, 190-191, 264
Young animals, effect of drugs on, 63

Z

Zantac; *see* Ranitidine
Zolazepam, 174, 178, 227

Terpin hydrate, 133

Testosterone, 160, 163, 164, 228

Tetracycline, 19, 89, 175, 217-220

Tetramethrin, 263

Theobromine, 136-139, 189-190

Theophylline, 90, 122, 136-139, 189

Therapeutic dehydration, 141

Therapeutic range, 30-31, 32

Therapeutic window, 30

Thiabendazole (Equizole; Tresaderm Otic), 249, 250

Thiacetarsamide sodium (Caparsolate), 254-255

Thiamin, 258

Thiamylal (Surital), 170, 173

Thiazide diuretics, 121, 152

Thiobarbiturates, 170-172

Thiopental (Pentothal), 52-53, 170

Thorazine; *see* Chlorpromazine

Thromboxanes, 274, 282

Thyroid disease, 146-151

   hyperthyroidism, 149-151

   hypothyroidism, 146-149

Thyroid extract, 148

Thyroid hormones, 146-147

Thyroid storms, 149

Thyroid supplements, 5-6

Thyroidectomy, 150

Thyroid-releasing hormone (TRH), 147, 148

Thyroid-stimulating hormone (TSH), 146-147, 148

Thyrotoxicosis, 149

Thyroxine (T_4), 147, 148

Ticarcillin, 203

Tight junctions, 50

Tiguvon, 262-263

Tiletamine, 173, 174, 178

Tilmicosin (Micotil), 224

Timolol, 111

Tincture, 5, 242

   of iodine, 242

   of opium, 84-85

Tissue perfusion, 49, 51-53, 54

T-max, 37

Tobramycin, 211, 215

Tocainide, 109

Tolazoline (Priscoline), 181, 190-191

Topical administration of drugs, 5, 34

Torbugesic; *see* Butorphanol

Torbutrol; *see* Butorphanol

Total daily dose, 33

Toxic synergism, 138

Trade name of drugs, 3, 6

Tranquilizers

   benzodiazepine, 178, 187, 227

   phenothiazine, 80, 81, 82, 152, 177, 178, 184

   and sedatives, 123, 169, 176, 177-181

      acepromazine, 177-178

      clonazepam, 178

      detomidine, 178-181

      diazepam, 178

      droperidol, 178

      medetomidine, 178-181

      midazolam, 178

      xylazine, 178-181

      zolazepam, 178

Transduction, 200

Transitional estrus, 159

Trematodes, 249

Tresaderm Otic; *see* Thiabendazole

TRH; *see* Thyroid-releasing hormone

Triamcinolone (Vetalog), 276

Tribrissen, 220

Trichlorfon, 251

Triiodothyronine (T_3), 146-147, 148

Trimethoprim, 220, 221-222

Troches, 4

Trough drug concentration, 67

TSH; *see* Thyroid-stimulating hormone

Tums, 89

Tylan; *see* Tylosin

Tylenol; *see* Acetaminophen

Tylosin (Tylan), 92, 223-224, 226

Tympany, 180

U

Ultane; *see* Sevoflurane

Unenveloped viruses, 238

Universal antidote, 81

Up-regulation of β-adrenergic receptors, 112

U.S. Department of Agriculture (USDA), 11

Utimox; *see* Amoxicillin